THE POCKET

calorie counter

the complete, discreet, and portable guide for managing your health

SUZANNE BEILENSON

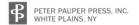
PETER PAUPER PRESS, INC.
WHITE PLAINS, NY

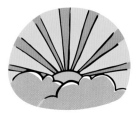

The publisher would like to thank Claudine Gandolfi for her essential and excellent contributions to the Introduction, and Christina Lundy for updating the 2012 edition.

Designed by Heather Zschock
Illustrations copyright © 2012 Kerren Barbas Steckler

Visit us at www.peterpauper.com

THE POCKET

calorie counter

the complete, discreet, and portable guide for managing your health

contents

introduction

It's all about choice. Every day, we have to choose what foods we are going to put into our bodies. And those decisions really matter because they affect our weight, our health, and our longevity.

It can be daunting to choose well when we have so many options. Not only are our kitchens full of different foods, but we have a huge variety of restaurant and take-out foods available. Did you know that supermarkets on average carry 45,000 items? (It's estimated that in 1949 supermarkets carried only 3,750 items.) The choices are overwhelming, and it's no wonder we have trouble making the right decisions.

That's where *The Pocket Calorie Counter* can help you simplify your life, lose weight, and become healthier. We've compiled information on the **calories**, **total fat**, **saturated fat**, **sodium**, **carbohydrates**, **fiber**, and **protein** for thousands and thousands of foods. Not only will you find this information on the foods that we buy and cook ourselves based on data provided by the United States Department of Agriculture (www.usda.gov), but you'll also find nutritional information from many popular **chain restaurants** and **fast-food outlets**. As you consider which foods to eat, simply look them up and find out which ones have fewer calories, less fat and sodium, and more fiber and protein.

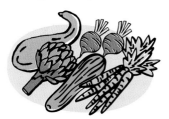

Bring *The Pocket Calorie Counter* with you wherever you go. It can help you make better choices. (And its discreet design lets you make those choices privately!)

understanding nutrition

As the saying goes, we are what we eat. But what exactly are we eating? A French fry may just be a fried potato (and a yummy one at that!), but at a chemical level, it's a combination of fat, carbohydrates, protein, sodium, and more.

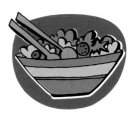

We can compare different foods by looking at the energy and nutrients they provide. Understanding the nutritional content of food is vital to ensure we provide our bodies with what they need to function properly. Since there's no one perfect food, we must eat a variety of foods to capture all the nutrients we need to stay healthy. It can be complicated, however, to follow a diet that's nutrient-rich, but not overloaded with calories.

energy and weight loss
CALORIES

Calories are the measure of energy contained in a food. Calories are not bad—in fact, they are essential. Our bodies need them to function properly, from taking a breath to running a marathon. Without calories, our bodies would come to a grinding halt.

Your body converts calories into physical energy. Any extra calories you consume that aren't used are stored as fat. If you consume fewer calories than your body needs, your body will start burning stored fat to get the energy it requires.

WEIGHT LOSS

For all the hype and fad diets that abound, weight loss really comes down to a simple equation. *Calories consumed minus calories used* determines whether you gain or lose weight. If you consume more calories than your body burns, you gain weight. If you burn more calories than you consume, you lose weight.

Every pound of fat on your body is equivalent to 3,500 calories that did not get used. So to lose a pound a week, divide 3,500 calories by 7 days, and reduce your intake by 500 calories per day or burn an extra 500 calories a day—or some combination of the two.

The bottom line? To lose weight, you have to eat less, burn more, or do both.

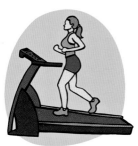

But note: Consuming too *few* calories will not necessarily get you to your goal faster! If you're not eating enough, your body will lower your BMR (Basal Metabolic Rate, *see page 12*) in order to conserve its fat stores. A lower BMR means that instead of needing perhaps 1,500 calories a day, you may only require 1,000. So if you're consuming 1,200, that may be 200 too many, and you may actually gain weight! See what a tricky business this can be?

It's also important to lose *no more than two pounds* per week. When you lose weight faster than that, you actually lose muscle, not fat. You definitely want to avoid doing that. Losing muscle tissue slows down your metabolism, making you work even harder to burn the same calories!

On the other hand, the more muscle you have, the more calories you burn and the easier it is to burn them. That's because the body uses up more calories to simply sustain muscle tissue. What a great reason to get to the gym!

Our best tips to tip the scale in the right direction:

- Get moving. The more you move, the more calories you burn. So, while it's terrific if you're working out at the gym, don't forget that you can add more activity to your day without "exercising." How? Take the stairs instead of the elevator. Walk the kids to school instead of driving them. Carry a basket while you shop for food instead of using a cart. (You'll buy less, too!) Any movement you can build into your daily routine can quickly add up to a surprising number of calories burned.

- Break up your exercise. Many people don't feel like they have an hour or more to spend exercising. So, take a 20-minute walk after every meal. It doesn't matter to your body whether you exercise all at once or split it up.

- Take ownership of your food. If you're a fast food junkie or always buying pre-made, pre-packaged food, consider a cooking class. A cooking class, and I'm trying to lose weight? Yup. Because when you cook for yourself, you are fully conscious of what's going into the food you eat, from the amount of salt you add to the type of oil you use. You can often prepare the same dish that you might have bought, but with fewer calories and more wholesome ingredients. And when you've gone to the trouble to cook, enjoy the fruits of your labor . . . which brings us to the next weight loss tip.

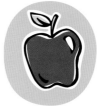

- Slow down. Don't be a turkey and gobble your food. Enjoy it. Savor it. Chew it thoroughly. Put your fork down between bites. It takes 15 minutes or more for your brain to get the message that you're full. Eating slower means you'll have consumed less by the time your brain realizes you're satisfied.

- Ditch the "grab" habit. A handful of chips here, a spoonful of ice cream there. When you grab a little food, it may seem like it doesn't count . . . but the calories do. Be aware that whether you eat at the table, in the car, or on the go, it all counts.

- Write it down. Keep a daily food diary, recording everything you eat *before* you eat it. Not only will writing down *everything* you eat help you say "no" to that handful of chips, it can also reveal your eating patterns and triggers. Are you eating the leftovers off your kids' plates because you hate waste? Has your late-morning coffee break turned into a coffee and muffin break? Are you eating after having a fight with your mother? Being aware of when and why you eat is the first step to making real changes in your diet.

- Snack! The reason we often "grab" food is because we're hungry. If you want to make good eating choices and lose weight, you can't be hungry! That's when the pangs in your stomach overpower your good intentions. So snack, but plan your snacks in advance and be sure to include some protein, which will leave you feeling fuller for longer. So, cut up extra celery sticks to have with low-fat peanut butter. Or have low-fat string cheese and a piece of fresh fruit. A couple of well-timed snacks each day will help keep you on track.

- Quit drinking up calories! Just because you're not chewing doesn't mean you're not swallowing. If you currently drink a can of regular soda or a glass of wine a day, and you replace it with water, you'll lose 10 pounds in a year.

- Use a plate! When you eat directly out of a bag of chips or a container of ice cream, it's difficult to know how much you're actually consuming. Put your food on a plate or in a bowl so that you can control your portion size.

- Now use a smaller plate—because the "eyes" have it. It's important that what you see looks satisfying. It's natural to want to fill up that plate. Just use a smaller one. The same portion of food that looked skimpy on a large dinner plate will seem far more generous on a smaller lunch plate. A similar strategy can work for dessert too. Fill half your bowl with fresh fruit before adding ice cream or frozen yogurt. You'll reduce the amount of high-calorie food, but it will be visually filling!

- Weigh yourself regularly. Get on the scale at least once a week. If you've had a small weight gain, it's easier to get back on track. If you've lost weight, it's a big motivator to keep up the good work!

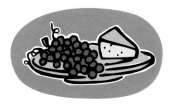

basal metabolic rate

Welcome to your Basal Metabolic Rate! Your BMR indicates the calories your body needs per day to survive without moving. First, calculate your BMR using the formula below. Now, multiply that number by 1.2—the result is the number of calories you need to maintain weight. If you don't ingest enough calories for the day, you'll do more harm than good. Cutting too many calories will lower your BMR. In general, if you're trying to lose weight, aim for a loss of 1 to 2 pounds a week, no more.

Here's the formula:

Women: BMR = 655 + (4.35 x weight in pounds) + (4.7 x height in inches) – (4.7 x age in years)

Men: BMR = 66 + (6.23 x weight in pounds) + (12.7 x height in inches) – (6.8 x age in years)

daily recommended caloric intake

According to American College of Sports Medicine (ACSM), calories consumed should be no less than 1,200 for women, and 1,800 for men.

If you reduce net calories (by eating 500 fewer calories a day and/or exercising), you'll be able to lose 1 pound a week. You need 3,500 fewer calories than required by your BMR to burn off one pound (500 x 7 days = 3,500 calories).

body mass index

The dreaded Body Mass Index! A good indicator of body fatness, your BMI should stay below 25. The formula below tells how to find yours. Height is measured without shoes and weight without clothes.

BMI = Weight in pounds divided by height in inches squared. Multiply result by 703. End product is your BMI.

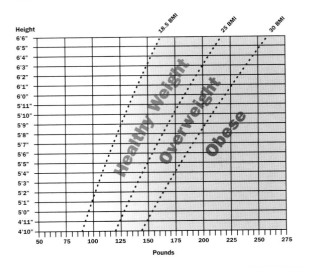

Here are guidelines for healthy body fat percentages, by age and gender. You can ascertain your body fat with a specialized scale or with help from a personal trainer.*

AGE	WOMEN	MEN
20-39	21% to 32%	8% to 19%
40-59	23% to 33%	11% to 21%
60 and up	24% to 35%	13% to 24%

*In addition, BMI should be between 18.5 and 24.9.

portion control

American food industry portions are out of control. Ask someone from another country what they think of an individual restaurant portion here and you'll likely hear it would feed their entire family!

Here are some USDA guidelines that may help you visualize proper portion sizes:

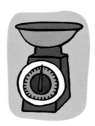

Protein/meat	3 oz (size of your palm or a deck of cards)
Carbs/pasta/rice	1/2 cup (size of a tennis ball or baseball cut in half)
Fruits	1 cup (size of a tennis ball or baseball)
Cheese	1 oz (size of 4 dice or your thumb)
Bagel	Average serving: hockey puck size
Potato	Medium serving: size of a computer mouse
Peanut butter/butter	1 tsp (the tip of your thumb)
Bread	1 slice
Pancake	1 (size of a CD/DVD)
Vegetables	1/2 cup cooked (size of a tennis ball or baseball cut in half)
Lettuce	1 cup (4 leaves)
Milk/yogurt	1 cup (size of a tennis ball or baseball)
Nuts	8 (handful)

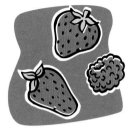

If you're having a hard time judging sizes, consider investing in a food scale. That way you can weigh and portion out food in advance. Do it when you get home from the grocery store. Try putting meats, veggies, and especially snacks in individual storage bags.

food groups

When it comes to supplying the calories our bodies need for fuel, there are three energy- and nutrient-loaded food groups: **fat**, **carbohydrates** (which include **fiber**), and **protein**. Fat provides nine calories per gram, while carbohydrates and protein provide four calories per gram. Fat, carbohydrates, and protein are sometimes called **macronutrients** because we require large quantities of them. Other substances like vitamins and minerals are considered **micronutrients** because, while necessary, we need far less of them in our diet.

FAT

You need fat. You really do. It's an important nutrient that ensures your body functions properly, from providing you with energy to helping you make estrogen, testosterone, and even Vitamin D. **In fact, it's recommended that 25% to 30% of your calories come from fat!**

So what's the problem? First, fat is a high-calorie nutrient. It doesn't take much fat to hit your recommended intake. Second, the foods found in nature contain two types of fat—saturated and unsaturated—and they're not created equal. Saturated fat is linked to a whole host of health problems, particularly coronary heart disease. What's more, your body can produce all of the saturated fat it requires, so there's no health benefit to eating it.

Luckily, *unsaturated* fats have great health benefits. These fats can improve cholesterol levels, reduce inflammation, and help your heart. Better yet, most people don't get enough unsaturated fats. So make it a habit to consume unsaturated fats while watching your overall calorie intake.

Tips for getting the right fats into your diet:

- Eat foods that are good sources of unsaturated fats. These include nuts, avocados, pumpkin and sesame seeds, flax seeds, and fish and vegetable oils (canola, peanut, olive, sunflower, corn, and soybean).

- Reduce saturated fat by avoiding these foods: butter, whole-fat milk, ice cream, palm and coconut oils, high-fat cheeses, and high-fat cuts of meat.

- Swap out solid fats like butter or stick margarine with liquid oils. Try dipping bread in olive oil rather than spreading on the butter.

- Check the label on pre-packaged food to avoid palm and coconut oils, which are often used in commercial bakeries.

- Replace whole milk with low-fat or skim milk.

- Ditch the skin on poultry. Don't eat the skin or leave it on when you cook.

- Eat more fish and less meat, and when you do go for red meat, opt for a leaner cut like sirloin.

CARBOHYDRATES

Carbohydrates come in all shapes, sizes, and colors, from red raspberries to milk, from orange sweet potatoes to wild rice. Of all the nutrients we need, carbs offer the greatest choice and provide our main source of energy, along with vitamins, minerals, and fiber. Talk about multitasking!

But different carbs are digested at different rates. Some are slowly processed into blood sugar, while others, such as potatoes, are quickly converted into blood sugar and give us quick bursts of energy. Diabetes, heart disease, and other conditions have been linked to diets high in these types of "fast" carbs.

About 50% of the calories you consume should come from carbohydrates, and complex, "slow" carbs should dominate your

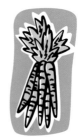

diet. "Slow" carbs keep you feeling fuller, and may improve your blood pressure and cholesterol. You can find these carbs (and not a lot of added calories!) in fruits, vegetables, beans, and whole-grain foods. See the next page for information about incorporating fiber—that carb essential for digestive health—into your diet.

Some good ideas to get good carbs:

- Make your diet colorful. Choose foods that are richly colored, from fuchsia beets and dark green broccoli to blueberries and peachy peaches.

- Skip the added sugar. Packaged foods often come with added sugar, not to mention added calories and fewer nutrients.

- Switch out potatoes with grains such as barley, quinoa, and millet.

- Less processing is better. The more processing a food has undergone before you eat it, the faster your body will convert it to blood sugar. So, skip the fruit juice and eat whole fruits instead. Also, stay away from "milled," "refined," or "finely ground" grains.

- Expand your horizons. Try whole-wheat pasta!

- Give beans a whirl. They'll keep you satisfied longer since your body digests them slowly.

FIBER

Fiber is the freebie of the carbohydrate world. The body can't digest fiber, so it passes through us, grabbing fatty substances as it goes, thus helping to reduce cholesterol levels. Fiber also gets things moving in the intestinal tract—say goodbye to constipation! And if that weren't enough, fiber keeps food in your stomach longer, thereby keeping you feeling fuller longer. Now that's a nutrient everyone can love. **Recommended amounts of fiber: 25–40 grams daily.**

How can you get recommended daily amounts of fiber?

- Eat "slow" carbs; fruits, vegetables, beans, and whole grains are good sources of fiber.

- Swap out those potato chips for popcorn!

- Make legumes the main course. Try black bean soup or chili made with beans for a high-fiber entrée.

- Throw a handful of rinsed chickpeas into your salad.

- Choose breads with a fiber content of more than 3 grams per slice.

PROTEIN

Protein is the one nutrient of which most people get enough. Eating a varied diet generally takes care of our protein needs. That's good news because proteins are found in every cell of our bodies.

So what exactly is protein? Proteins are strings of molecules known as amino acids. Our bodies can actually produce some of those amino acids. The others have to come from the foods we eat. Sometimes you'll hear a food called a "complete protein," which means that it contains all of the essential amino acids we need. Complete proteins are often found in animal-based foods like meat, chicken, fish, and dairy. Vegetarians have to be extra careful to get enough complete proteins. Many foods are high only in certain amino acids, but can provide a complete package when combined with other foods. For example, rice and beans is a power pair, as is peanut butter on whole wheat bread!

Protein is your friend. Eating protein keeps you feeling fuller longer than eating carbohydrates. The extra bonus? Your body burns more calories digesting protein than it does carbs! **Protein should make up 25%–35% of your daily caloric intake**. On a 1,500 calories a day plan, that would be 375–525 calories (or 94–132 grams/3.5–4 oz).

Take your pick of these excellent protein choices:

- Leaner cuts of meat
- Skinless chicken and turkey
- Low-fat or fat-free dairy products like milk, yogurt, or cheese
- Nuts, seeds, and legumes such as beans, lentils, or chickpeas
- Tofu, soybeans, or other soy-based foods

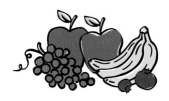

about sodium

When it comes to sodium, a little goes a long way. Sodium helps balance the amount of water in your cells, but too much sodium leads to excess fluid in your blood. Excess fluid makes your heart work harder, and that in turn can lead to hypertension, kidney disease, and even diabetes.

How much sodium do you need? **The experts now recommend a diet that contains just 1,500 milligrams per day**. One teaspoon of table salt contains over 2,300 milligrams of sodium! The average consumption is more than 3,400 milligrams daily.

For most people, though, overusing the salt shaker is not the problem. More than 70% of our sodium intake comes from processed and prepared food. When you're at the store, it's crucial to read the ingredient list! Also, many foods are packed *with* sodium even if they don't contain salt. Look out for any ingredient that contains the word *sodium* or *soda*, such as "monosodium glutamate," "baking soda," and "sodium nitrate."

Keep your sodium intake in check with these strategies:

- Condiments, salad dressings, and sauces are often high in sodium. Limit how much ketchup, mustard, and relish you use at your next barbecue.

- Wave bye-bye to breakfast meat. That bacon, sausage, or ham you're having with your omelet is shooting your sodium levels sky-high.

- Spice up your diet. Add flavor with herbs and spices, rather than salt.

- Be fresh. Fresh meats, fruits, and vegetables generally have lower sodium levels than their processed counterparts.

- Wash it. When you rinse canned food, you wash away some of the sodium.

- De-salt your fat! Substitute canola or olive oil for butter or margarine.

nutrition label tips

Nutrition labels contain a wealth of information. Here are things to note:

- Watch the serving size!

- 5% is low and 20% is high for all nutrients.

- 40 calories is low, 100 is moderate, and 400 is high.

- Keep saturated fats, sodium, and sugar LOW.

- Keep protein and fiber HIGH.

- Keep in mind that Nutrition Facts are based on a 2,000 calorie/day diet—adjust accordingly.

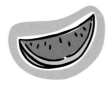

using *the pocket calorie counter*

For every food in *The Pocket Calorie Counter*, we've given the calorie and nutrient information for a designated portion size. However, you may want to use a different measure. The table below will help you easily convert one portion size to another.

Equivalents

Teaspoon	Tablespoon	Cup	Fluid Ounce	Pints+
1 tsp	1/3 tbsp			
3 tsp	1 tbsp			
	2 tbsp	1/8 cup	1 fl oz	
	4 tbsp	1/4 cup	2 fl oz	
	8 tbsp	1/2 cup	4 fl oz	
	12 tbsp	3/4 cup	6 fl oz	
	16 tbsp	1 cup	8 fl oz	1/2 pint
		2 cups	16 fl oz	1 pint
		4 cups	32 fl oz	1 quart
		16 cups	128 fl oz	1 gallon

setting goals: where we want to be

It's time to set some goals. Want to drop 20 pounds by summer? Want to firm up and lower your blood pressure? Find out where you need to be, then set small goals. Sometimes larger goals throw us off track because they seem so, well, big. Small steps help us get there without despair.

WEIGHT

Check out the accompanying government chart of healthy, overweight, and obese weights. Remember, these are only guidelines. Not everyone is made the same. Some people will be healthy at a higher weight than this suggests. Some may need to weigh less. Each of us is unique. Our cultural background can predetermine our body composition through DNA. Strive to be healthy, not thin.

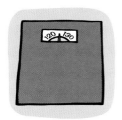

BMI	19	20	21	22	23	24	25	26	27	28	29	30	31	32	33	34	35
Height									Weight in pounds								
4'10"	91	96	100	105	110	115	119	124	129	134	138	143	148	153	158	162	167
4'11"	94	99	104	109	114	119	124	128	133	138	143	148	153	158	163	168	173
5'	97	102	107	112	118	123	128	133	138	143	148	153	158	163	168	174	179
5'1"	100	106	111	116	122	127	132	137	143	148	153	158	164	169	174	180	185
5'2"	104	109	115	120	126	131	136	142	147	153	158	164	169	175	180	186	191
5'3"	107	113	118	124	130	135	141	146	152	158	163	169	175	180	186	191	197
5'4"	110	116	122	128	134	140	145	151	157	163	169	174	180	186	192	197	204
5'5"	114	120	126	132	138	144	150	156	162	168	174	180	186	192	198	204	210
5'6"	118	124	130	136	142	148	155	161	167	173	179	186	192	198	204	210	216
5'7"	121	127	134	140	146	153	159	166	172	178	185	191	198	204	211	217	223
5'8"	125	131	138	144	151	158	164	171	177	184	190	197	203	210	216	223	230
5'9"	128	135	142	149	155	162	169	176	182	189	196	203	209	216	223	230	236
5'10"	132	139	146	153	160	167	174	181	188	195	202	209	216	222	229	236	243
5'11"	136	143	150	157	165	172	179	186	193	200	208	215	222	229	236	243	250
6'	140	147	154	162	169	177	184	191	199	206	213	221	228	235	242	250	258
6'1"	144	151	159	166	174	182	189	197	204	212	219	227	235	242	250	257	265
6'2"	148	155	163	171	179	186	194	202	210	218	225	233	241	249	256	264	272
6'3"	152	160	168	176	184	192	200	208	216	224	232	240	248	256	264	272	279
	Healthy						Overweight					Obese					

BLOOD PRESSURE

Your blood pressure should be below 120/80.

RESTING HEART RATE (RHR)

You should be aiming for a RHR between 60 and 80 beats per minute. In order to determine your RHR, first take your pulse, best done when you get up in the morning. Place your forefinger and middle finger on your wrist pulse point. Have a clock or watch with a second hand (or a digital version) nearby. Count the number of pulses in a given time period (i.e., count for 10 seconds, and multiply that number by 6 to get your beats per minute. Or count for 30 seconds and multiply by 2). That's your

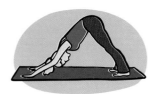

RHR. It should be between 50 and 100. Most people have a RHR around 70. The more active you are, the lower your RHR will get. The lower your RHR, the better your cardiovascular health.

You want to get your heart rate up during activity to burn more calories. Your Maximum Heart Rate is 220 minus your age. If you're 33, that would be 187 beats per minute (220 − 33 = 187 MHR). For optimum fat-burning benefits during exercise, keep that heart rate between 60% and 85% of your MHR. Do the math, multiplying your MHR by .6 or .85, to figure out where your heart rate should be for the best fat burn.

Now, while the "fat-burning zone" will burn a higher percentage of fat, the cardio zone will burn more calories and a higher *amount* of fat. Thus, if you can keep it up in the cardio zone, you'll see better results. The faster your heart beats, the speedier your metabolism. (That's why most "diet" pills have caffeine in them.)

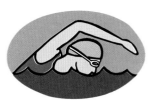

WAIST TO HIP RATIO

This is actually said to be one of the best indicators of overall health, as body fat stored around your midsection is a risk factor for heart disease. Work to get and keep this ratio low. To determine Waist to Hip Ratio, you'll need a tape measure. Measure your hips around the widest part of your buttocks. Then measure your waist where it's smallest, above the belly button. Divide the waist measurement by the hip measurement. Cardiovascular risk is higher for women with ratios higher than 0.85, and for men with ratios above 0.90.

getting started

First, take some time to check the nutritional information on the foods you eat on a regular basis. You may find some foods are more caloric than you realize or that your protein intake is too low. Armed with that knowledge, you can begin to make modifications to your diet that will get you healthier and more energetic. Most important, make changes that you can live

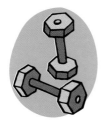

with over the long haul. Because it's not just about losing weight, adding fiber, or eating good fats in the short term. It's about being able to maintain a new style of eating for years to come.

You've already taken the first step. Now just turn the page and you'll be on your way to a more nutritious way of life!

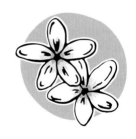

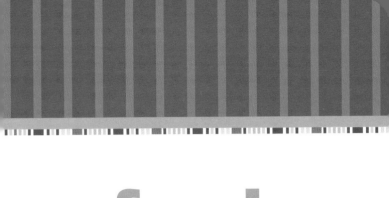

food

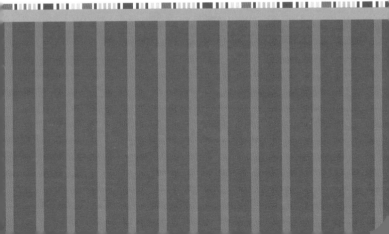

ITEM DESCRIPTION	Serving Size	Calories	Total Fat (g)	Saturated Fat (g)	Sodium (mg)	Carbohydrates (g)	Fiber (g)	Protein (g)
ABALONE (fried)	3 oz	161	6	1	502	9	0	17
ABIYUCH (fresh)	1/2 cup	79	0	0	23	20	6	2
ACAI JUICE	8 oz	98	0	0	85	23	n/a	0
ACEROLA (fresh)	1 fruit	2	0	0	0	0	0	0
ACEROLA JUICE (fresh)	1 cup	56	1	0	7	12	1	1
ACORN FLOUR	1 oz	142	9	1	0	15	0	2
ACORN SQUASH								
Baked, cubed	1 cup	115	0	0	8	30	9	2
Boiled, mashed	1 cup	83	0	0	7	22	6	2
Fresh, cubed	1 cup	56	0	0	4	15	2	1
ADOBO FRESCO	1 tbsp	49	4	1	3087	3	0	0
ADZUKI BEANS								
Canned, sweetened	1 cup	702	0	0	645	163	0	11
Dried, boiled	1 cup	294	0	0	18	57	17	17
Yokan	1 slice	36	0	0	12	9	0	0
ALFALFA SPROUTS (fresh)	1/4 cup	2	0	0	0	0	0	1
ALLSPICE (ground)	1 tbsp	16	1	0	5	4	1	0
ALMOND BUTTER								
Plain, w/o salt	1 tbsp	101	9	1	2	3	1	2
Plain, w/ salt	1 tbsp	101	9	1	72	3	1	2
ALMOND OIL	1 tbsp	120	14	1	0	0	0	0
ALMOND PASTE	1 oz	130	8	1	3	13	1	3
ALMONDS								
Blanched	1 oz	165	14	1	8	6	3	6
Dry roasted, w/o salt	1 oz	169	15	1	0	5	3	6
Dry roasted, w/ salt	1 oz	169	15	1	96	5	3	6
Honey roasted, unblanched	1 oz	168	14	1	37	8	4	5
Oil roasted, w/o salt	1 oz	172	16	1	0	5	3	6
Oil roasted, w/ salt	1 oz	172	16	1	96	5	3	6
Raw	10	69	6	0	0	3	2	3
Sugar coated	1 pc	17	1	0	0	2	0	0
AMARANTH								
Grain, cooked	1 cup	251	4	0	15	46	5	9
Leaves, boiled	1 cup	28	0	0	28	5	0	3

ITEM DESCRIPTION	Serving Size	Calories	Total Fat (g)	Saturated Fat (g)	Sodium (mg)	Carbohydrates (g)	Fiber (g)	Protein (g)
leaves, fresh	1 cup	6	0	0	6	1	0	1
ANCHOVY								
European, canned in oil	1 oz	60	3	1	1040	0	0	8
European, fresh	3 oz	111	4	1	88	0	0	17
ANISE SEED (whole)	1 tbsp	23	1	0	1	3	1	1
APPLE BUTTER	1 tbsp	29	0	0	3	7	0	0
APPLE CRISP	1/2 cup	227	5	1	495	43	2	2
APPLE DRINKS								
Apple cider-flavored drink, low calorie	8 fl oz	2	0	0	34	1	0	0
Apple-grape juice	8 fl oz	125	0	0	18	31	0	0
Apple-grape-pear juice	8 fl oz	130	0	0	13	32	0	0
APPLE JUICE								
Canned or bottled, (unsweetened)	8 fl oz	114	0	0	10	28	0	0
Concentrate, unsweetened, diluted	8 fl oz	112	0	0	17	28	0	0
Concentrate, unsweetened, undiluted	6 fl oz	350	1	0	53	87	0	1
APPLE PIE FILLING (canned)	1/8 can	74	0	0	35	19	1	0
APPLES								
Boiled, w/o skin, slices	1 cup	91	1	0	2	23	4	0
Canned, sweetened, slices	1 cup	137	1	0	6	34	4	0
Dried, stewed, w/ added sugar	1 cup	232	0	0	53	58	5	1
Dried, stewed, w/o added sugar	1 cup	145	0	0	51	39	5	1
Dried, uncooked	1 cup	209	0	0	75	57	7	1
Fresh, whole	1 med	72	0	0	1	19	3	0
Fresh, w/o skin, slices	1 cup	53	0	0	0	14	1	0
Fresh, w/ skin, slices	1 cup	57	0	0	1	15	3	0
Frozen, unsweetened, heated, slices	1 cup	97	1	0	6	25	4	1
Frozen, unsweetened, unheated, slices	1 cup	83	1	0	5	21	3	0
Microwaved, w/o skin, slices	1 cup	95	1	0	2	25	5	0
APPLESAUCE								
Sweetened, w/o salt	1 cup	167	0	0	5	43	3	0
Sweetened, w/ salt	1 cup	194	0	0	71	51	3	0
Unsweetened	1 cup	102	0	0	5	28	3	0

ITEM DESCRIPTION	Serving Size	Calories	Total Fat (g)	Saturated Fat (g)	Sodium (mg)	Carbohydrates (g)	Fiber (g)	Protein (g)
APPLE STRUDEL	1 pc	195	8	1	191	29	2	2
APPLE TURNOVERS (Pepperidge Farm, frozen)	1 serv	284	16	4	176	31	2	4
APRICOT NECTAR (canned)	1 cup	141	0	0	8	36	2	1
APRICOTS								
Canned in heavy syrup, halves, w/ skin	1 cup	214	0	0	10	55	4	1
Canned in juice, halves, w/ skin	1 cup	117	0	0	10	30	4	2
Canned in light syrup, halves, w/ skin	1 cup	159	0	0	10	42	4	1
Canned in water, halves, w/ skin	1 cup	66	0	0	7	16	4	2
Dehydrated, stewed	1 cup	314	1	0	12	81	0	5
Dehydrated, uncooked	1 cup	381	1	0	15	99	0	6
Dried, stewed, halves, w/o sugar	1 cup	212	0	0	10	55	7	3
Dried, stewed, halves, w/ sugar	1 cup	305	0	0	8	79	11	3
Dried, uncooked, halves	1 cup	313	1	0	13	81	9	4
Fresh, slices	1 cup	79	1	0	2	18	3	2
Fresh, whole	1 med	17	0	0	0	4	1	0
Frozen, sweetened	1 cup	237	0	0	10	61	5	2
ARROWHEAD (boiled)	1 corm	9	0	0	2	2	0	1
ARROWROOT (fresh, slices)	1 cup	78	0	0	31	16	2	5
ARROWROOT FLOUR	1 cup	457	0	0	3	113	4	0
ARTICHOKES								
Boiled	1 med	64	0	0	72	14	10	3
Canned or jarred, marinated	1/2 cup	58	3	0	244	7	2	2
Fresh, whole	1 med	60	0	0	120	13	7	4
Frozen, boiled	9 oz pkg	108	1	0	127	22	11	7
Jerusalem, fresh, slices	1 cup	110	0	0	6	26	2	3
ARUGULA (fresh)	1/2 cup	3	0	0	3	0	0	0
ASPARAGUS								
Boiled, cut	1/2 cup	20	0	0	13	4	2	2
Canned, drained	1/2 cup	23	0	0	347	3	1	3
Fresh, cut	1/2 cup	13	0	0	1	3	1	1
Frozen, boiled	10 oz pkg	53	1	0	9	6	5	9

ITEM DESCRIPTION	Serving Size	Calories	Total Fat (g)	Saturated Fat (g)	Sodium (mg)	Carbohydrates (g)	Fiber (g)	Protein (g)
AVOCADO								
California, fresh, whole	1 fruit	227	21	3	11	12	9	3
Common varieties, cubed	1 cup	240	22	3	10	13	10	3
Florida, fresh, whole	1 fruit	365	31	6	6	24	17	7
AVOCADO OIL	1 tbsp	124	14	2	0	0	0	0
BABASSU OIL	1 tbsp	120	14	11	0	0	0	0
BACON								
Baked	1 slice	44	4	1	178	0	0	3
Bits, meatless	1 tbsp	33	2	0	124	2	1	2
Broiled or roasted	1 slice	43	3	1	185	0	0	3
Broiled or roasted, reduced sodium	1 slice	43	3	1	82	0	0	3
Canadian style, grilled	1 slice (1 oz)	43	2	1	363	0	0	6
Grease	1 tsp	39	4	2	6	0	0	0
Hormel Canadian style	1 serv	68	3	1	569	1	0	9
Microwaved	1 slice	25	2	1	104	0	0	2
Pan fried	1 slice	42	3	1	192	0	0	3
BACON & BEEF STICKS	1 oz	145	12	4	398	0	0	8
BACON SUBSTITUTE								
Breakfast strips, pork, cooked	1 slice	52	4	1	238	0	0	3
Meatless, cooked	1 oz	50	5	1	234	1	0	2
Morningstar Farms Veggie Bacon Strips, frozen	2 strips	55	4	1	234	2	1	2
Worthington Stripples, frozen	2 strips	55	4	1	234	2	1	2
BAGELS								
Cinnamon-raisin (3" dia)	1 bagel	156	1	0	184	31	1	6
Egg (3" dia)	1 bagel	192	1	0	348	37	2	7
Oat bran (3" dia)	1 bagel	145	1	0	289	30	2	6
Onion (3" dia)	1 bagel	146	1	0	255	29	1	6
Plain (3" dia)	1 bagel	146	1	0	255	29	1	6
Poppy (3" dia)	1 bagel	146	1	0	255	29	1	6
Sesame (3" dia)	1 bagel	146	1	0	255	29	1	6
BAKED BEANS								
Campbell's, brown sugar & bacon	1 cup	320	5	1	941	60	16	10
Canned, w/ beef	1 cup	322	9	4	1264	45	0	17

ITEM DESCRIPTION	Serving Size	Calories	Total Fat (g)	Saturated Fat (g)	Sodium (mg)	Carbohydrates (g)	Fiber (g)	Protein (g)
Canned, w/ franks	1 cup	368	17	6	1114	40	18	17
Canned, w/o salt	1 cup	266	1	0	3	52	14	12
Canned, w/ pork	1 cup	268	4	2	1047	51	14	13
Canned, w/ pork & sweet sauce	1 cup	283	4	1	845	53	11	13
Canned, w/ pork & tomato sauce	1 cup	231	2	1	1075	46	10	13
Canned, w/ salt	1 cup	239	1	0	871	54	10	12
Homemade	1 cup	392	13	5	1068	55	14	14
Vegetarian	1 cup	339	3	0	441	65	15	15
BAKING CHOCOLATE								
Unsweetened, liquid	1 oz	134	14	7	3	10	5	3
Unsweetened, squares	1 sq	145	15	9	7	9	5	4
BAKING POWDER								
Sodium aluminum sulfate	1 tsp	2	0	0	488	1	0	0
Straight phosphate	1 tsp	2	0	0	363	1	0	0
Low sodium	1 tsp	5	0	0	4	2	0	0
BAKING SODA	1 tsp	0	0	0	1259	0	0	0
BALSAM PEAR								
Leafy tips, boiled	1 cup	20	0	0	8	4	1	2
Pods, boiled (1/2" pcs)	1 cup	24	0	0	7	5	3	1
BAMBOO SHOOTS								
Boiled (1/2" slices)	1 cup	14	0	0	5	2	1	2
Canned (1/8" slices)	1 cup	25	1	0	9	4	2	2
BANANA BREAD (Made w/margarine, homemade)	1 slice	196	6	1	181	33	1	3
BANANA CHIPS	1 oz	147	10	8	2	17	2	1
BANANA POWDER	1 tbsp	21	0	0	0	5	1	0
BANANAS								
Dehydrated	1 cup	346	2	1	3	88	10	4
Fresh, slices	1 cup	134	0	0	2	34	4	2
Fresh, whole	1 med	105	0	0	1	27	3	1
BARBEQUE SAUCE								
Low sodium	2 tbsp	52	0	0	46	13	0	0
Regular	2 tbsp	52	0	0	386	13	0	0
BARLEY (pearled, cooked)	1 cup	193	1	0	5	44	6	4

ITEM DESCRIPTION	Serving Size	Calories	Total Fat (g)	Saturated Fat (g)	Sodium (mg)	Carbohydrates (g)	Fiber (g)	Protein (g)
BARLEY FLOUR (or barley meal)								
w/o malt	1 cup	511	2	0	6	110	15	16
w/ malt	1 cup	585	3	1	18	127	12	17
BASIL								
Dried, leaves	1 tbsp	5	0	0	1	1	1	0
Fresh, chopped	2 tbsp	1	0	0	0	0	0	0
BASS								
Freshwater, cooked in dry heat	3 oz	124	4	1	76	0	0	21
Sea bass, cooked in dry heat	3 oz	105	2	1	74	0	0	20
BAY LEAF (crumbled)	1 tbsp	6	0	0	0	1	0	0
BEECHNUTS (dried)	1 oz	163	14	2	11	10	0	2
BEEF								
Bottom round, 0" fat, braised	3 oz	190	9	3	36	0	0	28
Bottom round, 0" fat, roasted	3 oz	190	8	3	30	0	0	23
Bottom round, 1/8" fat, braised	3 oz	210	11	4	36	0	0	28
Bottom round, 1/8" fat, roasted	3 oz	190	11	4	29	0	0	22
Bottom sirloin, tri-tip roast, 0" fat, all grades, roasted	3 oz	175	9	3	45	0	0	22
Bottom sirloin, tri-tip steak, 0" fat, all grades, roasted	3 oz	231	11	4	62	0	0	26
Brisket, flat half, 0" fat, all grades, braised	3 oz	175	7	3	46	0	0	28
Brisket, flat half, 1/8" fat, all grades, braised	3 oz	246	16	6	41	0	0	25
Brisket, point half, 0" fat, all grades, braised	3 oz	304	24	10	58	0	0	20
Brisket, point half, 1/8" fat, all grades, braised	3 oz	297	23	9	59	0	0	21
Brisket, whole, 0" fat, all grades, braised	3 oz	247	17	6	55	0	0	23
Brisket, whole, 1/8" fat, all grades, braised	3 oz	281	21	8	54	0	0	22
Chuck, arm pot roast, 0" fat, all grades, braised	3 oz	252	16	6	40	0	0	25
Chuck, arm pot roast, 1/8" fat, all grades, braised	3 oz	257	16	6	42	0	0	26

ITEM DESCRIPTION	Serving Size	Calories	Total Fat (g)	Saturated Fat (g)	Sodium (mg)	Carbohydrates (g)	Fiber (g)	Protein (g)
Chuck, blade roast, 0" fat, USDA Choice, braised	3 oz	296	22	9	55	0	0	23
Chuck, blade roast, 1/8" fat, all grades, braised	3 oz	290	21	9	55	0	0	23
Chuck, clod roast, 0" fat, all grades, roasted	3 oz	176	9	3	60	0	0	22
Chuck, clod steak, top & center, 0" fat, all grades, grilled	3 oz	155	7	2	51	0	0	22
Chuck, clod steak, top blade, 0" fat, all grades, grilled	3 oz	189	11	4	65	0	0	21
Chuck, mock tender steak, 0" fat, all grades, broiled	3 oz	136	5	2	60	0	0	22
Chuck, shoulder clod steak, top & center, 0" fat, USDA Choice, grilled	3 oz	155	7	2	51	0	0	22
Chuck, top blade, 0" fat, all grades, broiled	3 oz	184	10	3	57	0	0	22
Cured beef, corned beef brisket, cooked	3 oz	213	16	5	964	0	0	15
Cured beef, corned beef, canned	3 oz	213	13	5	856	0	0	23
Cured beef, dried	1 slice	4	0	0	78	0	0	1
Cured beef, luncheon meat, jellied	1 slice	31	1	0	375	0	0	5
Cured beef, pastrami	1 slice	41	2	1	248	0	0	6
Cured beef, sausage, smoked	3 oz	265	23	10	962	2	0	12
Cured beef, smoked, chopped beef	1 slice	37	1	1	352	1	0	6
Cured beef, thin slices	1 slice	4	0	0	30	0	0	1
Eye of round, 0" fat, all grades, roasted	3 oz	143	4	1	32	0	0	25
Eye of round, 1/8" fat, all grades, roasted	3 oz	177	8	3	31	0	0	24
Flank, 0" fat, all grades, broiled	3 oz	200	7	3	48	0	0	24
Full cut, 1/8" fat, USDA Choice, broiled	3 oz	230	11	4	53	0	0	23
Ground beef, 30% fat, crumbles, pan browned	3 oz	175	15	6	82	0	0	22
Ground beef, 30% fat, loaf, baked	3 oz	205	13	5	62	0	0	20
Ground beef, 30% fat, patty, broiled	3 oz	232	15	6	69	0	0	22

ITEM DESCRIPTION	Serving Size	Calories	Total Fat (g)	Saturated Fat (g)	Sodium (mg)	Carbohydrates (g)	Fiber (g)	Protein (g)
Ground beef, 30% fat, patty, pan browned	3 oz	202	13	5	78	0	0	19
Ground beef, 25% fat, crumbles, pan browned	3 oz	239	15	6	79	0	0	22
Ground beef, 25% fat, loaf, baked	3 oz	216	14	5	60	0	0	21
Ground beef, 25% fat, patty, broiled	3 oz	236	16	6	66	0	0	22
Ground beef, 25% fat, patty, pan broiled	3 oz	211	14	5	74	0	0	20
Ground beef, 20% fat, crumbles, pan browned	3 oz	231	15	6	77	0	0	23
Ground beef, 20% fat, loaf, baked	3 oz	216	14	5	57	0	0	21
Ground beef, 20% fat, patty, broiled	3 oz	230	15	6	64	0	0	22
Ground beef, 20% fat, patty, pan broiled	3 oz	209	14	5	71	0	0	20
Ground beef, 15% fat, crumbles, pan browned	3 oz	218	13	5	76	0	0	24
Ground beef, 15% fat, loaf, baked	3 oz	204	12	5	54	0	0	22
Ground beef, 15% fat, patty, pan broiled	3 oz	197	12	5	67	0	0	21
Ground beef, 10% fat, crumbles, pan browned	3 oz	196	10	4	74	0	0	24
Ground beef, 10% fat, loaf, baked	3 oz	182	9	4	52	0	0	23
Ground beef, 10% fat, patty, broiled	3 oz	184	10	4	58	0	0	22
Ground beef, 10% fat, patty, pan broiled	3 oz	173	9	4	64	0	0	21
Ground beef, 5% fat, crumbles, pan browned	3 oz	164	6	3	72	0	0	25
Ground beef, 5% fat, loaf, baked	3 oz	148	5	2	49	0	0	23
Ground beef, 5% fat, patty, broiled	3 oz	145	6	3	55	0	0	22
Ground beef, 5% fat, patty, pan browned	3 oz	139	5	2	60	0	0	22
Loin, bottom sirloin butt, tri-tip, 0" fat, all grades, roasted	3 oz	155	7	3	47	0	0	23
Outside round, bottom round steak, 0" fat, all grades, grilled	3 oz	155	6	2	49	0	0	23

ITEM DESCRIPTION	Serving Size	Calories	Total Fat (g)	Saturated Fat (g)	Sodium (mg)	Carbohydrates (g)	Fiber (g)	Protein (g)
Rib eye, small end, 0" fat, all grades, broiled	1 steak	576	34	13	130	0	0	64
Ribs, large end, 0" fat, USDA Choice, roasted	3 oz	316	26	10	54	0	0	19
Ribs, large end, 1/8" fat, all grades, broiled	3 oz	287	23	9	54	0	0	18
Ribs, large end, 1/8" fat, all grades, roasted	3 oz	302	24	10	54	0	0	20
Ribs, large end, 1/8" fat, USDA Prime, broiled	3 oz	343	30	12	53	0	0	18
Ribs, large end, 1/8" fat, USDA Prime, roasted	3 oz	334	28	12	54	0	0	19
Ribs, short ribs, USDA Choice, braised	3 oz	400	36	15	43	0	0	18
Ribs, small end, 0" fat, all grades, broiled	3 oz	212	13	5	48	0	0	23
Ribs, small end, 1/8" fat, all grades, broiled	3 oz	247	17	7	45	0	0	22
Ribs, small end, 1/8" fat, all grades, roasted	3 oz	290	23	9	54	0	0	19
Ribs, small end, 1/8" fat, USDA Prime, broiled	3 oz	301	24	10	54	0	0	21
Ribs, small end, 1/8" fat, USDA Prime, roasted	3 oz	349	30	12	55	0	0	19
Ribs, whole, 1/8" fat, all grades, broiled	3 oz	286	23	9	54	0	0	19
Ribs, whole, 1/8" fat, all grades, roasted	3 oz	298	24	10	54	0	0	19
Ribs, whole, 1/8" fat, USDA Prime, broiled	3 oz	328	28	11	53	0	0	19
Ribs, whole, 1/8" fat, USDA Prime, roasted	3 oz	340	29	12	55	0	0	19
Roast beef spread	1/4 cup	127	9	4	413	2	0	9
Round, knuckle, tip center steak, 0" fat, all grades, grilled	1 steak	266	10	4	78	0	0	41
Round, knuckle, tip side steak, 0" fat, all grades, grilled	3 oz	143	4	2	46	0	0	25
Short loin, Porterhouse steak, 0" fat, all grades, broiled	3 oz	235	16	6	55	0	0	20

ITEM DESCRIPTION	Serving Size	Calories	Total Fat (g)	Saturated Fat (g)	Sodium (mg)	Carbohydrates (g)	Fiber (g)	Protein (g)
Short loin, Porterhouse steak, 1/8" fat, all grades, broiled	3 oz	252	19	7	54	0	0	20
Short loin, T-bone steak, 0" fat, all grades, broiled	3 oz	210	14	5	57	0	0	21
Short loin, T-bone steak, 1/8" fat, all grades, broiled	3 oz	238	17	6	56	0	0	21
Short loin, top loin, 0" fat, all grades, broiled	3 oz	164	7	3	50	0	0	25
Short loin, top loin, 1/8" fat, all grades, broiled	3 oz	224	14	6	46	0	0	22
Short loin, top loin, 1/8" fat, USDA Prime, broiled	3 oz	264	19	8	54	0	0	22
Sirloin, tri-tip steak, 0" fat, all grades, broiled	3 oz	225	13	5	61	0	0	25
Skirt steak, 0" fat, all grades, broiled	3 oz	187	10	4	64	0	0	22
Skirt steak, outside, 0" fat, all grades, broiled	3 oz	217	15	6	78	0	0	20
Tenderloin, 0" fat, all grades, broiled	3 oz	185	9	4	48	0	0	23
Tenderloin, 1/8" fat, all grades, broiled	3 oz	227	15	6	46	0	0	22
Tenderloin, 1/8" fat, all grades, roasted	3 oz	275	21	8	48	0	0	20
Tenderloin, 1/8" fat, USDA Prime, broiled	3 oz	262	19	8	50	0	0	21
Tenderloin, 1/8" fat, USDA Prime, roasted	3 oz	292	23	9	47	0	0	20
Tip round, 0" fat, all grades, roasted	3 oz	160	7	3	30	0	0	23
Tip round, 1/8" fat, all grades, roasted	3 oz	186	10	4	54	0	0	23
Top round, 0" fat, all grades, braised	3 oz	178	5	2	38	0	0	30
Top round, 0" fat, all grades, broiled	3 oz	175	5	2	35	0	0	27
Top round, 1/8" fat, all grades, braised	3 oz	202	9	3	38	0	0	29
Top round, 1/8" fat, all grades, broiled	3 oz	173	8	3	35	0	0	26
Top round, 1/8" fat, USDA Choice, pan fried	3 oz	226	12	4	58	0	0	28
Top sirloin, 0" fat, all grades, broiled	3 oz	180	7	2	55	2	0	29
Top sirloin, 1/8" fat, all grades, broiled	3 oz	207	12	5	48	0	0	23
Top sirloin, 1/8" fat, USDA Choice, pan fried	3 oz	266	18	7	60	0	0	24

ITEM DESCRIPTION	Serving Size	Calories	Total Fat (g)	Saturated Fat (g)	Sodium (mg)	Carbohydrates (g)	Fiber (g)	Protein (g)
BEEF BOUILLON								
(powder, prepared w/ water)	1 cube	9	0	0	611	1	0	1
BEEF BROTH								
Broth & tomato juice, canned	1 cup	90	0	0	320	21	0	1
Campbell's Red & White, condensed	1 cup	15	0	0	636	1	0	3
Canned, ready to serve	1 cup	17	1	0	782	0	0	3
Cubed, prepared w/ water	1 cube	6	0	0	864	1	0	1
BEEF JERKY	1 lg pc	82	5	2	443	2	0	7
BEEF STEW								
Canned	1 serv	220	12	5	947	16	4	11
Hormel Dinty Moore, canned	1 cup	222	13	6	984	16	3	11
BEEF STICKS	1 stick	110	10	4	296	1	0	4
BEEF STOCK (homemade)	1 cup	31	0	0	475	3	0	5
BEEF SUBSTITUTE, BRAND NAME								
Carl Buddig Smoked Slices, beef	2 oz	79	4	1	816	0	0	11
Loma Linda Dinner Cuts, canned	2 slices	96	1	0	456	4	2	18
Loma Linda Swiss Stake, w/ gravy, canned	1 pc	130	6	1	433	10	3	9
Loma Linda Tender Bits, canned	6 pcs	115	4	1	521	7	4	13
Loma Linda Tender Rounds, w/ gravy, canned	6 pcs	116	5	1	354	6	3	13
Worthington Choplets, canned	2 slices	95	1	0	420	4	3	18
Worthington Prime Stakes, canned	1 pc	124	7	1	442	7	1	9
Worthington Stakelets, frozen	1 pc	150	7	1	462	7	2	14
Worthington Vegetable Steaks, canned	2 slices	81	1	0	300	4	2	15
BEER								
Bud Light	12 fl oz	110	0	12	11	7	0	1
Budweiser	12 fl oz	146	0	0	11	11	0	1
Budweiser Select	12 fl oz	99	0	0	11	3	0	1
Light, all	12 fl oz	103	0	0	14	6	0	1
Michelob Ultra Light	12 fl oz	96	0	0	11	3	0	1
Regular, all	12 fl oz	153	0	0	14	13	0	2

ITEM DESCRIPTION	Serving Size	Calories	Total Fat (g)	Saturated Fat (g)	Sodium (mg)	Carbohydrates (g)	Fiber (g)	Protein (g)
BEET GREENS								
Boiled (1" pcs)	1 cup	39	0	0	347	8	4	4
Fresh	1 cup	8	0	0	86	2	1	1
BEETS								
Boiled (2" dia)	1 beet	22	0	0	39	5	1	1
Canned, diced	1 cup	49	0	0	305	11	3	1
Canned, no salt	1 cup	69	0	0	52	16	3	2
Canned, reg	1 cup	74	0	0	352	18	3	2
Fresh (2" dia)	1 beet	35	0	0	64	8	2	1
Harvard, canned	1 cup	180	0	0	399	45	6	2
Pickled, canned	1 cup	148	0	0	599	37	6	2
BISCUITS								
Martha White Buttermilk Biscuit	1 serv	159	5	2	531	24	1	3
Mixed grain, refrigerated (2.5" dia)	1 biscuit	116	2	1	295	21	0	3
Pillsbury Buttermilk Biscuits, refrigerated	1 serv	150	2	0	570	29	1	4
Pillsbury Golden Layer Buttermilk Biscuits, refrigerated	1 serv	104	5	1	360	14	0	2
Pillsbury Grands Buttermilk Biscuits, refrigerated	1 serv	193	8	3	631	25	1	4
Plain or buttermilk, commercial 2.5" dia	1 biscuit	128	6	1	368	17	0	2
Plain or buttermilk, dry mix, prepared	1 oz	95	3	1	271	14	1	2
Plain or buttermilk, homemade 2.5" dia	1 biscuit	212	10	3	348	27	1	4
Plain or buttermilk, refrigerated 2.5" dia	1 biscuit	95	4	1	292	13	0	2
Plain or buttermilk, refrigerated, lower fat (2.25" dia)	1 biscuit	63	1	0	305	12	0	2
BLACK BEANS (boiled)	1 cup	227	1	0	2	41	15	15
BLACKBERRIES								
Canned in heavy syrup	1 cup	236	0	0	8	59	9	3
Fresh	1 cup	62	1	0	1	14	8	2
Frozen, unsweetened	1 cup	97	1	0	2	24	8	2
Juice, canned	1 cup	95	2	0	3	20	0	1

ITEM DESCRIPTION	Serving Size	Calories	Total Fat (g)	Saturated Fat (g)	Sodium (mg)	Carbohydrates (g)	Fiber (g)	Protein (g)
BLUEBERRIES								
Canned in heavy syrup	1 cup	225	1	0	8	56	4	2
Canned in light syrup	1 cup	215	1	0	7	55	6	3
Fresh	1 cup	84	0	0	1	21	4	1
Frozen, sweetened	1 cup	186	0	0	2	50	5	1
Frozen, unsweetened	1 cup	79	1	0	2	19	4	1
Frozen, wild	1 cup	71	0	0	4	19	6	0
Pie filling, canned	1 cup	474	1	0	31	116	7	1
BLUEFISH (cooked in dry heat)	3 oz	135	5	1	65	0	0	22
BOLOGNA								
Beef	1 oz slice	87	8	3	302	1	0	3
Beef & pork	1 oz slice	87	7	3	206	2	0	4
Beef & pork, low fat	1 oz slice	64	5	2	310	1	0	3
Beef, low fat	1 oz slice	57	4	2	330	1	0	3
Beef, reduced sodium	1 oz slice	88	8	3	191	1	0	3
Chicken & pork	1 oz slice	94	9	3	347	1	0	3
Chicken, pork, beef	1 oz slice	76	6	2	314	2	0	3
Chicken, turkey, pork	1 oz slice	83	7	2	258	2	0	3
Oscar Mayer, beef	1 oz slice	88	8	4	330	1	0	3
Oscar Mayer, beef, light	1 oz slice	56	4	2	322	2	0	3
Oscar Mayer, chicken, pork & beef	1 oz slice	89	8	3	289	1	0	3
Oscar Mayer, fat free	1 oz slice	22	0	0	274	2	0	4
Oscar Mayer, light	1 oz slice	57	4	2	313	2	0	3
Pork	1 oz slice	69	6	2	332	0	0	4
Pork & turkey lite	1 oz slice	59	5	2	200	1	0	4
Pork, turkey & beef	1 oz slice	95	8	3	299	2	0	3
Turkey	1 oz slice	59	4	1	351	1	0	3
BOYSENBERRIES								
Canned, heavy syrup	1 cup	225	0	0	8	57	7	3
Frozen, unsweetened	1 cup	66	0	0	1	16	7	1
BRAN								
Corn, crude	1 cup	170	1	0	5	65	60	6
Wheat, crude	1 cup	125	2	0	1	37	25	9

ITEM DESCRIPTION	Serving Size	Calories	Total Fat (g)	Saturated Fat (g)	Sodium (mg)	Carbohydrates (g)	Fiber (g)	Protein (g)
BRAZIL NUTS								
(Dried, unblanched, whole)	1 cup	874	89	20	4	16	10	19
BREAD								
Arnold, 100% whole wheat	1 slice	110	1	0	170	20	3	5
Arnold, 12 grain	1 slice	110	1.5	0	170	21	3	5
Arnold, Multi-Grain Sandwich Thins	1	100	1	0	230	22	5	5
Arnold, oatnut	1 slice	120	2.5	0	170	22	2	4
Boston brown	1 slice	88	1	0	284	19	2	2
Cracked wheat	1 slice	65	1	0	135	12	1	2
Egg	1 slice	113	2	1	197	19	1	4
French or Vienna (2" slice)	1 slice	92	1	0	208	18	1	4
Irish soda	1 oz	82	1	0	113	16	1	2
Italian	1 slice	54	1	0	117	10	1	2
Multi-grain	1 slice	69	1	0	109	11	2	3
Oat bran	1 slice	71	1	0	122	12	1	3
Oat bran, reduced calorie	1 slice	46	1	0	81	10	3	2
Oatmeal	1 slice	70	1	0	121	12	1	3
Oatmeal, reduced calorie	1 slice	48	1	0	89	10	1	2
Pepperidge Farm, 100% whole wheat	1 slice	100	1.5	.5	105	20	4	5
Pepperidge Farm, 9 grain	1 slice	100	1.5	0	110	17	3	4
Pepperidge Farm Crusty Italian Bread, garlic	1 serv	186	10	2	200	21	0	4
Pepperidge Farm Hearty White	1 slice	120	1.5	.5	210	22	1	4
Pillsbury Crusty French Loaf, refrigerated	1 serv	149	2	1	358	29	1	5
Pita, white (4" dia)	1 pita	77	0	0	150	16	1	3
Pita, whole wheat (4" dia)	1 pita	74	1	0	149	15	2	3
Protein, including gluten	1 slice	47	0	0	104	8	1	2
Pumpernickel	1 slice	65	1	0	174	12	2	2
Raisin	1 slice	71	1	0	101	14	1	2
Rice bran	1 slice	66	1	0	119	12	1	2
Rye	1 slice	83	1	0	211	15	2	3
Rye, reduced calorie	1 slice	47	1	0	93	9	3	2
Sourdough (2" slice)	1 slice	92	1	0	208	18	1	4

ITEM DESCRIPTION	Serving Size	Calories	Total Fat (g)	Saturated Fat (g)	Sodium (mg)	Carbohydrates (g)	Fiber (g)	Protein (g)
Wheat	1 slice	66	1	0	130	12	1	3
Wheat bran	1 slice	89	1	0	175	17	1	3
Wheat, reduced calorie	1 slice	46	1	0	118	10	3	2
White, commercial	1 slice	66	1	0	170	13	1	2
White, commercial, low sodium	1 slice	67	1	0	7	13	0	2
White, homemade, w/ lowfat milk	1 slice	120	2	0	151	21	1	3
White, homemade, w/ nonfat dry milk	1 slice	121	1	0	148	24	1	3
White, reduced calorie	1 slice	48	1	0	104	10	2	2
Whole wheat, commercial	1 slice	69	1	0	132	12	2	4
Whole wheat, homemade	1 slice	128	2	0	159	24	3	4
Wonder Bread, whole grain	1 slice	80	1	0	150	15	2	3
BREAD CRUMBS								
Dry, grated, plain	1 cup	427	6	1	791	78	5	14
Dry, grated, seasoned	1 cup	460	7	2	2111	82	6	17
Kraft Shake 'n' Bake Original Recipe, coating for pork	1 serv	106	1	0	795	22	0	2
White, commercial	1 cup	120	1	0	306	23	1	3
White, commercial, low sodium	1 cup	120	2	0	12	22	1	4
BREAD STICKS plain (4.25")	1 stick	21	0	0	33	3	0	1
BREAD STUFFING								
Dry mix, prepared	1 oz	50	2	0	154	6	1	1
Cornbread, prepared	1 oz	51	2	0	129	6	1	1
BREAKFAST STRIPS								
(Cured beef, cooked)	1 slice	51	4	2	255	0	0	4
BROAD BEANS (boiled)	1 cup	187	1	0	8	33	9	13
BROCCOLI								
Boiled, chopped	1/2 cup	27	0	0	32	6	3	2
Fresh, chopped	1 cup	31	0	0	30	6	2	3
Fresh, flowers	1 cup	20	0	0	19	4	0	2
Frozen, boiled, chopped	1 cup	20	0	0	20	10	6	6
Frozen, boiled, spears	10 oz pkg	70	0	0	60	13	8	8
Green Giant Broccoli in Cheese Flavored Sauce, frozen	1 cup	113	4	1	806	15	0	4

ITEM DESCRIPTION	Serving Size	Calories	Total Fat (g)	Saturated Fat (g)	Sodium (mg)	Carbohydrates (g)	Fiber (g)	Protein (g)
Stalks, fresh	1 stalk	32	0	0	31	6	0	3
BROCCOLI RABE								
Cooked	1 cup	144	2	0	245	14	12	17
Fresh, chopped	1 cup	9	0	0	13	1	1	1
BROWNIES								
Commercial (2-3/4" sq)	1	227	9	2	175	36	1	3
Homemade (2" sq)	1	112	7	2	82	12	0	1
Martha White Chewy Fudge Brownies	1 serv	114	2	0	128	23	1	1
Pillsbury Traditional Fudge Brownies	1 serv	132	4	1	88	23	0	1
BRUSSELS SPROUTS								
Boiled	1/2 cup	28	0	0	16	6	2	2
Frozen, boiled	1/2 cup	33	0	0	12	6	3	3
BUCKWHEAT								
Flour, whole groat	1 cup	402	4	1	13	85	15	15
Groats, roasted, cooked	1 cup	155	1	0	7	34	5	6
Groats, roasted, dry	1 cup	567	4	1	18	123	17	19
BULGUR (cooked)	1 cup	151	0	0	9	34	8	6
BURBOT (cooked in dry heat)	3 oz	98	1	0	105	0	0	21
BURDOCK ROOT								
Boiled (1" pcs)	1 cup	110	0	0	5	26	2	3
Fresh (1" pcs)	1 cup	85	0	0	6	20	4	2
BURRITO								
Bean & cheese, microwavable	1	309	9	2	758	48	12	10
Beef & bean, frozen	1	332	13	4	816	43	6	10
BUTTER								
No salt	1 tbsp	102	12	7	2	0	0	0
Salted	1 tbsp	102	12	7	82	0	0	0
Whipped, w/ salt	1 tbsp	67	8	5	78	0	0	0
BUTTER BLEND								
Butter-margarine, stick, w/o salt	1 tbsp	101	11	4	4	0	0	0
Butter-vegetable oil, spread, reduced calorie, w/ salt	1 tbsp	63	7	2	85	0	0	0
Butter-vegetable oil, spread, w/ salt	1 tbsp	51	6	1	110	0	0	0
BUTTERBUR (canned, chopped)	1 cup	4	0	0	5	0	0	0

ITEM DESCRIPTION	Serving Size	Calories	Total Fat (g)	Saturated Fat (g)	Sodium (mg)	Carbohydrates (g)	Fiber (g)	Protein (g)
BUTTERFISH (cooked in dry heat)	3 oz	159	9	0	97	0	0	0
BUTTERMILK								
Low fat	1 cup	98	2	1	257	12	0	8
Reduced fat	1 cup	137	5	3	211	13	0	10
BUTTERMILK SQUASH (baked, cubed)	1 cup	82	0	0	8	22	0	2
BUTTERNUTS (dried)	1 cup	734	68	2	1	14	6	30
BUTTERNUT SQUASH (frozen, boiled, mashed)	1 cup	94	0	0	5	24	0	3
BUTTER OIL	1 tbsp	112	13	8	0	0	0	0
BUTTER REPLACEMENT (powder, no fat)	1 cup	298	1	0	960	71	0	2
BUTTERSCOTCH TOPPING	2 tbsp	103	0	0	143	27	0	1
CABBAGE								
Chinese (bok choy), boiled, shredded	1 cup	20	0	0	58	3	2	3
Chinese (bok choy), fresh, shredded	1 cup	9	0	0	46	2	1	1
Chinese (pe tsai), boiled, shredded	1 cup	17	0	0	11	3	2	2
Chinese (pe tsai), fresh, shredded	1 cup	12	0	0	7	2	1	1
Common, fresh, shredded	1 cup	17	0	0	13	4	2	1
Japanese style, fresh, pickled	1 cup	45	0	0	416	9	5	2
Mustard, boiled, shredded	1 cup	36	0	0	13	7	4	1
Napa, cooked	1 cup	13	0	0	12	2	0	1
Red, boiled, shredded	1 cup	44	0	0	42	10	4	2
Red, fresh, shredded	1 cup	22	0	0	19	5	1	1
Savoy, boiled, shredded	1 cup	35	0	0	35	8	4	3
Savoy, fresh, shredded	1 cup	19	0	0	20	4	2	1
CAKE								
Angelfood, commercial (12 oz cake)	1/12 cake	72	0	0	210	16	0	2
Angelfood, from mix (10" dia cake)	1/12 cake	129	0	0	255	29	0	3
Betty Crocker Super Moist Party Cake Swirl	1 serv	178	3	1	266	35	0	2
Betty Crocker Super Moist Yellow Cake	1 serv	178	3	1	289	35	0	2

ITEM DESCRIPTION	Serving Size	Calories	Total Fat (g)	Saturated Fat (g)	Sodium (mg)	Carbohydrates (g)	Fiber (g)	Protein (g)
Boston cream pie, commercial	1/6 pie	232	8	2	132	39	1	2
Cheesecake, commercial (17 oz cake)	1/6 cake	257	18	8	166	20	0	4
Cheesecake, from no-bake mix (9" dia)	1/12 cake	271	13	7	376	35	2	5
Cherry fudge, w/ chocolate frosting	1/8 cake	187	9	4	160	27	1	2
Chocolate, commercial, w/ chocolate frosting (18 oz cake)	1/8 cake	235	10	3	214	35	2	3
Chocolate, from pudding-type mix	1 oz	112	3	1	253	22	1	1
Chocolate, homemade w/o frosting (9" dia)	1/12 cake	352	14	5	299	51	2	5
Coffee cake, cheese (16 oz cake)	1/6 cake	258	12	4	258	34	1	5
Coffee cake, cinnamon w/ crumb topping, commercial (20 oz cake)	1/9 cake	263	15	4	221	29	1	4
Coffee cake, cinnamon w/ crumb topping, from mix	1/8 cake (2 oz)	178	5	1	236	30	1	3
Coffee cake, crème filled, w/ chocolate frosting (19 oz cake)	1/6 cake	298	10	3	291	48	2	5
Coffee cake, fruit	1/8 cake	156	5	1	193	26	1	3
Fruitcake, commercial	1 pc	139	4	0	116	26	2	1
German chocolate, from pudding-type mix	1 oz	114	3	1	182	23	1	1
Gingerbread, homemade (8" sq cake)	1/9 cake	101	5	1	93	14	0	1
Pineapple upside-down, homemade (8" sq cake)	1/9 cake	367	14	3	367	58	1	4
Pound, commercial, fat free (12 oz cake)	1/12 cake	80	0	0	97	17	0	2
Pound, commercial, w/ butter (12 oz cake)	1/12 cake	109	6	3	111	14	0	2
Pound, commercial, w/o butter (12 oz cake)	1/12 cake	109	5	1	112	15	0	1
Shortcake, biscuit, homemade (12 oz cake)	1/12 cake	98	4	1	143	14	0	2
Snackwell's Fat Free Devil's Food Cookie Cakes	1 serv	49	0	0	28	12	0	1

ITEM DESCRIPTION	Serving Size	Calories	Total Fat (g)	Saturated Fat (g)	Sodium (mg)	Carbohydrates (g)	Fiber (g)	Protein (g)
Sponge, commercial (16 oz cake)	1/12 cake	110	1	0	93	23	0	2
Sponge, homemade (10" dia)	1/12 cake	187	3	1	144	36	0	5
White, homemade w/ coconut frosting (9" dia)	1/12 cake	399	12	4	318	71	1	5
White, homemade, w/o frosting (9" dia)	1/12 cake	264	9	2	242	42	1	4
Yellow, commercial, w/ chocolate frosting (18 oz cake)	1/8 cake	243	11	3	216	35	1	2
Yellow, commercial, w/ vanilla frosting (18 oz cake)	1/8 cake	239	9	2	220	38	0	2
Yellow, homemade w/o frosting (8" dia)	1/12 cake	245	10	3	233	36	0	4
CALABASH GOURD								
Boiled, cubed	1 cup	22	0	0	3	5	0	1
Fresh (1" pcs)	1 cup	16	0	0	2	4	0	1
CANDY								
Butterscotch	1 pc	21	0	0	21	5	0	0
Candy corn	1 oz	105	0	0	57	27	0	0
Caramels	1 pc	39	1	0	25	8	0	0
Caramels, chocolate-flavored roll	1 pc	26	0	0	3	6	0	0
Caramels, w/ nuts, chocolate covered	1 pc	66	3	1	3	8	1	1
Carob, unsweetened	3 oz bar	470	27	25	93	49	3	7
Coffee beans, dark chocolate coated	1 pc	8	0	0	0	1	0	0
Divinity, homemade	1 pc	40	0	0	4	10	0	0
Gumdrops, dietetic, w/ Sorbitol	1 pc	8	0	0	0	4	1	0
Gumdrops, starch jelly pieces	1 pc	14	0	0	2	4	0	0
Hard	1 pc	24	0	0	2	6	0	0
Hard, dietetic, w/ Sorbitol	1 pc	11	0	0	0	3	0	0
Jellybeans	10 sml	41	0	0	6	10	0	0
Milk chocolate, w/ almonds	1.45 oz bar	216	14	7	30	22	3	4
Milk chocolate, w/ rice cereal	1.45 oz bar	230	13	7	39	27	1	3
Nougat, w/ almonds	1 pc	56	0	0	5	13	0	0
Peanut bar	1.4 oz bar	209	13	2	62	19	2	6
Peanuts, milk chocolate coated	1 pc	21	1	1	2	2	0	1

ITEM DESCRIPTION	Serving Size	Calories	Total Fat (g)	Saturated Fat (g)	Sodium (mg)	Carbohydrates (g)	Fiber (g)	Protein (g)
Praline, homemade	1 pc	189	10	1	19	23	1	1
Raisins, milk chocolate coated	10 pcs	39	1	1	4	7	0	0
Sesame crunch	1 pc	10	1	0	3	1	0	0
Taffy, homemade	1 pc	60	0	0	8	14	0	0
Toffee, homemade	1 pc	67	4	2	16	8	0	0
Truffles, homemade	1 pc	61	4	2	8	5	0	1
CANDY, BRAND NAME								
100 Grand Bar	1.5 oz bar	201	8	5	87	31	0	1
3 Musketeers Bar	2.13 oz bar	259	8	5	117	47	1	2
5th Avenue Candy Bar	2 oz bar	270	13	4	126	35	2	5
After Eight Thin Mints	5 mints	170	5	3	0	32	1	1
Almond Joy Bites	18 pcs	218	14	8	16	23	2	2
Almond Joy Candy Bar	1.76 oz pkg	235	13	9	70	29	2	2
Baby Ruth Bar	2.1 oz bar	273	13	7	137	39	1	3
Bit-O-Honey Candy Chews	6 pcs	150	3	2	118	32	0	1
Butterfinger Bar	2.1 oz bar	273	11	6	137	43	1	3
Caramello Candy Bar	1.25 oz bar	162	7	4	43	22	0	2
Chunky Bar	1.4 oz bar	190	11	5	15	24	1	3
Dove Dark Chocolate	1.3 oz bar	192	12	7	1	22	3	2
Dove Milk Chocolate	1.3 oz bar	201	12	7	23	22	1	2
Golden Almond Solitaires	13 pcs	234	15	6	21	19	2	5
Goobers Chocolate Covered Peanuts	1.375 oz pkg	200	13	5	14	21	4	4
Heath Bites	15 pcs	207	12	6	96	25	1	2
Hershey's Nuggets	17 pcs	215	14	7	29	20	1	4
Hershey's Skor Toffee Bar	1.4 oz bar	209	13	7	124	24	1	1
Hershey's Special Dark Chocolate Bar	1.45 oz bar	228	13	0	2	25	3	2
Hershey's Symphony Milk Chocolate Bar	1.5 oz bar	223	13	8	42	24	1	4
Kit Kat Bites	15 pcs	199	10	7	26	25	1	3
Kit Kat, big bar	1.94 oz bar	286	15	10	35	35	1	3
Kit Kat, wafer bar	1.5 oz bar	218	11	8	23	27	0	3
Krackel Chocolate Bar	1.45 oz bar	210	11	7	80	26	1	3

ITEM DESCRIPTION	Serving Size	Calories	Total Fat (g)	Saturated Fat (g)	Sodium (mg)	Carbohydrates (g)	Fiber (g)	Protein (g)
M&M's Almond Chocolate Candies	1.31 oz bar	189	10	4	17	22	2	3
M&M's Milk Chocolate Candies	1.48 oz box	207	9	5	26	30	1	2
M&M's Minis Milk Chocolate Candies	1 oz tube	151	7	4	20	21	1	1
M&M's Peanut Butter Chocolate Candies	1.63 oz bag	244	14	9	98	26	2	5
M&M's Peanut Chocolate Candies	1 bag	280	14	6	27	33	2	5
Mars Almond Bar	1.76 oz bar	234	12	4	85	31	1	4
Milky Way Bar	2.05 oz bar	263	10	7	97	41	1	2
Milky Way Midnight Bar	1.76 oz bar	221	9	6	84	36	1	2
Milky Way Minis, dark chocolate covered	5 pcs	202	9	6	108	30	1	2
Milky Way Minis, milk chocolate covered	5 pcs	204	8	6	120	30	0	2
Mounds Candy Bar, snack size	1 bar	92	5	4	28	11	1	1
Mr. Goodbar Chocolate Bar	1.75 oz bar	264	16	7	20	27	2	5
Nestle Crunch Bar & Dessert Topping	1.55 oz bar	220	11	7	66	29	1	2
Oh Henry! Bar	2 oz bar	263	13	5	110	37	1	4
Pop'ables 3 Musketeers Bite Size	15 pcs	182	6	4	71	31	1	1
Pop'ables Milky Way Brand Bite Size	13 pcs	177	7	3	57	28	0	1
Pop'ables Snickers Brand Bite Size	13 pcs	187	9	4	87	24	1	3
Raisinets Chocolate Covered Raisins	1.58 oz bag	189	8	5	15	32	1	2
Reese's Bites	16 pcs	203	12	7	70	22	1	4
Reese's Fast Break	1 bar	277	13	5	180	36	2	5
Reese's Fast Break, milk chocolate, peanut butter	2 oz bar	265	13	5	185	34	2	5
Reese's NutRageous	1.92 oz bar	281	17	5	77	29	2	6
Reese's Peanut Butter Cups	1 PB cup	88	5	2	53	9	1	2
Reese's Pieces	10 pcs	40	2	1	16	5	0	1
Reesesticks Crispy Wafers, peanut butter, milk chocolate	1.5 oz	219	13	6	111	23	1	4
Rolo Caramels, milk chocolate	7 pcs	199	9	6	79	29	0	2

ITEM DESCRIPTION	Serving Size	Calories	Total Fat (g)	Saturated Fat (g)	Sodium (mg)	Carbohydrates (g)	Fiber (g)	Protein (g)
Skittles Original Bite Size Candies	2.17 oz pk	249	3	3	9	56	0	0
Skittles Sours Original	1.8 oz bag	202	2	2	7	44	0	0
Skittles Tropical Bite Size Candies	2.1 oz bag	249	3	0	9	56	0	0
Skittles Wild Berry Bite Size	2.1 oz bag	249	3	3	9	56	0	0
Snickers Almond Bar	1.76 oz bar	236	11	4	78	32	1	3
Snickers Bar	2 oz bar	271	14	5	140	35	1	4
Snickers Cruncher	1.66 oz bar	230	11	6	89	30	1	3
Snickers Munch Bar	1.42 oz bar	216	15	4	144	18	2	6
Starburst Fruit Chews, original	8 chews	163	3	3	1	33	0	0
Starburst Fruit Chews, tropical	8 chews	164	3	3	1	33	0	0
Starburst Sour Fruit Chews	2.07 oz pk	235	5	4	52	47	0	0
Tootsie Roll, chocolate-flavored roll	6 pcs	155	1	0	18	35	0	1
Twix Caramel Cookie Bars	2 oz pkg	286	14	11	113	37	1	3
Twix Peanut Butter Cookie Bars	2 bars	289	18	9	122	29	2	5
Twizzlers Cherry Bites	18 pcs	135	1	0	104	32	0	1
Twizzlers Nibs Cherry Bits	27 pcs	139	1	0	78	32	0	1
Twizzlers Strawberry Twists Candy	4 pcs	133	1	0	109	30	0	1
Whatchamacallit Candy Bar	1.7 oz bar	237	11	8	144	30	1	4
York Bites	15 pcs	154	3	2	18	32	1	1
York Peppermint Pattie	1.5 oz patty	163	3	2	12	34	1	1
CANDY COATING								
Butterscotch	1 oz	153	8	7	25	19	0	1
Peanut butter	1 oz	153	8	4	71	13	1	5
Yogurt	1 oz	153	8	7	25	18	0	2
CANOLA OIL								
Canola oil	1 tbsp	124	14	1	0	0	0	0
Natreon	1 tbsp	124	14	1	0	0	0	0
CANTALOUPE (fresh, cubed)	1 cup	54	0	0	26	13	1	1
CAPERS (canned)	1 tbsp	2	0	0	255	0	0	0
CARAMBOLA (STARFRUIT) (fresh, cubed)	1 cup	41	0	0	3	9	4	1
CARAMEL CUSTARD FLAN (homemade)	1/2 cup	223	6	3	81	35	0	7

ITEM DESCRIPTION	Serving Size	Calories	Total Fat (g)	Saturated Fat (g)	Sodium (mg)	Carbohydrates (g)	Fiber (g)	Protein (g)
CARAMEL TOPPING	2 tbsp	103	0	0	143	27	0	1
CARDAMOM (ground)	1 tbsp	18	0	0	1	4	2	1
CARDOON (fresh, shredded)	1 cup	30	0	0	303	7	3	1
CAROB FLOUR	1 cup	229	1	0	36	92	41	5
CARP (cooked in dry heat)	3 oz	138	6	1	54	0	0	19
CARROT JUICE (canned)	1 cup	94	0	0	68	22	2	2
CARROTS								
Baby, fresh	1 med	4	0	0	8	1	0	0
Boiled, slices	1/2 cup	27	0	0	45	6	2	1
Canned, w/o salt	1/2 cup	18	0	0	31	4	1	0
Canned, w/ salt	1/2 cup	18	0	0	177	4	1	0
Dehydrated	1/2 cup	126	1	0	102	29	9	3
Fresh, whole	1 med	25	0	0	42	6	2	1
Frozen, boiled	1/2 cup	27	0	0	43	6	2	0
CASABA MELON								
(fresh, cubed)	1 cup	48	0	0	15	11	2	2
CASHEW BUTTER								
Plain, w/o salt	1 tbsp	94	8	2	2	4	0	3
Plain, w/ salt	1 tbsp	94	8	2	98	4	0	3
CASHEW NUTS								
Dry roasted, w/o salt, halves	1 cup	786	64	13	22	45	4	21
Dry roasted, w/ salt, halves	1 cup	786	64	13	877	45	4	21
Fresh	1 oz	157	12	2	3	9	1	5
Oil roasted, w/o salt, whole	1 cup	748	62	11	17	39	4	22
Oil roasted, w/ salt, whole	1 cup	750	62	11	397	39	4	22
CASSAVA (fresh)	1 cup	330	1	0	29	78	4	3
CATFISH								
Channel, breaded & fried	3 oz	195	11	3	238	7	1	15
Channel, farmed, cooked in dry heat	3 oz	129	7	2	68	0	0	16
Channel, wild, cooked in dry heat	3 oz	89	2	1	42	0	0	16
CAULIFLOWER								
Boiled (1" pcs)	1/2 cup	14	0	0	9	3	1	1
Fresh	1 cup	25	0	0	30	5	3	2
Frozen, boiled (1" pcs)	1/2 cup	17	0	0	16	3	2	1

ITEM DESCRIPTION	Serving Size	Calories	Total Fat (g)	Saturated Fat (g)	Sodium (mg)	Carbohydrates (g)	Fiber (g)	Protein (g)
CAULIFLOWER GREENS								
Cooked	1/5 head	29	0	0	21	6	3	3
Fresh	1 cup	20	0	0	15	4	2	2
CAVIAR (black & red, granular)	1 tbsp	40	3	1	240	1	0	4
CELERIAC								
Boiled	1 cup	42	0	0	95	9	2	1
Fresh	1 cup	66	0	0	156	14	3	2
CELERY								
Boiled, diced	1 cup	27	0	0	136	6	2	1
Fresh, chopped	1 cup	16	0	0	81	3	2	1
Seed	1 tbsp	25	2	0	10	3	1	1
CEREAL								
Bran flakes	3/4 cup	96	1	0	220	24	5	3
Bran, malted flour	1/3 cup	83	1	0	121	23	8	4
Chocolate flavored rings, presweetened	3/4 cup	112	2	0	128	22	2	1
Corn flakes, low sodium	1 cup	100	0	0	2	22	0	2
Corn flakes, plain	1 cup	101	0	0	266	24	1	2
Corn, rice, wheat, oat, presweetened, w/ fruit & almonds	1-1/4 cup	211	2	0	266	43	2	4
Crispy brown rice	1 cup	124	1	0	4	28	2	2
Farina, cooked w/ water	1 cup	112	0	0	5	24	1	3
Muesli, dried fruit & nuts	1 cup	289	4	1	196	66	6	8
Oat cereal, frosted w/ marshmallows	1 cup	109	1	0	158	24	1	2
Oat, corn & wheat squares, presweetened, maple flavored	1 cup	129	3	0	130	27	1	2
Oats, instant, cinnamon & spice, cooked w/ water	1 cup	257	3	1	362	52	4	6
Oats, instant, plain, cooked w/ water	1 cup	159	3	1	115	27	4	6
Oats, instant, raisins & spice, cooked w/ water	1 cup	240	3	0	362	49	4	5
Oats, reg & quick & instant, cooked w/ water	1 cup	166	4	1	9	28	4	6
Puffed corn, chocolate frosted	1 cup	122	1	0	201	26	1	1

ITEM DESCRIPTION	Serving Size	Calories	Total Fat (g)	Saturated Fat (g)	Sodium (mg)	Carbohydrates (g)	Fiber (g)	Protein (g)
Puffed oats, corn mixture, presweetened	1 cup	130	1	0	212	27	1	3
Puffed oats, corn, presweetened, w/ marshmallows	1 cup	115	1	0	206	25	0	2
Puffed rice	1 cup	56	0	0	0	13	0	1
Puffed rice, presweetened, fruit flavored	3/4 cup	108	1	0	158	24	0	1
Puffed rice, presweetened, w/ cocoa	3/4 cup	115	1	1	157	25	1	1
Puffed wheat	1 cup	44	0	0	0	10	1	2
Puffed wheat, presweetened	3/4 cup	107	0	0	40	25	0	1
Shredded wheat bran, plain, salt & sugar free	1-1/4 cup	197	1	0	3	47	8	7
Shredded wheat, plain, salt & sugar free	2 biscuits	155	1	0	3	36	6	5
Shredded wheat, plain, salt & sugar free, spoon size	1 cup	167	1	0	3	41	6	5
Shredded wheat, presweetened	1 cup	183	1	0	10	44	5	4
Shredded whole wheat, presweetened	1 cup	200	2	0	11	42	4	5
Wheat & bran, presweetened, w/ nuts & fruit	1 cup	212	3	0	280	42	5	4
Wheat & malt barley flakes	3/4 cup	106	1	0	140	24	3	3
Wheat germ, toasted, plain	1 cup	432	12	2	5	56	17	33
Whole wheat & oats, presweetened, w/ nuts & fruit	2/3 cup	204	5	1	156	40	4	4
Whole wheat & oats, presweetened, w/ pecans	2/3 cup	216	6	1	214	38	4	5
Whole wheat & oats, presweetened, w/ walnuts & fruit	1 cup	249	6	1	253	44	4	5
Whole wheat, corn & oats, presweetened, w/ almonds	3/4 cup	126	3	0	187	24	1	2
Whole wheat, hot natural cereal, cooked w/ water	1 cup	150	1	0	0	33	4	5
Whole wheat, oats & rice, maple flavored, w/ pecans	1 serv	219	5	2	145	40	3	4

ITEM DESCRIPTION	Serving Size	Calories	Total Fat (g)	Saturated Fat (g)	Sodium (mg)	Carbohydrates (g)	Fiber (g)	Protein (g)
CEREAL BARS								
Kashi TLC (Tasty Little Cereal) Bars, Blackberry Graham	1 bar	110	3	0	125	21	3	2
Kellogg's Nutri-Grain Cereal Bars, fruit filled	1 bar	139	3	0	110	27	1	2
Rice & wheat	1 bar	90	2	0	110	16	0	2
CEREAL, BRAND NAME								
Alpen	2/3 cup	200	3	0	30	41	4	6
Cream of Rice, cooked w/ water	1 cup	127	0	0	2	28	0	2
Cream of Wheat, instant, cooked w/ water	1 cup	149	1	0	10	32	1	4
Cream of Wheat, Mix 'n Eat, apple, banana & maple flavored	1 packet	132	0	0	242	29	1	2
Cream of Wheat, Mix 'n Eat, plain, cooked w/ water	1 packet	102	0	0	241	21	0	3
Cream of Wheat, quick, cooked w/ water	1 cup	129	0	0	139	27	1	4
Cream of Wheat, reg, cooked w/ water	1 cup	131	1	0	8	28	1	4
Familia	1/2 cup	220	7	2	125	36	4	5
General Mills Apple Cinnamon Cheerios	3/4 cup	120	2	0	120	25	1	2
General Mills Basic 4	1 cup	210	3	1	320	44	3	4
General Mills Berry Berry Kix	3/4 cup	104	1	0	139	23	1	1
General Mills Berry Burst Cheerios, all flavors	3/4 cup	99	1	0	162	22	2	3
General Mills Cheerios	1 cup	103	2	0	186	21	3	3
General Mills Chocolate Lucky Charms	1 cup	120	1	0	160	26	1	1
General Mills Cinnamon Grahams	3/4 cup	113	1	0	237	26	1	2
General Mills Cinnamon Toast Crunch	3/4 cup	134	3	0	217	25	1	2
General Mills Cocoa Puffs	3/4 cup	108	1	0	144	23	1	1
General Mills Cookie Crisp	1 cup	120	2	0	170	26	1	1
General Mills Cookie Crisp, peanut butter	3/4 cup	130	4	1	135	23	1	2

ITEM DESCRIPTION	Serving Size	Calories	Total Fat (g)	Saturated Fat (g)	Sodium (mg)	Carbohydrates (g)	Fiber (g)	Protein (g)
General Mills Corn Chex	1 cup	114	1	0	289	26	1	2
General Mills Count Chocula	3/4 cup	108	1	0	171	24	1	1
General Mills Country Corn Flakes	1 cup	110	1	0	270	25	1	2
General Mills Fiber One	1/2 cup	60	1	0	105	25	14	2
General Mills French Toast Crunch	3/4 cup	136	3	0	223	24	1	2
General Mills Frosted Cheerios	3/4 cup	110	1	0	200	23	1	2
General Mills Frosted Chex	3/4 cup	110	1	0	180	27	0	1
General Mills Golden Grahams	3/4 cup	120	1	0	270	26	1	1
General Mills Harmony	1-1/4 cup	201	1	0	355	43	2	6
General Mills Honey Nut Cheerios	3/4 cup	110	2	0	190	22	2	3
General Mills Honey Nut Chex	3/4 cup	128	1	0	235	28	0	2
General Mills Honey Nut Clusters	1 cup	218	3	0	290	48	3	4
General Mills Kix	1-1/4 cup	110	1	0	199	25	3	2
General Mills Lucky Charms	3/4 cup	110	1	0	183	22	1	2
General Mills Multi-Bran Chex	3/4 cup	154	1	0	292	40	6	3
General Mills Multi-Grain Cheerios	1 cup	114	1	0	207	25	3	2
General Mills Nature Valley Low Fat Fruit Granola	2/3 cup	212	3	0	207	44	3	4
General Mills Oatmeal Crisp, apple cinnamon	1 cup	210	2	1	270	46	4	4
General Mills Oatmeal Crisp, raisin	1 cup	237	2	1	248	50	4	6
General Mills Oatmeal Crisp, triple berry	1 cup	210	3	1	260	45	5	5
General Mills Oatmeal Crisp, w/ almonds	1 cup	240	5	1	273	46	5	5
General Mills Para Su Familia Raisin Bran	1-1/3 cup	170	1	0	300	42	7	4
General Mills Peanut Butter Toast Crunch	3/4 cup	130	4	1	135	23	1	2
General Mills Raisin Nut Bran	3/4 cup	200	4	1	250	42	5	4
General Mills Reese's Puffs	3/4 cup	126	3	0	193	22	1	2
General Mills Rice Chex	1 cup	103	0	0	240	23	0	2
General Mills Team Cheerios	3/4 cup	100	1	0	180	22	2	2
General Mills Total Corn Flakes	1-1/3 cup	112	0	0	209	26	1	2
General Mills Total Raisin Bran	1 cup	170	1	0	240	42	5	3

ITEM DESCRIPTION	Serving Size	Calories	Total Fat (g)	Saturated Fat (g)	Sodium (mg)	Carbohydrates (g)	Fiber (g)	Protein (g)
General Mills Trix	1 cup	128	2	0	180	28	1	1
General Mills Wheat Chex	3/4 cup	169	1	0	395	38	5	5
General Mills Wheaties	3/4 cup	99	1	0	189	22	3	3
General Mills Wheaties Raisin Bran	1 cup	183	1	0	251	45	5	4
General Mills Whole Grain Total	3/4 cup	100	1	0	190	23	3	2
General Mills Yogurt Burst Cheerios	3/4 cup	120	2	1	190	25	2	2
Health Valley Organic Fiber 7 Flakes	3/4 cup	109	0	0	16	24	4	4
Health Valley Organic Oat Bran Flakes	1 cup	166	1	0	17	37	6	5
Kashi 7 Whole Grain Flakes	1 cup	175	1	0	152	41	6	6
Kashi 7 Whole Grain Honey Puffs	1 cup	114	1	0	6	25	2	3
Kashi 7 Whole Grain Nuggets	1/2 cup	206	2	0	260	47	7	7
Kashi Cinnamon-Raisin Crunch	1 cup	165	1	0	104	41	8	4
Kashi Go Lean	1 cup	148	1	0	86	30	10	14
Kashi Go Lean Crunch!	1 cup	200	3	0	204	36	8	9
Kashi Go Lean Crunch!, honey almond flax	1 cup	202	4	0	138	36	9	9
Kashi Good Friends	1 cup	167	2	0	129	43	12	5
Kashi Granola, Cocoa Beach	1/2 cup	226	9	2	118	34	7	6
Kashi Granola, Mountain Medley	1/2 cup	218	7	1	110	37	6	6
Kashi Granola, Orchard Spice	1/2 cup	222	7	1	129	37	6	6
Kashi Granola, Summer Berry	1/2 cup	214	6	1	132	37	7	7
Kashi Heart to Heart, honey toasted oat	3/4 cup	118	2	0	79	25	5	4
Kashi Heart to Heart, wild blueberry	1 cup	204	3	0	133	42	4	6
Kashi Mighty Bites, cinnamon	1 cup	117	1	0	162	23	3	6
Kashi Mighty Bites, honey crunch	1 cup	116	1	0	159	23	3	6
Kashi Organic Promise Autumn Wheat	1 cup	191	1	0	5	45	6	5
Kashi Organic Promise Cinnamon Harvest	1 cup	184	1	0	5	44	6	4
Kashi Organic Promise Cranberry Sunshine	1 cup	116	1	0	21	26	3	2

ITEM DESCRIPTION	Serving Size	Calories	Total Fat (g)	Saturated Fat (g)	Sodium (mg)	Carbohydrates (g)	Fiber (g)	Protein (g)
Kashi Organic Promise Strawberry Fields	1 cup	118	0	0	200	28	1	3
Kashi Puffs	1 cup	75	1	0	2	15	1	2
Kashi Seven in the Morning	1/2 cup	178	1	0	224	41	6	6
Kellogg's All-Bran Bran Buds	1/3 cup	75	1	0	203	24	13	2
Kellogg's All-Bran Complete Wheat Flakes	3/4 cup	92	1	0	207	23	5	3
Kellogg's All-Bran, original	1/2 cup	81	2	0	75	23	9	4
Kellogg's All-Bran Yogurt Bites	1-1/4 cup	192	3	2	235	44	10	6
Kellogg's Apple Jacks	1 cup	129	0	0	146	30	1	1
Kellogg's Apple Jacks Cereal Straws	3 straws	136	4	2	16	24	0	2
Kellogg's Berry Rice Krispies	1 cup	115	0	0	218	26	0	2
Kellogg's Cocoa Krispies	3/4 cup	118	1	1	197	27	1	2
Kellogg's Cocoa Krispies Cereal Straws	3 straws	136	4	2	16	24	1	2
Kellogg's Corn Flakes	1 cup	101	0	0	202	24	1	2
Kellogg's Corn Flakes, w/ real bananas	3/4 cup	108	2	2	118	22	1	1
Kellogg's Corn Pops	1 cup	117	0	0	120	28	0	1
Kellogg's Cracklin' Oat Bran	3/4 cup	197	7	3	151	35	6	4
Kellogg's Crispix	1 cup	109	0	0	222	25	0	2
Kellogg's Cruncheroos	1 cup	110	2	0	240	22	3	4
Kellogg's Eggo Crunch Cereal, maple syrup	1 cup	124	1	0	158	27	2	2
Kellogg's Froot Loops	1 cup	118	1	1	141	26	1	1
Kellogg's Froot Loops Cereal Straws	3 straws	136	4	2	15	24	0	2
Kellogg's Froot Loops, marshmallow	1 cup	118	1	0	108	27	1	1
Kellogg's Froot Loops, reduced sugar	1-1/4 cup	126	1	0	180	28	1	2
Kellogg's Frosted Flakes	3/4 cup	110	0	0	139	27	1	1
Kellogg's Frosted Flakes, reduced sugar	1 cup	117	0	0	178	28	0	2

ITEM DESCRIPTION	Serving Size	Calories	Total Fat (g)	Saturated Fat (g)	Sodium (mg)	Carbohydrates (g)	Fiber (g)	Protein (g)
Kellogg's Frosted Krispies	3/4 cup	115	0	0	193	27	0	2
Kellogg's Frosted Mini-Wheats, bite size	24 biscuits	203	1	0	5	48	6	6
Kellogg's Frosted Mini-Wheats, bite size maple & brown sugar	24 biscuits	185	1	0	1	43	5	4
Kellogg's Frosted Mini-Wheats, bite size strawberry	24 biscuits	180	1	0	0	43	5	4
Kellogg's Frosted Mini-Wheats, bite size vanilla	24 biscuits	180	1	0	1	43	5	4
Kellogg's Frosted Mini-Wheats, original	5 biscuits	175	1	0	5	42	5	5
Kellogg's Fruit Harvest, apple cinnamon	1 cup	206	3	0	255	43	3	4
Kellogg's Fruit Harvest, banana berry	3/4 cup	119	2	1	136	26	2	2
Kellogg's Fruit Harvest, peach strawberry	3/4 cup	110	0	0	165	26	2	2
Kellogg's Fruit Harvest, strawberry blueberry	3/4 cup	107	0	0	137	25	1	2
Kellogg's Healthy Choice, almond crunch w/raisins	1 cup	198	3	0	215	43	5	5
Kellogg's Honey Crunch Corn Flakes	3/4 cup	116	1	0	210	26	1	2
Kellogg's Honey Smacks	3/4 cup	104	0	0	50	24	1	2
Kellogg's Just Right Fruit & Nut	3/4 cup	194	2	0	243	43	3	4
Kellogg's Just Right, w/crunchy nuggets	1 cup	204	1	0	338	46	3	4
Kellogg's Low Fat Granola, w/o raisins	1/2 cup	190	3	1	107	40	3	4
Kellogg's Low Fat Granola, w/raisins	2/3 cup	230	3	1	148	49	4	5
Kellogg's Mini-Wheats, apple cinnamon	3/4 cup	182	1	0	20	44	5	4
Kellogg's Mini-Wheats, strawberry	1 cup	184	1	0	16	44	5	5
Kellogg's Mueslix	2/3 cup	196	3	0	170	40	4	5
Kellogg's Product 19	1 cup	100	0	0	207	25	1	2
Kellogg's Puffed Wheat	3/4 cup	29	0	0	0	7	1	1

ITEM DESCRIPTION	Serving Size	Calories	Total Fat (g)	Saturated Fat (g)	Sodium (mg)	Carbohydrates (g)	Fiber (g)	Protein (g)
Kellogg's Raisin Bran	1 cup	190	1	0	342	46	7	5
Kellogg's Raisin Bran Crunch	1 cup	188	1	0	209	45	4	3
Kellogg's Raisin Mini-Wheats	3/4 cup	188	1	0	3	44	5	5
Kellogg's Rice Krispies	1-1/4 cup	128	0	0	299	28	0	2
Kellogg's Rice Krispies Treats Cereal	3/4 cup	120	1	0	166	25	0	1
Kellogg's Robots	1 cup	113	1	0	157	25	1	2
Kellogg's Scooby-Doo! Berry Bones	1 cup	127	1	0	233	28	1	2
Kellogg's Shredded Wheat Miniatures	30 biscuits	102	1	0	0	24	4	3
Kellogg's Smart Start Strong Heart, antioxidant cereal	1 cup	182	1	0	275	43	3	4
Kellogg's Smart Start Strong Heart, brown sugar	1-1/4 cup	220	2	0	140	47	5	6
Kellogg's Smart Start Strong Heart, original	1-1/4 cup	220	2	0	140	47	5	6
Kellogg's Smorz	1 cup	122	2	1	137	25	1	1
Kellogg's Special K	1 cup	117	0	0	224	22	1	7
Kellogg's Special K, fruit & yogurt	3/4 cup	122	1	0	137	28	2	2
Kellogg's Special K, protein plus	3/4 cup	101	3	1	110	14	5	10
Kellogg's Special K, red berries	1 cup	114	0	0	220	25	1	4
Kellogg's Special K, vanilla almond	3/4 cup	115	1	0	164	25	2	2
Kellogg's SpongeBob Squarepants Cereal	1 cup	118	1	0	121	26	1	2
Kellogg's Star Wars Cereal	1 cup	109	1	0	182	24	2	2
Kellogg's Tiger Power	1 cup	105	1	0	253	21	3	6
Kellogg's Tony's Cinnamon Krunchers	3/4 cup	130	3	1	154	23	0	1
Malt-O-Meal Apple Cinnamon Toasty O's	3/4 cup	123	2	0	162	25	2	2
Malt-O-Meal Apple Zings	1 cup	130	1	0	170	29	1	2
Malt-O-Meal Berry Colossal Crunch	3/4 cup	124	2	0	247	26	1	1
Malt-O-Meal Blueberry Muffin Tops Cereal	3/4 cup	133	3	1	124	24	1	1

ITEM DESCRIPTION	Serving Size	Calories	Total Fat (g)	Saturated Fat (g)	Sodium (mg)	Carbohydrates (g)	Fiber (g)	Protein (g)
Malt-O-Meal Chocolate, cooked w/ water	1 serv	118	0	0	8	25	1	3
Malt-O-Meal Cinnamon Toasters	3/4 cup	129	3	1	138	24	1	2
Malt-O-Meal Cocoa Dyno-Bites	3/4 cup	117	1	1	177	26	0	1
Malt-O-Meal Coco Roos	3/4 cup	119	1	0	170	27	1	1
Malt-O-Meal Colossal Crunch	3/4 cup	124	2	0	197	26	0	1
Malt-O-Meal Corn Bursts	1 cup	122	0	0	124	29	1	1
Malt-O-Meal Corn Flakes	1 cup	114	0	0	306	26	1	2
Malt-O-Meal Crispy Rice	1 cup	126	0	0	297	29	0	2
Malt-O-Meal Frosted Flakes	3/4 cup	116	0	0	172	27	1	2
Malt-O-Meal Fruity Dyno-Bites	3/4 cup	109	1	0	173	24	0	1
Malt-O-Meal Golden Puffs	3/4 cup	107	0	0	48	24	1	2
Malt-O-Meal High Fiber Bran Flakes	3/4 cup	113	1	0	195	23	4	3
Malt-O-Meal Honey Buzzers	1-1/3 cup	115	1	0	206	25	1	2
Malt-O-Meal Honey Graham Cereal	3/4 cup	114	1	0	273	25	2	2
Malt-O-Meal Original, cooked w/ water	1 serv	113	0	0	8	23	1	4
Malt-O-Meal Puffed Rice Cereal	1 cup	60	0	0	1	14	0	1
Malt-O-Meal Puffed Wheat Cereal	1 cup	59	0	0	2	12	1	2
Malt-O-Meal Raisin Bran Cereal	1 cup	213	1	0	392	45	8	5
Malt-O-Meal Tootie Fruities	1 cup	128	1	0	148	28	1	2
Mother's Cinnamon Oat Crunch	1 cup	228	3	0	251	48	5	6
Mother's Cocoa Bumpers	1 cup	124	1	0	180	29	1	2
Mother's Instant Oatmeal	1/4 cup	144	3	1	1	26	4	5
Mother's Oat Bran	1/2 cup	146	3	1	2	25	6	7
Mother's Peanut Butter Bumpers Cereal	1 cup	133	2	0	266	26	1	3
Mother's Toasted Oat Bran Cereal, brown sugar	3/4 cup	119	2	0	202	24	3	4
Nature's Path, Optimum Slim	1 cup	180	3	0	250	38	11	9
Post 100% Bran Cereal	1/3 cup	83	1	0	121	23	8	4
Post Alpha-Bits Cereal	1 cup	130	1	0	212	27	1	3
Post Bran Flakes	3/4 cup	96	1	0	220	24	5	3
Post Cocoa Pebbles Cereal	3/4 cup	115	1	1	157	25	1	1

ITEM DESCRIPTION	Serving Size	Calories	Total Fat (g)	Saturated Fat (g)	Sodium (mg)	Carbohydrates (g)	Fiber (g)	Protein (g)
Post Frosted Shredded Wheat Spoon Size Cereal	1 cup	183	1	0	10	44	5	4
Post Fruit & Fiber Dates, raisins & walnuts	1 cup	212	3	0	280	42	5	4
Post Fruity Pebbles Cereal	3/4 cup	108	1	0	158	24	0	1
Post Golden Crisp Cereal	3/4 cup	107	0	0	40	25	0	1
Post Grape-Nuts Cereal	1/2 cup	208	1	0	317	46	5	7
Post Grape-Nuts Flakes	3/4 cup	106	1	0	140	24	3	3
Post Honey Bunches of Oats, honey roasted	3/4 cup	118	1	0	180	25	1	2
Post Honey Bunches of Oats, w/ almonds	3/4 cup	126	3	0	187	24	1	2
Post Honey Nut Shredded Wheat Spoon Size	1 cup	190	1.5	0	70	44	5	4
Post Honeycomb Cereal	1-1/3 cup	115	1	0	215	26	1	2
Post Marshmallow Alpha-Bits Cereal	1 cup	115	1	0	206	25	1	2
Post Oreo O's Cereal	3/4 cup	112	2	0	128	22	2	1
Post Original Shredded Wheat 'n Bran	1-1/4 cup	197	1	0	3	47	8	7
Post Original Shredded Wheat Spoon Size	1 cup	167	1	0	3	41	6	5
Post Raisin Bran Cereal	1 cup	178	1	0	274	43	7	5
Post Selects Banana Nut Crunch Cereal	1 cup	249	6	1	253	44	4	5
Post Selects Blueberry Morning Cereal	1-1/4 cup	211	2	0	266	43	2	4
Post Selects Cranberry Almond Crunch	1 cup	220	3	0	200	45	3	4
Post Selects Great Grains Crunchy Pecan Cereal	2/3 cup	216	6	1	214	38	4	5
Post Selects Great Grains Raisin, Date & Pecan Cereal	2/3 cup	204	5	1	156	40	4	4
Quaker 100% Natural Granola, w/ oats & honey	1/2 cup	206	6	4	24	35	3	5
Quaker 100% Natural Granola, w/ oats, honey, & raisins	1/2 cup	213	6	4	28	38	3	5

ITEM DESCRIPTION	Serving Size	Calories	Total Fat (g)	Saturated Fat (g)	Sodium (mg)	Carbohydrates (g)	Fiber (g)	Protein (g)
Quaker 100% Natural Granola, w/ raisins, low fat	2/3 cup	214	3	1	139	45	3	4
Quaker Apple Zaps	3/4 cup	118	1	0	135	27	1	1
Quaker Cap'n Crunch	3/4 cup	109	2	1	202	23	1	1
Quaker Cap'n Crunch Chocolatey Peanut Butter Crunch Cereal	3/4 cup	112	2	1	141	21	1	2
Quaker Cap'n Crunch Crunch Berries	3/4 cup	105	1	1	182	22	1	1
Quaker Cap'n Crunch Peanut Butter Crunch	3/4 cup	112	2	1	200	21	1	2
Quaker Christmas Crunch	3/4 cup	104	1	1	184	22	1	1
Quaker Cocoa Blasts	1 cup	130	1	0	135	29	1	1
Quaker Cranberry Macadamia Nut Cereal	1 cup	245	6	1	251	46	4	4
Quaker Crunchy Bran	3/4 cup	90	1	1	235	23	5	2
Quaker Fruitangy Oh!s	1 cup	122	1	0	152	27	1	2
Quaker Honey Graham Life Cereal	3/4 cup	119	1	0	156	25	2	3
Quaker Honey Graham Oh!s	3/4 cup	111	2	2	166	23	1	1
Quaker Instant Oatmeal Express, baked apple, cooked w/ water	1 packet	208	3	0	322	42	4	4
Quaker Instant Oatmeal Express, golden brown sugar, cooked w/ water	1 packet	209	3	0	294	42	4	5
Quaker Instant Oatmeal, apples & cinnamon, cooked w/ water	1 packet	130	1	0	165	26	3	3
Quaker Instant Oatmeal, brown sugar cinnamon, cooked w/ water	1 packet	199	4	2	251	38	3	4
Quaker Instant Oatmeal, cinnamon & spice, cooked w/ water	1 packet	177	2	0	249	36	3	4
Quaker Instant Oatmeal, cinnamon roll, cooked w/ water	1 packet	209	3	0	249	41	4	5
Quaker Instant Oatmeal, fruit & cream variety, cooked w/ water	1 packet	139	3	1	181	26	2	3
Quaker Instant Oatmeal, honey nut, cooked w/ water	1 packet	173	4	0	238	31	3	4

ITEM DESCRIPTION	Serving Size	Calories	Total Fat (g)	Saturated Fat (g)	Sodium (mg)	Carbohydrates (g)	Fiber (g)	Protein (g)
Quaker Instant Oatmeal, maple & brown sugar, cooked w/ water	1 packet	157	2	0	253	31	3	4
Quaker Instant Oatmeal, Nutrition for Women, applespice, cooked w/ water	1 packet	178	2	0	319	35	3	5
Quaker Instant Oatmeal, Nutrition for Women, brown sugar, cooked w/ water	1 packet	173	2	0	328	33	3	5
Quaker Instant Oatmeal, raisins & spice, cooked w/ water	1 packet	162	2	0	245	33	3	3
Quaker Instant Oatmeal, vanilla cinnamon, cooked w/ water	1 packet	165	2	0	249	33	3	4
Quaker King Vitaman	1-1/2 cup	120	1	0	259	26	1	2
Quaker Kretschmer Honey Crunch Toasted Wheat Germ	1-2/3 tbsp	52	1	0	2	8	1	4
Quaker Kretschmer Toasted Wheat Bran	1/4 cup	32	1	0	1	10	7	3
Quaker Kretschmer Wheat Germ, reg	1-2/3 tbsp	51	1	0	1	7	2	4
Quaker Life, cinnamon	3/4 cup	119	1	0	153	25	2	3
Quaker Life, original	3/4 cup	119	1	0	164	25	2	3
Quaker Life Vanilla Yogurt Crunch Cereal	1-1/4 cup	210	3	1	248	43	4	5
Quaker Marshmallow Safari	3/4 cup	119	2	0	192	25	1	2
Quaker Oat Bran Cereal	1-1/4 cup	212	3	1	207	43	6	7
Quaker Oatmeal Cereal, brown sugar bliss	1 cup	188	3	1	249	39	4	4
Quaker Oatmeal Squares	1 cup	212	2	1	269	44	4	6
Quaker Oatmeal Squares, cinnamon	1 cup	227	3	0	264	48	5	6
Quaker Puffed Rice	1 cup	54	0	0	1	12	0	1
Quaker Puffed Wheat	1-1/4 cup	55	0	0	1	11	1	2
Quaker Quisp	1 cup	109	2	1	200	23	1	1
Quaker Superman Life Cereal	3/4 cup	112	1	0	167	24	2	3
Quaker Sweet Puffs	1 cup	133	1	0	80	30	1	2
Quaker Toasted Oatmeal Cereal	1 cup	188	2	1	274	39	3	5

ITEM DESCRIPTION	Serving Size	Calories	Total Fat (g)	Saturated Fat (g)	Sodium (mg)	Carbohydrates (g)	Fiber (g)	Protein (g)
Quaker Toasted Oatmeal Cereal, honeynut	1 cup	188	2	1	228	40	3	4
Weetabix Whole Grain Cereal	1 cup	213	2	0	221	44	7	7
CHAYOTE								
Boiled (1" pcs)	1 cup	38	1	0	2	8	5	1
Fresh (1" pcs)	1 cup	25	0	0	3	6	2	1
CHEESE								
American, pasteurized, processed	3/4 oz slice	79	7	4	313	0	0	5
American, pasteurized, processed, low fat	3/4 oz slice	38	1	1	300	1	0	5
Blue	1 oz	100	8	5	395	1	0	6
Brick	1 oz	105	8	5	159	1	0	7
Brie	1 oz	95	8	5	178	0	0	6
Camembert	1 oz	84	7	4	236	0	0	6
Caraway	1 oz	107	8	5	196	1	0	7
Cheddar	1 oz slice	113	9	6	174	0	0	7
Cheddar, low fat	1 oz slice	48	2	1	171	1	0	7
Cheddar, low sodium	1 oz slice	105	9	6	6	1	0	7
Cheddar or American, pasteurized, processed, fat free	3/4 oz slice	31	0	0	321	3	0	5
Cheddar or American, pasteurized, processed, low sodium	3/4 oz slice	79	7	4	1	0	0	5
Cheshire	1 oz	110	9	6	198	1	0	7
Colby	1 oz slice	110	9	6	169	1	0	7
Colby, low fat	1 oz slice	48	2	1	171	1	0	7
Colby, low sodium	1 oz slice	111	9	6	6	1	0	7
Edam	1 oz	101	8	5	274	0	0	7
Feta	1 oz	75	6	4	316	1	0	4
Fontina	1 oz slice	109	9	5	224	0	0	7
Gjetost	1 oz	132	8	5	170	12	0	3
Goat, hard	1 oz	128	10	7	98	1	0	9
Goat, semisoft	1 oz	103	8	6	146	1	0	6
Goat, soft	1 oz	76	6	4	104	0	0	5
Gouda	1 oz	101	8	5	232	1	0	7

ITEM DESCRIPTION	Serving Size	Calories	Total Fat (g)	Saturated Fat (g)	Sodium (mg)	Carbohydrates (g)	Fiber (g)	Protein (g)
Gruyere	1 oz slice	116	9	5	94	0	0	8
Kraft Free Singles, American, nonfat, pasteurized, processed	1 slice	31	0	0	273	2	0	5
Limburger	1 oz	93	8	5	227	0	0	6
Mexican, queso anejo	1 oz	106	8	5	321	1	0	6
Mexican, queso asadero	1 oz	101	8	5	186	1	0	6
Mexican, queso Chihuahua	1 oz	106	9	5	175	2	0	6
Monterey	1 oz slice	104	8	5	150	0	0	7
Monterey, low fat	1 oz slice	88	6	4	158	0	0	8
Mozzarella, low sodium	1 oz	78	5	3	4	1	0	8
Mozzarella, nonfat	1 oz	42	0	0	211	1	1	9
Mozzarella, part skim milk	1 oz	72	5	3	175	1	0	7
Mozzarella, part skim milk, low moisture	1 oz	86	6	4	150	1	0	7
Mozzarella, whole milk	1 oz	85	6	4	178	1	0	6
Mozzarella, whole milk, low moisture	1 oz	90	7	4	118	1	0	6
Muenster	1 oz slice	103	8	5	176	0	0	7
Muenster, low fat	1 oz slice	105	5	3	168	1	0	7
Neufchatel	1 oz	77	6	4	95	1	0	3
Parmesan, dry grated, reduced fat	1 tbsp	13	1	1	76	0	0	1
Parmesan, grated	1 tbsp	22	1	1	76	0	0	2
Parmesan, hard	1 oz	111	7	5	454	1	0	10
Parmesan, low sodium	1 tbsp	23	2	1	3	0	0	2
Parmesan, shredded	1 tbsp	21	1	1	85	0	0	2
Pimento, pasteurized, processed	1 oz	106	9	6	405	0	0	6
Port de Salut	1 oz	100	8	5	151	0	0	7
Provolone	1 oz slice	98	7	5	245	1	0	7
Provolone, reduced fat	1 oz slice	77	5	3	245	1	0	7
Ricotta, part skim milk	1 oz	39	2	1	35	1	0	3
Ricotta, whole milk	1 oz	49	4	2	24	1	0	3
Romano	1 oz	110	8	5	340	1	0	9
Roquefort	1 oz	105	9	5	513	1	0	6

ITEM DESCRIPTION	Serving Size	Calories	Total Fat (g)	Saturated Fat (g)	Sodium (mg)	Carbohydrates (g)	Fiber (g)	Protein (g)
Swiss	1 oz slice	106	8	5	54	2	0	8
Swiss, low fat	1 oz slice	50	1	1	73	1	0	8
Swiss, low sodium	1 oz slice	105	8	5	4	1	0	8
Swiss, pasteurized, processed	3/4 oz slice	70	5	3	288	1	0	5
Swiss, pasteurized, processed, low fat	3/4 oz slice	36	1	1	300	1	0	5
Tilsit	1 oz	96	7	5	213	1	0	7
CHEESE FONDUE	1/2 cup	247	15	9	143	4	0	15
CHEESE FOOD								
American, cold packed	1 oz	94	7	4	274	2	0	6
American, pasteurized, processed	3/4 oz slice	79	7	4	313	1	0	5
Swiss, pasteurized, processed	1 oz	92	7	4	440	1	0	6
CHEESE PUFFS (corn based, low fat)	1 oz	122	3	1	364	21	3	2
CHEESE SAUCE								
Homemade	1 cup	479	36	20	1198	13	0	25
Kraft Cheez Whiz	2 tbsp	75	3	2	597	6	0	6
Ready to serve	1/4 cup	110	8	4	522	4	0	4
CHEESE SPREAD								
Cream cheese base	1 oz	84	8	5	191	1	0	2
Kraft Cheez Whiz	2 tbsp	91	7	4	541	3	0	4
Kraft Velveeta Light	1 oz	62	3	2	444	3	0	5
Kraft Velveeta	1 oz	85	6	4	420	3	0	5
Pasteurized, processed, American	1 oz	82	6	4	381	2	0	5
CHEESE SUBSTITUTE								
American cheddar imitation	1 slice	50	3	2	282	2	0	4
American or cheddar imitation, low cholesterol	1" cube	70	6	1	121	0	0	5
Mozzarella	1 oz	70	3	1	194	7	0	3
CHEESE TWISTS (corn based, low fat)	1 oz	122	3	1	364	21	3	2
CHERIMOYA (fresh, w/o skin)	1 fruit	231	2	0	12	55	7	5
CHERRIES								
Maraschino, canned	1 cherry	8	0	0	0	2	0	0
Sour, red, canned in ex heavy syrup	1 cup	298	0	0	18	76	2	2

ITEM DESCRIPTION	Serving Size	Calories	Total Fat (g)	Saturated Fat (g)	Sodium (mg)	Carbohydrates (g)	Fiber (g)	Protein (g)
Sour, red, canned in heavy syrup	1 cup	233	0	0	18	60	3	2
Sour, red, canned in light syrup	1 cup	189	0	0	18	49	2	2
Sour, red, canned in water	1 cup	88	0	0	17	22	3	2
Sour, red, fresh	1 cup	78	0	0	5	19	3	2
Sour, red, frozen, unsweetened	1 cup	71	1	0	2	17	3	1
Sweet, canned in ex heavy syrup	1 cup	266	0	0	8	68	4	2
Sweet, canned in heavy syrup	1 cup	210	0	0	8	54	4	2
Sweet, canned in juice	1 cup	135	0	0	8	35	4	2
Sweet, canned in light syrup	1 cup	169	0	0	8	44	4	2
Sweet, canned in water	1 cup	114	0	0	2	29	4	2
Sweet, fresh	1 cup	87	0	0	0	22	3	1
Sweet, frozen, sweetened	1 cup	231	0	0	3	58	5	3
CHERRY JUICE (from concentrate)	1 cup	140	0	0	25	34	0	1
CHERRY PIE FILLING								
Cherry pie filling	1/8 can	85	0	0	13	21	0	0
Low calorie	1 cup	140	0	0	32	32	3	2
CHERVIL (dried)	1 tbsp	5	0	0	2	1	0	0
CHESTNUTS								
Chinese, boiled & steamed	1 oz	43	0	0	1	10	0	1
Chinese, dried	1 oz	103	1	0	1	23	0	2
Chinese, fresh	1 oz	64	0	0	1	14	0	1
Chinese, roasted	1 oz	68	0	0	1	15	0	1
European, boiled & steamed	1 oz	37	0	0	8	8	0	1
European, dried, peeled	1 oz	105	1	0	10	22	0	1
European, dried, unpeeled	1 oz	106	1	0	10	22	3	2
European, fresh, peeled	1 oz	56	0	0	1	13	0	0
European, roasted	1 oz	69	1	0	1	15	1	1
Japanese, boiled & steamed	1 oz	16	0	0	1	4	0	0
Japanese, dried	1 oz	102	0	0	10	23	0	1
Japanese, fresh	1 oz	44	0	0	4	10	0	1
Japanese, roasted	1 oz	57	0	0	5	13	0	1
CHICKEN								
Breast, fat free mesquite flavored, slices	2 slices	34	0	0	437	1	0	7

EM DESCRIPTION	Serving Size	Calories	Total Fat (g)	Saturated Fat (g)	Sodium (mg)	Carbohydrates (g)	Fiber (g)	Protein (g)
east, oven roasted, fat free, ces	2 slices	33	0	0	457	1	0	7
oiler/fryer, back, w/ skin, ewed & chopped	1 cup	413	29	8	102	0	0	35
oiler/fryer, breast, meat only, fried	1 breast	322	8	2	136	1	0	58
oiler/fryer, breast, meat only, asted & chopped	1 cup	231	5	1	104	0	0	43
oiler/fryer, breast, meat only, ewed & chopped	1 cup	211	4	1	88	0	0	41
roiler/fryer, breast, w/ skin, oneless, fried, battered	1 breast	728	37	10	770	25	1	70
roiler/fryer, breast, w/ skin, oneless, fried, w/ flour	1 breast	435	17	5	149	3	0	62
roiler/fryer, breast, w/ skin, asted & chopped	1 cup	276	11	3	99	0	0	42
roiler/fryer, breast, w/ skin, tewed & chopped	1 cup	258	10	3	87	0	0	38
roiler/fryer, dark meat, meat only, fried	1 cup	335	16	4	136	4	0	41
oiler/fryer, dark meat, meat only, roasted & chopped	1 cup	287	14	4	130	0	0	38
roiler/fryer, dark meat, meat only, stewed & chopped	1 cup	269	13	3	104	0	0	36
Broiler/fryer, drumstick, meat only, fried	1 drumstick	82	3	1	40	0	0	12
Broiler/fryer, drumstick, meat only, roasted & chopped	1 cup	241	8	2	133	0	0	40
Broiler/fryer, drumstick, meat only, stewed & chopped	1 cup	270	9	2	128	0	0	44
Broiler/fryer, drumstick, w/ skin, oneless, fried, battered	1 drumstick	193	11	3	194	6	0	16
Broiler/fryer, drumstick, w/ skin, boneless, fried w/ flour	1 drumstick	120	7	2	44	1	0	13
Broiler/fryer, drumstick, w/ skin, roasted & chopped	1 cup	302	16	4	126	0	0	38
Broiler/fryer, drumstick, w/ skin, stewed & chopped	1 cup	286	15	4	106	0	0	35

ITEM DESCRIPTION	Serving Size	Calories	Total Fat (g)	Saturated Fat (g)	Sodium (mg)	Carbohydrates (g)	Fiber (g)	Protein (g)
Broiler/fryer, giblets, cooked, simmered	1 cup	228	7	2	97	0	0	39
Broiler/fryer, leg, meat only, fried	1 leg	196	9	2	90	1	0	27
Broiler/fryer, leg, meat only, roasted & chopped	1 cup	267	12	3	127	0	0	38
Broiler/fryer, leg, meat only, stewed & chopped	1 cup	296	13	4	125	0	0	42
Broiler/fryer, leg, w/ skin, boneless, fried, battered	1 leg	431	26	7	441	14	0	34
Broiler/fryer, leg, w/ skin, boneless, fried w/ flour	1 leg	284	16	4	99	3	0	30
Broiler/fryer, leg, w/ skin, roasted & chopped	1 cup	325	19	5	122	0	0	36
Broiler/fryer, leg, w/ skin, stewed & chopped	1 cup	308	18	5	102	0	0	34
Broiler/fryer, light meat, meat only, fried	1 cup	269	8	2	113	1	0	46
Broiler/fryer, light meat, meat only, roasted & chopped	1 cup	242	6	2	108	0	0	43
Broiler/fryer, light meat, meat only, stewed & chopped	1 cup	223	6	2	91	0	0	40
Broiler/fryer, meat only, stewed & chopped	1 cup	248	9	3	98	0	0	38
Broiler/fryer, meat only, fried	1 cup	307	13	3	127	2	0	43
Broiler/fryer, meat only, roasted & chopped	1 cup	266	10	3	120	0	0	41
Broiler/fryer, neck, meat only, fried	1 neck	50	3	1	22	0	0	6
Broiler/fryer, neck, meat only, simmered	1 neck	32	1	0	12	0	0	4
Broiler/fryer, neck, w/ skin, boneless, fried, battered	1 neck	172	12	3	144	5	0	10
Broiler/fryer, neck, w/ skin, boneless, fried w/ flour	1 neck	120	9	2	30	2	0	9
Broiler/fryer, neck, w/ skin, boneless, simmered	1 neck	94	7	2	20	0	0	7
Broiler/fryer, thigh, meat only, fried	1 thigh	113	5	1	49	1	0	15

ITEM DESCRIPTION	Serving Size	Calories	Total Fat (g)	Saturated Fat (g)	Sodium (mg)	Carbohydrates (g)	Fiber (g)	Protein (g)
Broiler/fryer, thigh, meat only, roasted & chopped	1 cup	293	15	4	123	0	0	36
Broiler/fryer, thigh, meat only, stewed & chopped	1 cup	273	14	4	105	0	0	35
Broiler/fryer, thigh, w/ skin, boneless, fried, battered	1 thigh	238	14	4	248	8	0	19
Broiler/fryer, thigh, w/ skin, boneless, fried w/ flour	1 thigh	162	9	3	55	2	0	17
Broiler/fryer, thigh, w/ skin, boneless, stewed	1 thigh	158	10	3	48	0	0	16
Broiler/fryer, thigh, w/ skin, roasted & chopped	1 cup	346	22	6	118	0	0	35
Broiler/fryer, wing, meat only, fried	1 wing	42	2	1	18	0	0	6
Broiler/fryer, wing, meat only, roasted	1 wing	43	2	0	19	0	0	6
Broiler/fryer, wing, meat only, stewed & chopped	1 cup	253	10	3	102	0	0	38
Broiler/fryer, wing, w/ skin, boneless, fried, battered	1 wing	159	11	3	157	5	0	10
Broiler/fryer, wing, w/ skin, boneless, fried w/ flour	1 wing	103	7	2	25	1	0	8
Broiler/fryer, wing, w/ skin, roasted & chopped	1 cup	406	27	8	115	0	0	38
Broiler/fryer, wing, w/ skin, stewed & chopped	1 cup	349	24	7	94	0	0	32
Broiler/fryer, w/ skin, roasted & chopped	1 cup	335	19	5	115	0	0	38
Broiler/fryer, w/ skin, stewed & chopped	1 cup	307	18	5	94	0	0	35
Canned, meat only, w/ broth	5 oz can	234	11	3	714	0	0	31
Canned, w/o broth	1 cup	377	17	5	277	2	0	52
Capons, giblets, simmered & chopped	1 cup	238	8	3	80	1	0	38
Chicken breast roll, oven roasted	2 oz	75	4	1	494	1	0	8
Chicken nuggets, boneless, breaded & fried	6 pieces	285	18	4	551	16	1	15
Chicken roll, light meat	2 slices	63	2	0	604	3	0	9

ITEM DESCRIPTION	Serving Size	Calories	Total Fat (g)	Saturated Fat (g)	Sodium (mg)	Carbohydrates (g)	Fiber (g)	Protein (g)
Chicken spread	1 serv	88 *	10	2	404	2	0	10
Cornish game hens, meat only, roasted	1 hen	295	9	2	139	0	0	51
Cornish game hens, w/ skin, roasted	1 hen	668	47	13	164	0	0	57
Fajita strips, frozen	1 strip	13	1	0	75	0	0	2
Ground, crumbles, pan browned	3 oz	161	9	3	64	0	0	20
Roasting, dark meat, meat only, roasted & chopped	1 cup	249	12	3	133	0	0	33
Roasting, giblets, simmered & chopped	1 cup	239	8	2	87	1	0	39
Roasting, light meat, meat only, roasted & chopped	1 cup	214	6	2	71	0	0	38
Roasting, meat only, roasted & chopped	1 cup	234	9	3	105	0	0	35
Stewing, dark meat, meat only, stewed & chopped	1 cup	361	21	6	133	0	0	39
Stewing, giblets, simmered & chopped	1 cup	281	13	4	81	0	0	37
Stewing, light meat, meat only, stewed & chopped	1 cup	298	11	3	81	0	0	46
Stewing, meat only, stewed & chopped	1 cup	332	17	4	109	0	0	43
Stewing, meat, skin, giblets & neck, stewed & chopped	1 cup	342	19	5	107	0	0	40
Wings, frozen, glazed, BBQ flavored	1 pc	61	4	1	178	1	0	6
Wings, frozen, glazed, BBQ flavored, heated in oven	1 serv	232	14	4	537	3	1	21
Wings, frozen, glazed, BBQ flavored, microwaved	1 serv	184	10	3	619	3	1	19
CHICKEN, BRAND NAME								
Carl Buddig Smoked Slices Chicken, light & dark meat	2 oz	94	6	1	544	0	0	10
Louis Rich Chicken Breast Classic, baked/grilled, Carving Board	1 slice	22	0	0	251	1	0	4
Louis Rich Chicken Breast, oven roasted deluxe	1 serv	28	1	0	333	1	0	5

ITEM DESCRIPTION	Serving Size	Calories	Total Fat (g)	Saturated Fat (g)	Sodium (mg)	Carbohydrates (g)	Fiber (g)	Protein (g)
Louis Rich Chicken, white, oven roasted	1 serv	36	2	0	335	1	0	5
Oscar Mayer Chicken Breast, honey glazed	4 slices	57	1	0	748	2	0	10
Oscar Mayer Chicken Breast, oven roasted, fat free	1 slice	11	0	0	161	0	0	2
CHICKEN BROTH								
Campbell's Red & White, condensed	4 fl oz	20	1	0	770	1	0	1
Canned, condensed	4 fl oz	39	1	0	786	1	0	6
Canned, condensed, prepared w/ water	8 fl oz	39	1	0	776	1	0	5
Canned, low sodium	8 fl oz	38	1	0	72	3	0	5
Canned, reduced sodium	8 fl oz	17	0	0	554	1	0	3
Cube, dry, prepared w/ water	8 fl oz	12	0	0	792	2	0	1
Swanson Chicken Broth	8 fl oz	9	0	0	928	0	0	1
CHICKEN ENTRÉE, BRAND NAME								
Bertolli Chicken Alfredo & Fettuccine	1 serv	630	32	17	1200	50	4	0
Bertolli Chicken Florentine & Farfalle	1 serv	570	31	17	1040	40	3	25
Bertolli Chicken, Rigatoni & Broccoli	1 serv	390	15	4	970	37	4	22
Bertolli Grilled Chicken & Roasted Vegetables	1 serv	400	18	2.5	950	33	4	22
Campbell's Supper Bakes Meal Kits, garlic chicken w/ pasta	1/6 box	227	1	1	763	44	2	10
Campbell's Supper Bakes Meal Kits, herb chicken w/ rice	1/6 box	185	1	1	780	40	1	4
Campbell's Supper Bakes Meal Kits, lemon chicken w/ herb rice	1 serv	197	1	1	780	43	2	4
Campbell's Supper Bakes Meal Kits, Southwest-style chicken w/ rice	1/6 box	153	1	0	600	32	2	4
Campbell's Supper Bakes Meal Kits, traditional roast chicken w/ stuffing	1 serv	162	3	1	740	29	2	5
Lean Cuisine Chicken Tuscan	1	280	6	2	780	34	4	22
Lean Cuisine Chicken Chow Mein w/ rice	1	240	4	1	550	39	3	13
Lean Cuisine Orange Peel Chicken	1	380	9	2	720	60	4	14
Swanson Chicken a la King	1 can	212	12	3	1371	12	2	14
Swanson Chicken & Dumplings	1 cup	230	10	5	990	24	2	11

ITEM DESCRIPTION	Serving Size	Calories	Total Fat (g)	Saturated Fat (g)	Sodium (mg)	Carbohydrates (g)	Fiber (g)	Protein (g)
Weight Watchers Smart Ones, chicken tenderloins w/ BBQ sauce	1 pkg	242	4	1	638	34	4	17
CHICKEN FAT	1 tbsp	115	13	4	0	0	0	0
CHICKEN STOCK (homemade)	1 cup	86	3	1	343	8	0	6
CHICKEN SUBSTITUTE								
Loma Linda Fried Chik'n w/ Gravy, canned	2 pcs	145	10	1	358	4	2	11
Meatless substitute	1 cup	376	21	3	1191	6	6	40
Meatless substitute, breaded, fried, diced	1 cup	304	17	1	520	11	6	28
Morningstar Farms Chik'n Nuggets, frozen	4 pcs	187	8	1	565	18	2	12
Morningstar Farms Chik Patties Original, frozen	1 patty	140	5	1	593	16	2	8
Morningstar Farms Italian Herb Chik Patties, frozen	1 patty	168	5	1	484	22	2	10
Morningstar Farms Meal Starters Chik'n Strips, frozen	12 strips	139	3	1	507	6	1	23
Morningstar Farms Meatfree Buffalo Wings, frozen	5 pcs	196	8	1	658	20	3	12
Morningstar Farms Original Chik'n Tenders, frozen	2 pcs	189	7	1	578	20	3	12
Morningstar Farms Roasted Herb Chik'n w/ Organic Soy, frozen	1 patty	107	3	0	340	9	2	12
Worthington Chic-Ketts, frozen	1 slice	112	5	1	405	3	2	14
Worthington Diced Chik, canned	1/4 cup	44	0	0	189	2	1	8
Worthington Frichik, canned	2 pcs	144	9	1	361	3	1	12
Worthington Low Fat Frichik, canned	2 pcs	87	2	0	354	4	1	12
CHICKPEA FLOUR (besan)	1 cup	356	6	1	59	53	10	21
CHICKPEAS								
Boiled	1 cup	269	4	0	11	45	13	15
Canned	1 cup	286	3	0	718	54	11	12
Fresh	1 cup	728	12	1	48	121	35	39
CHICORY (fresh)	1 head	9	0	0	1	2	2	0

ITEM DESCRIPTION	Serving Size	Calories	Total Fat (g)	Saturated Fat (g)	Sodium (mg)	Carbohydrates (g)	Fiber (g)	Protein (g)
CHICORY GREENS (fresh, chopped)	1 cup	7	0	0	13	1	1	0
CHICORY ROOTS (fresh)	1 root	44	0	0	30	11	0	1
CHILI								
BBQ w/ beans, ranch style, cooked	1 cup	245	3	0	1834	43	11	13
Beans included, canned	1 cup	287	14	6	1336	30	11	15
Campbell's Chunky Soups Firehouse Hot Spicy Beef Bean Chili	1 cup	233	8	4	870	25	8	15
Con carne, w/ beans, canned	1 cup	298	13	4	1043	28	10	17
Hormel Chili, w/ beans, canned	1 cup	240	4	2	1163	34	8	17
Hormel Chili, w/o beans, canned	1 cup	194	7	2	970	18	3	17
Hormel Vegetarian Chili, w/ beans, canned	1 cup	205	1	0	778	38	10	12
Nalley Chili Con Carne, w/ beans, canned	1 serv	281	8	3	1231	12	13	40
Nestle Chef-Mate Chili, w/ beans, canned	1 cup	420	24	10	1280	34	8	18
Nestle Chef-Mate Chili, w/o beans, canned	1 cup	368	23	8	1400	20	4	23
Old El Paso Chili, w/ beans, canned	1 serv	249	10	2	588	22	10	18
Stagg Classic Chili, w/ beans, canned	1 cup	324	16	7	825	29	7	17
Stagg Country Chili, w/ beans, canned	1 cup	319	16	7	1131	29	6	15
Stagg Dynamite Chili, w/ beans, canned	1 cup	333	15	6	862	31	8	18
Stagg Ranchhouse Chili, w/ beans, canned	1 cup	284	9	3	813	32	9	19
Stagg Silverado Chili, w/ beans, canned	1 cup	227	3	1	864	33	8	18
Worthington Chili, canned	1 cup	283	10	2	1042	25	8	24
CHILI POWDER	1 tbsp	24	1	0	76	4	3	1
CHITTERLINGS (pork, variety meat, simmered)	3 oz	198	17	8	15	0	0	11

ITEM DESCRIPTION	Serving Size	Calories	Total Fat (g)	Saturated Fat (g)	Sodium (mg)	Carbohydrates (g)	Fiber (g)	Protein (g)
CHIVES								
Freeze-dried	1 tbsp	1	0	0	0	0	0	0
Fresh, chopped	1 tbsp	1	0	0	0	0	0	0
CHOCOLATE								
Baking, M&M's Milk Chocolate Mini Baking Bits	1/2 oz	70	3	2	10	10	0	1
Baking, M&M's Semisweet Chocolate Mini Baking Bits	1/2 oz	72	4	2	0	9	1	1
Baking, Mexican, squares	1 tablet	85	3	2	1	15	1	1
Dark	1 oz	155	9	5	7	17	2	1
Dark, 45-59% cacao solid	1 oz	154	9	5	7	18	2	1
Dark, 60-69% cacao solid	1 oz	164	11	6	3	15	2	2
Dark, 70-85% cacao solid	1 oz	170	12	7	6	13	3	2
Sweet	1 oz	143	10	6	5	17	2	1
CHOCOLATE CHIPS								
Milk chocolate	1 cup	899	50	31	133	100	6	13
Semisweet	1 cup	805	50	30	18	106	10	7
Semisweet, made w/ butter	1 cup	811	50	30	19	108	10	7
White chocolate	1 cup	916	55	33	153	101	0	10
CHOCOLATE DRINK MIX								
Powder, prepared w/ whole milk	1 cup	225	9	5	159	30	1	9
Powder, w/ added nutrients, prepared w/ whole milk	1 serv	234	8	5	136	31	0	9
Reduced calorie, dairy powder prepared w/ water & ice	1 serv	70	1	0	148	11	2	5
Whey & milk based	1 cup	120	1	1	222	26	2	2
CHOCOLATE-HAZELNUT SPREAD	2 tbsp	200	11	11	15	23	2	2
CHOCOLATE MILK								
Commercial	1 cup	208	8	5	150	26	2	8
Commercial, low fat	1 cup	158	3	2	152	26	1	8
Commercial, reduced fat	1 cup	190	5	3	165	30	2	7
CHOCOLATE MOUSSE (homemade)	1/2 cup	454	32	18	77	32	1	8
CHOCOLATE SYRUP								
Fudge	2 tbsp	133	3	2	131	24	1	2

ITEM DESCRIPTION	Serving Size	Calories	Total Fat (g)	Saturated Fat (g)	Sodium (mg)	Carbohydrates (g)	Fiber (g)	Protein (g)
Hershey's Genuine Chocolate FlavorLite Syrup	2 tbsp	50	0	0	35	12	0	0
Hershey's Genuine Chocolate Flavor Syrup	2 tbsp	50	0	0	35	12	0	0
Prepared w/ whole milk	1 cup	254	8	5	133	36	1	9
Regular	2 tbsp	109	0	0	28	25	1	1
CHRYSANTHEMUM								
Leaves, fresh, chopped	1 cup	12	0	0	60	2	2	2
Garland, boiled (1" pcs)	1 cup	20	0	0	53	4	2	2
Garland, fresh (1" pcs)	1 cup	6	0	0	30	1	1	1
CILANTRO (fresh)	5 sprigs	1	0	0	3	0	0	0
CINNAMON (ground)	1 tbsp	19	0	0	1	6	4	0
CISCO (smoked)	3 oz	150	10	1	409	0	0	14
CITRUS FRUIT JUICE DRINK (frozen concentrate, prepared w/ water)	8 fl oz	114	0	0	10	28	0	1
CLAM & TOMATO JUICE (canned)	5.5 oz	80	0	0	601	18	1	1
CLAMS								
Breaded & fried	3 oz	172	9	2	309	9	0	12
Canned, drained	3 oz	126	2	0	95	4	0	22
Canned, liquid	3 oz	2	0	0	183	0	0	0
Cooked in moist heat	3 oz	126	2	0	95	4	0	22
CLEMENTINES (fresh, whole)	1 fruit	35	0	0	1	9	1	1
CLOVES (ground)	1 tbsp	21	1	0	16	4	2	0
COCOA								
Cocoa, hot, homemade	1 cup	192	6	4	110	27	3	9
Hershey's European Style Cocoa, powder, unsweetened	1 tbsp	84	1	0	0	3	1	1
Nestle Rich Chocolate	1 envelope	80	3	2	170	15	1	1
Nestle Rich Chocolate, w/ marshmallows	1 envelope	80	3	3	160	15	1	1
Powder, high fat, plain	1 tbsp	16	1	1	1	3	2	1
Powder, prepared w/ water	6 fl oz	113	1	1	150	24	1	2
Powder, unsweetened	1 tbsp	12	1	0	1	3	2	1
Powder w/ aspartame, prepared w/ water	6 fl oz	56	0	0	138	11	1	2

ITEM DESCRIPTION	Serving Size	Calories	Total Fat (g)	Saturated Fat (g)	Sodium (mg)	Carbohydrates (g)	Fiber (g)	Protein (g)
Swiss Miss, no sugar added, powder	1 envelope	57	0	0	131	11	1	2
COCOA BUTTER OIL	1 tbsp	120	14	8	0	0	0	0
COCONUT CREAM								
Canned, sweetened	1 cup	1057	48	46	107	158	1	3
Fresh liquid from grated meat	1 cup	792	83	74	10	16	5	9
COCONUT MEAT								
Dried, creamed	1 oz	194	20	17	10	6	0	2
Dried, sweetened, flaked, canned	1 cup	341	24	22	15	32	4	3
Dried, sweetened, flaked, packaged	1 cup	388	24	22	242	44	8	3
Dried, sweetened, shredded	1 cup	466	33	29	244	44	4	3
Dried, toasted	1 oz	168	13	12	10	13	0	2
Dried, unsweetened	1 oz	187	18	16	10	7	5	2
Fresh, shredded	1 cup	283	27	24	16	12	7	3
COCONUT MILK								
Canned liquid from grated meat & water	1 cup	445	48	43	29	6	0	5
Fresh liquid from grated meat & water	1 cup	552	57	51	36	13	5	6
Frozen liquid	1 cup	485	50	44	29	13	0	4
COCONUT OIL	1 tbsp	117	14	12	0	0	0	0
COCONUT WATER	1 cup	46	0	0	252	9	3	2
COD								
Atlantic, canned, solids & liquid	3 oz	89	1	0	185	0	0	19
Atlantic, cooked in dry heat	3 oz	89	1	0	66	0	0	19
Atlantic, dried & salted	1 oz	82	1	0	1992	0	0	18
Pacific, cooked in dry heat	3 oz	89	1	0	77	0	0	20
COD LIVER OIL	1 tbsp	123	14	3	0	0	0	0
COFFEE								
Brewed, prepared w/ water	8 fl oz	2	0	0	5	0	0	0
Espresso, restaurant	1 fl oz	1	0	0	4	0	0	0
Instant, decaffeinated, prepared w/ water	6 fl oz	4	0	0	7	1	0	0
Instant, reg, prepared w/ water	6 fl oz	4	0	0	7	1	0	0

ITEM DESCRIPTION	Serving Size	Calories	Total Fat (g)	Saturated Fat (g)	Sodium (mg)	Carbohydrates (g)	Fiber (g)	Protein (g)
Instant, w/ chicory, prepared w/ water	6 fl oz	5	0	0	13	1	0	0
Instant, w/ sugar, cappuccino flavor	4 tsp	53	1	0	23	11	0	0
Instant, w/ sugar, French flavor	4 tsp	63	3	1	72	9	0	1
Instant, w/ sugar, mocha flavor	2 tbsp	60	2	1	41	10	0	1
COFFEE LIQUEUR								
53 proof	1 fl oz	113	0	0	3	16	0	0
63 proof	1 fl oz	107	0	0	3	11	0	0
34 proof, w/ cream	1 fl oz	102	5	3	29	7	0	1
COFFEE SUBSTITUTE								
Natural Touch Kaffree Roma, powder	1 tsp, rounded	7	0	0	3	2	0	0
Prepared w/ water	6 fl oz	11	0	0	9	2	1	0
Prepared w/ whole milk	6 fl oz	120	6	4	91	10	0	6
COLESLAW	1 tbsp	62	5	1	114	4	0	0
Coleslaw, reduced fat	1 tbsp	56	3	1	272	7	0	0
COLLARDS								
Boiled, chopped	1 cup	49	1	0	30	9	5	4
Fresh, chopped	1 cup	11	0	0	7	2	1	1
Frozen, boiled, chopped	1 cup	61	1	0	85	12	5	5
CONCH (baked or broiled, slices)	1 cup	165	2	0	194	2	0	33
COOKIES								
Animal Crackers	1	11	0	0	10	2	0	0
Arrowroot	1	22	1	0	18	4	0	0
Butter, commercial	1	23	1	1	18	3	0	0
Chocolate chip, commercial, higher fat, (2.25" dia)	1	48	2	1	32	7	0	1
Chocolate chip, commercial, lower fat	1	45	2	1	38	7	0	1
Chocolate chip, commercial, soft	1	55	3	1	33	8	0	1
Chocolate chip, homemade, made w/ butter (2.25" dia)	1	78	5	2	55	9	0	1
Chocolate chip, homemade, made w/ margarine (2.25" dia)	1	78	5	1	58	9	0	1
Chocolate chip, refrigerated dough	1 oz	126	6	2	59	17	0	1
Chocolate chip, refrigerated dough, baked (2.25" dia)	1	59	3	1	28	8	0	1

ITEM DESCRIPTION	Serving Size	Calories	Total Fat (g)	Saturated Fat (g)	Sodium (mg)	Carbohydrates (g)	Fiber (g)	Protein (g)
Chocolate sandwich, w/ creme filling, chocolate coated	1	82	4	1	55	11	1	1
Chocolate sandwich, w/ creme filling, reg	1	54	2	1	58	8	0	1
Chocolate sandwich, w/ extra creme filling	1	65	3	1	46	9	0	1
Chocolate wafers	1	26	1	0	35	4	0	0
Coconut macaroons, homemade (2" dia)	1	97	3	3	59	17	0	1
Fig bars	1	56	1	0	56	11	1	1
Fortune	1	30	0	0	22	7	0	0
Fudge, cake type	1	73	1	0	40	16	1	1
Gingersnaps	1	29	1	0	46	5	0	0
Graham crackers, chocolate coated (2.5" sq)	1	68	3	2	41	9	0	1
Graham crackers, plain, honey, or cinnamon (2.5" sq)	1	30	1	0	42	5	0	0
Ladyfingers, w/ lemon juice & rind	1	40	1	0	16	7	0	1
Ladyfingers, w/o lemon juice & rind	1	40	1	0	16	7	0	1
Marshmallow, chocolate-coated (1.75" dia)	1	55	2	1	22	9	0	1
Molasses (3.5" dia)	1	138	4	1	147	24	0	2
Oatmeal, commercial (3.5" dia)	1	112	5	1	96	17	1	2
Oatmeal, commercial, fat free (3.5" dia)	1	113	0	0	75	20	2	1
Oatmeal, commercial, soft	1	61	2	1	52	10	0	1
Oatmeal, homemade, w/o raisins (2-5/8" dia)	1	67	3	1	90	10	0	1
Oatmeal, homemade, w/ raisins (2-5/8" dia)	1	65	2	0	81	10	0	1
Oatmeal, refrigerated dough	1 oz	120	5	1	83	17	1	2
Oatmeal, refrigerated dough, baked	1	57	3	1	39	8	0	1
Peanut butter, commercial	1	72	4	1	62	9	0	1
Peanut butter, commercial, soft	1	69	4	1	50	9	0	1
Peanut butter, homemade	1	95	5	1	104	12	0	2
Peanut butter, refrigerated dough	1 oz	130	7	2	113	15	0	2

ITEM DESCRIPTION	Serving Size	Calories	Total Fat (g)	Saturated Fat (g)	Sodium (mg)	Carbohydrates (g)	Fiber (g)	Protein (g)
Peanut butter, refrigerated dough, baked	1	60	3	1	52	7	0	1
Peanut butter sandwich	1	67	3	1	52	9	0	1
Raisin, soft	1	60	2	1	51	10	0	1
Shortbread, pecan, commercial (2" dia)	1	76	5	1	39	8	0	1
Shortbread, plain, commercial (1-5/8" sq)	1	40	2	0	36	5	0	0
Sugar, commercial	1	72	3	1	54	10	0	1
Sugar, homemade, made w/ margarine (3" dia)	1	66	3	1	69	8	0	1
Sugar, refrigerated dough	1 oz	124	6	1	120	17	0	1
Sugar, refrigerated dough, baked	1	73	3	1	70	10	0	1
Sugar wafers w/ creme filling (3.5" x 1")	1	46	2	0	13	6	0	0
Tea biscuits	1	22	1	0	19	4	0	0
Vanilla sandwich w/ creme filling (1.75" dia)	1	48	2	0	35	7	0	0
Vanilla wafers, higher fat	1	28	1	0	18	4	0	0
Vanilla wafers, lower fat	1	28	1	0	19	4	0	0
COOKIES, BRAND NAME								
Archway Home Style Cookies, chocolate chip drop	1 serv	102	4	1	98	16	0	1
Archway Home Style Cookies, chocolate chip ice box	1 serv	119	6	2	65	16	1	1
Archway Home Style Cookies, iced oatmeal	1 serv	122	5	1	106	19	1	1
Archway Home Style Cookies, oatmeal	1 serv	105	4	1	98	17	1	1
Archway Home Style Cookies, oatmeal raisin	1 serv	106	3	1	88	18	1	1
Archway Home Style Cookies, old fashioned molasses	1 serv	106	3	1	146	18	0	1
Archway Home Style Cookies, old fashioned windmill	1 serv	94	4	1	94	14	0	1
Archway Home Style Cookies, peanut butter	1 serv	101	5	1	85	12	1	2

ITEM DESCRIPTION	Serving Size	Calories	Total Fat (g)	Saturated Fat (g)	Sodium (mg)	Carbohydrates (g)	Fiber (g)	Protein (g)
Archway Home Style Cookies, sugar	1 serv	99	3	1	154	17	0	1
Archway Home Style Cookies, sugar free, chocolate chip	1 serv	117	5	2	64	16	0	1
Archway Home Style Cookies, sugar free, oatmeal	1 serv	106	5	1	74	16	1	1
Famous Amos® Chocolate Chip	4	150	7	3	105	20	<1	1
Keebler Chocolate Graham Selects	1 serv	144	5	1	111	22	0	2
Keebler Fudge Shoppe Fudge Stripes	3	150	7	4.5	110	21	<1	1
Keebler Golden Vanilla Wafers	2	147	6	1	120	22	0	2
Keebler Vienna Fingers	2	150	6	2	95	23	1	1
Little Debbie Nut Bar, wafer w/ peanut butter, chocolate covered	1 serv	312	19	4	127	31	0	5
Nabisco Chips Ahoy Chocolate Chip Cookies	3	160	8	2.5	105	21	1	2
Nabisco Chips Ahoy Chunky Chocolate Chip Cookies	3	80	4.5	1.5	55	11	1	1
Nabisco Graham Crackers	1 serv	119	3	0	185	21	1	2
Nabisco Oreo Crunchies, cookie crumb topping	1 serv	52	2	0	58	8	0	1
Nabisco Oreo Sandwich Cookie	2	160	7	2	160	25	1	1
Nestle Toll House Chocolate Chip Cookies, refrigerated dough	1 serv	130	6	2.5	90	17	<1	1
Pepperidge Farm Bordeaux	4	130	5	3.5	95	19	1	2
Pepperidge Farm Chocolate Chunk	1	140	8	3.5	80	16	0	2
Pepperidge Farm Milano	3	180	10	5	80	21	1	2
Pillsbury Chocolate Chip Cookies, refrigerated dough	1 serv	135	7	2	85	17	1	1
CORIANDER								
Leaves, dried	1 tbsp	5	0	0	4	1	0	0
Leaves, fresh	1/4 cup	1	0	0	2	0	0	0
Seed	1 tbsp	15	1	0	2	3	2	1
CORN								
White	1 cup	184	8	1	58	123	0	16
Yellow	1 cup	184	8	1	58	123	12	16

ITEM DESCRIPTION	Serving Size	Calories	Total Fat (g)	Saturated Fat (g)	Sodium (mg)	Carbohydrates (g)	Fiber (g)	Protein (g)
RN & CANOLA OIL	1 tbsp	124	14	1	0	0	0	0
RN BRAN	1 cup	170	1	0	5	65	60	6
RNBREAD								
mix, prepared	1 pc	188	6	2	467	29	1	4
memade, made w/ 2% milk	1 pc	173	5	1	428	28	0	4
RN CAKES (very low sodium)	1 cake	35	0	0	3	8	0	1
RN CHIPS (BBQ flavor, enriched masa flour)	1 oz	148	9	1	216	16	0	2
RNED BEEF								
rl Buddig Cooked Corned Beef, opped, pressed	2 oz serv	81	4	2	765	1	0	11
rmel Corned Beef Hash, canned	1 cup	387	24	10	1003	22	3	21
af, jellied	1 slice	43	2	1	267	0	0	6
stle Chef-Mate Corned Beef Hash, nned	1 cup	455	30	14	1619	28	3	21
bstitute, Worthington Meatless orned Beef, frozen	1 slice	46	3	0	144	2	1	4
ORN FLOUR								
egermed, unenriched, yellow	1 cup	472	2	0	1	104	2	7
asa, white	1 cup	416	4	1	6	87	11	11
asa, yellow	1 cup	416	4	1	6	87	0	11
hole grain, blue	100 grams	364	5	0	5	74	9	10
hole grain, white	1 cup	422	5	1	6	90	9	8
hole grain, yellow	1 cup	422	5	1	6	90	9	8
ORNMEAL								
egermed, white	1 cup	587	3	0	11	126	6	12
egermed, yellow	1 cup	587	3	0	11	126	6	12
elf-rising, bolted, plain, yellow	1 cup	407	4	1	1521	86	8	10
elf-rising, bolted, / wheat flour, white	1 cup	592	5	1	2242	125	11	14
elf-rising, degermed, white	1 cup	490	2	0	1860	103	10	12
elf-rising, degermed, yellow	1 cup	490	2	0	1860	103	10	12
hole grain, white	1 cup	442	4	1	43	94	9	10
hole grain, yellow	1 cup	442	4	1	43	94	9	10
ORN MUFFIN MIX	1 oz	119	3	1	315	20	2	2

ITEM DESCRIPTION	Serving Size	Calories	Total Fat (g)	Saturated Fat (g)	Sodium (mg)	Carbohydrates (g)	Fiber (g)	Protein (g)
CORNNUTS								
BBQ flavor	1 oz	124	4	1	277	20	2	3
Nacho flavor	1 oz	124	4	1	180	20	2	3
Plain	1 oz	126	4	1	156	20	2	2
CORN OIL (all purpose)	1 tbsp	120	14	2	0	0	0	0
CORN PUDDING (homemade)	1 cup	328	13	6	702	43	3	11
CORN SALAD (fresh)	1/2 cup	112	2.6	0	94	22	3	4
CORNSTARCH	1 cup	488	0	0	12	117	1	0
CORN, SWEET								
White, canned, cream style, reg	1/2 cup	92	1	0	365	23	2	2
White, canned, vacuum packed, no salt	1/2 cup	83	1	0	3	20	2	3
White, canned, vacuum packed, reg	1/2 cup	83	1	0	286	20	2	3
White, canned, whole kernel	1/2 cup	66	1	0	265	15	2	2
White, canned, whole kernel, no salt	1/2 cup	82	1	0	15	20	1	2
White, canned, whole kernel, reg	1/2 cup	82	1	0	273	20	2	2
White, fresh (6" long)	1 ear	63	1	0	11	14	2	2
White, frozen, kernels, boiled	1/2 cup	66	0	0	4	16	2	2
Yellow, boiled (6" long)	1 ear	96	1	0	0	22	2	3
Yellow, canned, cream style, no salt	1/2 cup	92	1	0	4	23	2	2
Yellow, canned, cream style, reg	1/2 cup	92	1	0	365	23	2	2
Yellow, canned in brine, reg	1/2 cup	82	1	0	273	20	2	2
Yellow, canned, no salt	1/2 cup	82	1	0	15	20	2	2
Yellow, canned, vacuum packed, no salt	1/2 cup	83	1	0	3	20	2	3
Yellow, canned, vacuum packed, reg	1/2 cup	83	1	0	286	20	2	3
Yellow, canned, whole kernel	1/2 cup	66	1	0	265	15	2	2
Yellow, fresh	1/2 cup	66	1	0	12	15	2	2
Yellow, frozen, kernels, boiled	1/2 cup	66	1	0	1	16	2	2
CORN SYRUP								
Dark	1 tbsp	57	0	0	31	16	0	0
High fructose	1 tbsp	53	0	0	0	14	0	0
Light	1 tbsp	62	0	0	14	17	0	0

ITEM DESCRIPTION	Serving Size	Calories	Total Fat (g)	Saturated Fat (g)	Sodium (mg)	Carbohydrates (g)	Fiber (g)	Protein (g)
COTTAGE CHEESE								
creamed, small curd	1/2 cup	110	5	2	410	4	0	13
creamed, w/ fruit	1/2 cup	110	4	3	389	5	0	12
low fat, 1% milkfat	1/2 cup	81	1	1	459	3	0	14
low fat, 1% milkfat, lactose reduced	1/2 cup	84	1	1	250	4	1	14
low fat, 1% milkfat, no sodium	1/2 cup	81	1	1	15	3	0	14
low fat, 2% milkfat	1/2 cup	97	3	1	373	4	0	13
nonfat, dry, large or small curd	1/2 cup	52	0	0	239	5	0	8
COTTONSEED FLOUR								
low fat	1 oz	94	0	0	10	10	0	14
part defatted	1 cup	337	6	1	33	38	3	39
part defatted, meal	1 oz	104	1	0	10	11	0	14
COTTONSEED OIL (all purpose)	1 tbsp	120	14	4	0	0	0	0
COUSCOUS (cooked)	1 cup	176	0	0	8	36	2	6
COWPEAS								
catjang, boiled	1 cup	200	1	0	32	35	6	14
catjang, fresh	1 cup	573	3	1	97	100	18	40
common, boiled	1 cup	200	1	0	7	36	11	13
common, canned, plain	1 cup	185	1	0	718	33	8	11
common, canned w/ pork	1 cup	199	4	1	840	40	8	7
common, fresh	1 cup	561	2	1	27	100	18	39
fresh	1 cup	131	1	0	6	27	7	4
fresh, boiled	1 cup	160	1	0	7	34	8	5
frozen, boiled	1 cup	224	1	0	8	40	11	14
leafy tips, boiled, chopped	1 cup	12	0	0	3	1	0	2
leafy tips, fresh, chopped	1 cup	10	0	0	3	2	0	1
young pods w/ seeds, boiled	1 cup	32	0	0	3	7	0	2
young pods w/ seeds, fresh	1 cup	41	0	0	4	9	0	3
CRAB								
Alaska King, cooked in moist heat	3 oz	82	1	0	911	0	0	16
blue, canned	1 cup	134	2	0	450	0	0	28
blue, crab cakes	1 cake	93	5	1	198	0	0	12
blue, flaked, cooked in moist heat	1 cup	120	2	0	329	0	0	24

ITEM DESCRIPTION	Serving Size	Calories	Total Fat (g)	Saturated Fat (g)	Sodium (mg)	Carbohydrates (g)	Fiber (g)	Protein (g)
Dungeness, cooked in moist heat	3 oz	94	1	0	321	1	0	19
Imitation Alaska King, made from surimi	3 oz	81	0	0	715	13	0	6
Queen, cooked in moist heat	3 oz	98	1	0	587	0	0	20
CRABAPPLES (fresh, slices)	1 cup	84	0	0	1	22	0	0
CRACKER MEAL	1 cup	440	2	0	32	93	3	11
CRACKERS								
Cheese, low sodium (1" sq)	1	5	0	0	5	1	0	0
Cheese, regular (1" sq)	1	5	0	0	10	1	0	0
Cheese, sandwich type, w/ peanut butter filling	1 sandwich	32	2	0	46	4	0	1
Crispbread, rye	1 crispbread	37	0	0	26	8	2	1
Matzo, egg	1 matzo	109	1	0	6	22	1	3
Matzo, egg & onion	1 matzo	109	1	0	80	22	1	3
Matzo, plain	1 matzo	111	0	0	1	23	1	3
Matzo, whole wheat	1 matzo	98	0	0	1	22	3	4
Melba toast, plain	1 toast	20	0	0	41	4	0	1
Melba toast, plain, w/o salt	1 toast	20	0	0	1	4	0	1
Melba toast, rye (includes pumpernickel)	1 toast	19	0	0	45	4	0	1
Melba toast, wheat	1 toast	19	0	0	42	4	0	1
Milk	1 cracker	50	2	0	65	8	0	1
Oyster	5 crackers	21	0	0	56	4	0	0
Oyster, low salt	5 crackers	21	0	0	32	4	0	0
Oyster, unsalted	5 crackers	21	0	0	32	4	0	0
Ritz Crackers	1 cracker	16	1	0	29	2	0	0
Rusk toast	1 rusk	41	1	0	25	7	0	1
Rye, sandwich, w/ cheese filling	1 sandwich	34	2	0	73	4	0	1
Rye, wafers, plain	1 cracker	37	0	0	87	9	3	1
Rye, wafers, seasoned (triple crackers)	1 triple	84	2	0	195	16	5	2
Saltines	5 crackers	63	1	0	167	11	0	1
Saltines, fat free, low sodium	5 crackers	59	0	0	95	12	0	2
Saltines, low salt	5 crackers	63	1	0	95	11	0	1

ITEM DESCRIPTION	Serving Size	Calories	Total Fat (g)	Saturated Fat (g)	Sodium (mg)	Carbohydrates (g)	Fiber (g)	Protein (g)
Saltines, unsalted tops	5 crackers	65	2	0	115	11	0	1
Sandwich, w/ cheese filling	1 sandwich	33	1	0	98	4	0	1
Sandwich, w/ peanut butter filling	1 sandwich	35	2	0	50	4	0	1
Wheat	1 cup, crushed	393	17	4	660	54	4	7
Wheat, low salt	1 cup, crushed	393	17	0	235	54	4	7
Wheat, sandwich, w/ cheese filling	1 sandwich	35	2	0	64	4	0	1
Wheat, sandwich, w/ peanut butter filling	1 sandwich	35	2	0	56	4	0	1
Whole wheat	1 cracker	18	1	0	26	3	0	0
Whole wheat, low salt	1 cracker	18	1	0	10	3	0	0
CRANBERRIES								
Dried, sweetened	1/3 cup	123	1	0	1	33	2	0
Fresh	1 cup	46	0	0	2	12	5	0
CRANBERRY-APPLE JUICE								
Bottled	8 fl oz	154	0	0	5	39	0	0
Low calorie	8 fl oz	46	0	0	12	11	0	0
CRANBERRY-APRICOT JUICE								
(bottled)	8 fl oz	157	0	0	5	40	0	0
CRANBERRY BEANS								
Boiled	1 cup	241	1	0	2	43	18	17
Canned	1 cup	216	1	0	863	39	16	14
Fresh	1 cup	653	2	1	12	117	48	45
CRANBERRY-GRAPE JUICE								
(bottled)	8 fl oz	137	0	0	7	34	0	0
CRANBERRY JUICE								
(unsweetened)	1 cup	116	0	0	5	31	0	1
CRANBERRY JUICE COCKTAIL								
Bottled	8 fl oz	137	0	0	5	34	0	0
Frozen concentrate, prepared w/ water	8 fl oz	111	0	0	9	28	0	0
CRANBERRY-ORANGE RELISH								
(canned)	1 cup	490	0	0	88	127	0	1
CRANBERRY SAUCE								
(canned, sweetened)	1 cup	418	0	0	80	108	3	1

ITEM DESCRIPTION	Serving Size	Calories	Total Fat (g)	Saturated Fat (g)	Sodium (mg)	Carbohydrates (g)	Fiber (g)	Protein (g)
CRAYFISH								
Farmed, cooked in moist heat	3 oz	74	1	0	82	0	0	15
Wild, cooked in moist heat	3 oz	70	1	0	80	0	0	14
CREAM								
Half & half	1 tbsp	20	2	1	6	1	0	0
Light	1 tbsp	29	3	2	6	1	0	0
CREAM CHEESE								
Cream cheese	1 tbsp	50	5	3	47	1	0	1
Low fat	1 tbsp	30	2	1	70	1	0	1
CREAM OF TARTAR	1 tsp	8	0	0	2	2	0	0
CREAM PUFFS								
Homemade, shell & custard filling	1 puff	335	20	5	443	30	1	9
Homemade, shell only	1 puff	239	17	4	368	15	0	6
CREAM SUBSTITUTE								
Liquid, light	1 fl oz	21	1	0	18	3	0	0
Powder, light	1 packet	13	0	0	7	2	0	0
CRÈME DE MENTHE (72 proof)	1 fl oz	125	0	0	2	14	0	0
CRESS								
Garden, boiled	1 cup	31	1	0	11	5	1	3
Garden, fresh	1 cup	16	0	0	7	3	1	1
CROAKER (Atlantic, breaded & fried)	3 oz	188	11	3	296	6	0	15
CROISSANTS								
Apple	1 med	145	5	3	156	21	1	4
Butter	1 med	231	12	7	424	26	1	5
Cheese	1 med	236	12	6	316	27	1	5
CROOKNECK & STRAIGHTNECK SQUASH								
Boiled, slices	1 cup	36	1	0	0	8	3	2
Canned, w/o salt, slices	1 cup	28	0	0	11	6	3	1
Fresh, slices	1 cup	25	0	0	3	5	2	1
Frozen, boiled, slices	1 cup	48	0	0	12	11	3	2
CROUTONS								
Pepperidge Farm Classic Style Croutons, seasoned	1 serv	33	1	0	97	4	0	1
Plain	1 cup	122	2	0	209	22	1	4

ITEM DESCRIPTION	Serving Size	Calories	Total Fat (g)	Saturated Fat (g)	Sodium (mg)	Carbohydrates (g)	Fiber (g)	Protein (g)
seasoned	1 cup	186	7	2	495	25	2	4
CUCUMBER								
peeled, fresh, slices	1 cup	14	0	0	2	3	1	1
w/ peel, fresh, slices	1 cup	16	0	0	2	4	1	1
CUMIN SEED	1 tbsp	22	1	0	10	3	1	1
CUPCAKES (chocolate, w/ frosting)	1 cupcake	131	2	0	178	29	2	2
CURRANTS								
European black, fresh	1 cup	71	0	0	2	17	0	2
Red & white, fresh	1 cup	63	0	0	1	15	5	2
Zante, dried	1 cup	408	0	0	12	107	10	6
CURRY POWDER	1 tbsp	20	1	0	3	4	2	1
CUSK (cooked in dry heat)	3 oz	95	1	0	34	0	0	21
CUTTLEFISH (cooked in moist heat)	3 oz	134	1	0	632	1	0	28
DAIQUIRI								
Canned	6 fl oz	229	0	0	73	29	0	0
Homemade	6 fl oz	337	0	0	9	13	0	0
DANDELION GREENS								
Boiled, chopped	1 cup	35	1	0	46	7	3	2
Fresh, chopped	1 cup	25	0	0	42	5	2	1
DANISH PASTRY								
Almond (4.25" dia)	1 pastry	280	16	4	236	30	1	5
Cheese	1 pastry	266	16	5	320	26	1	6
Cinnamon (4.25" dia)	1 pastry	262	15	4	241	29	1	5
Fruit (4.25" dia)	1 pastry	263	13	3	251	34	1	4
Kellogg's Pop-Tarts Pastry Swirls, apple cinnamon	1 pastry	256	11	3	190	37	1	3
Kellogg's Pop-Tarts Pastry Swirls, cheese	1 pastry	252	11	3	180	37	0	3
Kellogg's Pop-Tarts Pastry Swirls, strawberry	1 pastry	254	11	3	170	37	1	3
Lemon	1 pastry	263	13	2	251	34	1	4
DATES								
Deglet Noor	1 date	20	0	0	0	5	1	0
Medjool	1 date	66	0	0	0	18	2	0

ITEM DESCRIPTION	Serving Size	Calories	Total Fat (g)	Saturated Fat (g)	Sodium (mg)	Carbohydrates (g)	Fiber (g)	Protein (g)
DILL SEED	1 tbsp	20	1	0	1	4	1	1
DILL WEED								
Dried	1 tbsp	8	0	0	6	2	0	1
Sprigs, fresh	5 sprigs	0	0	0	1	0	0	0
DOLPHINFISH								
(cooked in dry heat)	3 oz	93	1	0	96	0	0	20
DOUGHNUTS								
Cake type, chocolate, sugared or glazed (3" dia)	1	175	8	2	143	24	1	2
Cake type, plain (3.25" dia)	1	226	13	4	301	25	1	3
Cake type, plain, chocolate coated or frosted (3" dia)	1	194	11	6	178	22	1	2
Cake type, plain, sugared or glazed (3" dia)	1	192	10	3	181	23	1	2
Cake type, wheat, sugared or glazed (3" dia)	1	162	9	1	160	19	1	3
French crullers, glazed (3" dia)	1	169	8	2	141	24	0	1
Holes, glazed	1	52	2	1	50	7	0	1
Honey buns, glazed, enriched (4" x 3")	1	259	12	4	252	33	1	4
Honey buns, glazed, unenriched (3.25" dia)	1	242	14	3	205	27	1	4
Old fashioned, plain (3.25" dia)	1	226	13	4	301	25	1	3
Yeast leavened, glazed, enriched (3" dia)	1	124	6	2	120	16	1	2
Yeast leavened, glazed, unenriched (3.25" dia)	1	242	14	3	205	27	1	4
Yeast leavened, w/ creme filling (3-1/2" x 2-1/2")	1	307	21	5	263	26	1	5
Yeast leavened, w/ jelly filling (3-1/2" x 2-1/2")	1	289	16	4	249	33	1	5
DOVE cooked (includes squab), diced	1 cup	307	18	5	80	0	0	33
DRUM (freshwater, cooked in dry heat)	3 oz	130	5	1	82	0	0	19
DUCK								
Meat only, roasted, chopped	1 cup	281	16	6	91	0	0	33
w/ skin, roasted, chopped	1 cup	472	40	14	83	0	0	27
DUCK EGGS (whole, fresh)	1	130	10	3	102	1	0	9

ITEM DESCRIPTION	Serving Size	Calories	Total Fat (g)	Saturated Fat (g)	Sodium (mg)	Carbohydrates (g)	Fiber (g)	Protein (g)
DUCK FAT	1 tbsp	113	13	4	0	0	0	0
DURIAN (fresh or frozen, chopped)	1 cup	357	13	0	5	66	9	4
ECLAIRS								
Custard filled, w/ chocolate glaze, homemade	1	262	16	4	337	24	1	6
Weight Watchers, frozen	1	142	4	1	177	24	1	3
EDAMAME (frozen)	1 cup	189	8	1	9	15	8	17
EEL (boneless, cooked in dry heat)	3 oz	201	13	3	55	0	0	20
EGG CUSTARD								
Baked, homemade	1/2 cup	148	6	3	86	15	0	7
Dry mix, prepared w/ 2% milk	100 grams	111	3	1	89	17	0	4
EGGNOG								
Eggnog	8 fl oz	343	19	11	137	34	0	10
Mix prepared w/ whole milk	8 fl oz	258	8	5	150	39	0	8
EGGPLANT								
Boiled, cubed	1 cup	35	0	0	1	9	3	1
Fresh, cubed	1 cup	20	0	0	2	5	3	1
Pickled	1 cup	67	1	0	2277	13	3	1
EGG ROLLS								
Chicken, refrigerated, heated	1	158	4	1	448	23	2	8
Pork, refrigerated, heated	1	189	6	1	446	25	2	8
Vegetable, refrigerated, heated	1	153	4	1	438	25	2	5
EGG ROLL WRAPPERS	1	93	0	0	183	19	1	3
EGGS								
Cooked, omelet	1 lg	96	7	2	98	0	0	6
Fresh	1 lg	72	5	2	70	0	0	6
Fried	1 lg	90	7	2	94	0	0	6
Hard-boiled	1 lg	78	5	2	62	1	0	6
Poached	1 lg	71	5	2	147	0	0	6
Scrambled	1 lg	102	7	2	171	1	0	7
EGG SUBSTITUTE								
Frozen	1/4 cup	96	7	1	119	2	0	7
Liquid	1 tbsp	13	1	0	28	0	0	2
Powder	7/10 oz	89	3	1	160	4	0	11

ITEM DESCRIPTION	Serving Size	Calories	Total Fat (g)	Saturated Fat (g)	Sodium (mg)	Carbohydrates (g)	Fiber (g)	Protein (g)
EGG WHITE	1/4 cup	30	0	0	0	0	0	6
EGG YOLK								
Fresh	1 lg	54	5	2	8	1	0	
Frozen	100 grams	303	26	8	67	1	0	16
Frozen, sugared	100 grams	307	23	7	67	11	0	14
ELDERBERRIES (fresh)	1 cup	106	1	0	9	27	10	1
ENCHILADA SAUCE (Pace)	1 serv	24	0	0	520	5	1	1
ENDIVE (fresh)	1 head	87	1	0	113	17	16	6
ENERGY DRINK, BRAND NAME								
Red Bull	8.3 fl oz	115	0	0	214	28	0	1
Red Bull, sugar free	8.3 fl oz	12	0	0	210	2	0	1
ENGLISH MUFFINS								
Apple-cinnamon, toasted	1	144	1	0	192	29	2	5
Mixed grain, toasted	1	156	1	0	276	31	2	6
Plain, toasted	1	140	1	0	248	27	2	5
Raisin-cinnamon, toasted	1	144	1	0	192	29	2	5
Sourdough, toasted	1	140	1	0	248	27	2	5
Thomas' English Muffins	1 serv	132	1	0	197	26	0	5
Wheat, toasted	1	160	1	0	216	25	3	5
Whole wheat, toasted	1	135	1	0	422	27	5	6
FALAFEL (homemade)	1 patty	57	3	0	50	5	0	2
FAVA BEANS								
Boiled	1 cup	187	1	0	8	33	9	13
Canned	1 cup	182	1	0	1160	32	10	14
Fresh beans	1 cup	512	2	0	20	87	38	39
Fresh, in pod	1 cup	111	1	0	32	22	0	10
FENNEL								
Bulb, fresh, slices	1 cup	27	0	0	45	6	3	1
Seed, whole	1 tbsp	20	1	0	5	3	2	1
FENUGREEK (seed)	1 tbsp	36	1	0	7	6	3	3
FIGS								
Canned in ex heavy syrup	1 cup	279	0	0	3	73	0	1
Canned in heavy syrup	1 cup	228	0	0	3	59	6	1

ITEM DESCRIPTION	Serving Size	Calories	Total Fat (g)	Saturated Fat (g)	Sodium (mg)	Carbohydrates (g)	Fiber (g)	Protein (g)
Canned in light syrup	1 cup	174	0	0	3	45	6	1
Canned in water	1 cup	131	0	0	2	35	5	1
Dried, stewed	1 cup	277	1	0	10	71	11	4
Dried, uncooked	1 fruit	21	0	0	1	5	1	0
Fresh, whole	1 lg	47	0	0	1	12	2	0
FISH BROTH	1 cup	39	1	0	776	1	0	5
FISH OIL								
Menhaden	1 tbsp	123	14	4	0	0	0	0
Menhaden, fully hydrogenated	1 tbsp	113	13	12	0	0	0	0
FISH SAUCE	1 tbsp	6	0	0	1390	1	0	1
FISH STICKS								
Frozen, preheated	1 stick	70	4	1	118	6	0	3
Meatless	1 stick	81	5	1	137	3	2	6
FISH STOCK (homemade)	1 cup	40	2	0	363	0	0	5
FLATFISH (flounder & sole, cooked in dry heat)	3 oz	99	1	0	89	0	0	21
FLAXSEED								
Oil	1 tbsp	120	14	1	0	0	0	0
Seeds, whole	1 tbsp	55	4	0	3	3	3	2
FLOUNDER (flounder & sole cooked in dry heat)	3 oz	99	1	0	89	0	0	21
FRANKFURTERS								
Beef (5" long x 3/4" dia)	1	148	13	5	513	2	0	5
Beef & pork	1	137	12	5	504	1	0	5
Beef & pork, low fat	1	88	6	2	716	3	0	6
Beef, low fat	1	133	11	5	593	1	0	7
Beef, pork, & turkey, fat free	1	62	1	0	455	6	0	7
Chicken	1 link	100	7	2	380	1	0	7
Low sodium	1	180	16	7	177	1	0	7
Meat & poultry, low fat	1 cup, slices	182	4	1	1406	12	0	22
Pork	1 link	204	18	7	620	0	0	10
Turkey	1	100	8	2	485	2	0	6
FRANKFURTERS, BRAND NAME								
Ball Park Beef Franks	1	190	16	7	550	4	0	7

ITEM DESCRIPTION	Serving Size	Calories	Total Fat (g)	Saturated Fat (g)	Sodium (mg)	Carbohydrates (g)	Fiber (g)	Protein (g)
Ball Park Turkey Franks	1	110	7	2	580	6	0	6
Boar's Head Beef Frankfurters w/ natural casing	1	160	14	6	440	1	0	7
Butcher Boy Meats Turkey Franks	1 serv	134	10	3	651	3	0	8
Hebrew National Beef Franks	1 serv	150	14	6	460	1	0	6
Hebrew National Beef Franks reduced fat	1 serv	110	9	3.5	490	2	0	5
Hormel Wrangler Beef Franks	1	162	14	6	557	1	0	7
Kanh's Beef Franks, bun size	1	180	17	7	530	3	0	6
Louis Rich Franks, turkey & chicken	1 serv	85	6	2	511	2	0	5
Oscar Mayer Little Wieners, pork & turkey	1 serv	177	16	6	592	1	0	6
Oscar Mayer Wieners, beef	1 serv	147	14	6	461	1	0	5
Oscar Mayer Wieners, beef, bun length	1 link	185	17	7	584	2	0	6
Oscar Mayer Wieners, beef, fat free	1 serv	39	0	0	464	3	0	7
Oscar Mayer Wieners, beef, light	1 serv	110	8	4	615	2	0	6
Oscar Mayer Wieners, light pork, turkey & beef	1 serv	111	8	3	591	2	0	7
Oscar Mayer Wieners, pork & turkey	1 link	147	13	4	445	1	0	5
Oscar Mayer Wieners, turkey & cheese	1 serv	143	13	5	514	1	0	5
Sabrett Beef Frankfurters	1	140	12	5	410	1	0	6
FRANKFURTERS SUBSTITUTE								
Frankfurter, meatless	1	163	10	1	330	5	3	14
Loma Linda Big Franks, canned	1 link	111	6	1	217	3	2	11
Loma Linda Linketts, canned	1 link	73	4	1	140	2	1	7
Loma Linda Little Links, canned	2 links	102	6	1	217	3	2	9
Loma Linda Low Fat Big Franks, canned	1 link	79	2	0	245	3	2	12
Morningstar Farms America's Original Veggie Dog, frozen	1 link	75	1	0	609	7	2	11
Morningstar Farms Meatless Corn Dogs, frozen	1 pc	162	4	1	466	22	3	8
Morningstar Farms Meatless Mini Corn Dogs, frozen	4 pcs	174	5	1	515	22	3	10

ITEM DESCRIPTION	Serving Size	Calories	Total Fat (g)	Saturated Fat (g)	Sodium (mg)	Carbohydrates (g)	Fiber (g)	Protein (g)
Morningstar Farms Veggie Corn Dogs, frozen	1 pc	164	5	1	522	22	2	8
Worthington Super Links, canned	1 link	105	7	1	340	3	1	7
FRENCH BEANS								
Boiled	1 cup	228	1	0	11	43	17	12
Fresh	1 cup	631	4	0	33	118	46	35
FRENCH TOAST								
Frozen	1 pc	126	4	1	292	19	1	4
Homemade, w/ 2% milk	1 slice	149	7	2	311	16	0	5
FROSTING								
Chocolate, creamy, ready to eat	2 tbsp	163	7	2	75	26	0	0
Coconut, ready to eat	2 oz	250	14	5	113	30	1	1
Cream cheese, ready to eat	2 tbsp	137	6	2	63	22	0	0
Vanilla, creamy, ready to eat	2 oz	241	9	2	106	39	0	0
White, fluffy, dry mix, prepared w/ water	1/8 pkg	211	3	0	7	48	0	0
FROZEN BREAKFAST ITEMS								
Breakfast burrito, ham & cheese, frozen	1 serv	212	7	2	405	28	1	10
Cinnamon swirl French toast w/ sausage, frozen	1 serv	415	23	7	502	38	2	13
Scrambled eggs & sausage w/ hashed brown potatoes, frozen	1 serv	361	27	7	772	17	1	13
FROZEN YOGURT								
Chocolate	1/2 cup	110	3	2	55	19	1	3
Chocolate, nonfat milk, sweetened w/o sugar	1/2 cup	100	1	0	75	18	1	4
Chocolate, soft serve	1/2 cup	115	4	3	71	18	2	3
Flavors other than chocolate	1/2 cup	110	3	2	55	19	0	3
Vanilla, soft serve	1/2 cup	117	4	2	63	17	0	3
FRUIT & VEGETABLE JUICE DRINK								
(w/ added nutrients)	8 fl oz	72	0	0	52	18	0	0
FRUIT COCKTAIL								
Canned in ex heavy syrup	1 cup	229	0	0	16	60	3	1

ITEM DESCRIPTION	Serving Size	Calories	Total Fat (g)	Saturated Fat (g)	Sodium (mg)	Carbohydrates (g)	Fiber (g)	Protein (g)
Canned in ex light syrup	1 cup	111	0	0	10	29	3	1
Canned in heavy syrup	1 cup	181	0	0	15	47	2	1
Canned in heavy syrup, drained	1 cup	150	0	0	13	40	4	1
Canned in juice	1 cup	109	0	0	9	28	2	1
Canned in light syrup	1 cup	138	0	0	15	36	2	1
Canned in water	1 cup	76	0	0	9	20	2	1
FRUIT DRINKS								
Fruit-flavored drink mix powder, low calorie, w/ aspartame	1 tsp	17	0	0	32	7	0	0
Fruit-flavored drink mix powder, unsweetened	2 tbsp	56	0	0	682	23	0	0
FRUIT LEATHER								
Betty Crocker Fruit Roll Ups, berry flavored	2 rolls	104	1	0	89	24	0	0
Pieces	1 pkg	97	1	0	109	22	0	0
Rolls	1 lg	78	1	0	67	18	0	0
FRUIT PUNCH								
Canned	8 fl oz	117	0	0	94	30	0	0
Frozen concentrate	1 fl oz	56	0	0	3	14	0	0
Frozen concentrate, prepared w/ water	8 fl oz	114	0	0	12	29	0	0
Juice drink, frozen concentrate	1 fl oz	62	0	0	4	15	0	0
Juice drink, frozen concentrate, prepared w/ water	8 fl oz	98	0	0	12	24	0	0
Powder, w/o sodium, prepared w/ water	8 fl oz	97	0	0	18	25	0	0
FRUIT SALAD								
Canned in ex heavy syrup	1 cup	228	0	0	13	59	3	1
Canned in heavy syrup	1 cup	186	0	0	15	49	3	1
Canned in juice	1 cup	124	0	0	12	32	3	1
Canned in light syrup	1 cup	146	0	0	15	38	3	1
Canned in water	1 cup	74	0	0	7	19	3	1
Tropical, canned in heavy syrup	1 cup	221	0	0	5	57	3	1
FUDGE								
Chocolate marshmallow, homemade	1 pc	91	4	2	17	14	0	0

ITEM DESCRIPTION	Serving Size	Calories	Total Fat (g)	Saturated Fat (g)	Sodium (mg)	Carbohydrates (g)	Fiber (g)	Protein (g)
chocolate, homemade	1 pc	70	2	1	8	13	0	0
peanut butter, homemade	1 pc	62	1	0	19	12	0	1
GARBANZO BEANS								
Boiled	1 cup	269	4	0	11	45	13	15
Canned	1 cup	286	3	0	718	54	11	12
Fresh	1 cup	728	12	1	48	121	35	39
GARLIC								
Fresh	1 tsp	4	0	0	0	1	0	0
Powder	1 tbsp	28	0	0	2	6	1	1
GEFILTE FISH (sweet)	1 pc	35	1	0	220	3	0	4
GELATIN DESSERT								
Dry mix, prepared w/ water	1/2 cup	84	0	0	101	19	0	2
Dry mix, w/ aspartame, prepared w/ water	1/2 cup	23	0	0	56	5	0	1
GIN								
80 proof	1 fl oz	64	0	0	0	0	0	0
86 proof	1 fl oz	70	0	0	0	0	0	0
90 proof	1 fl oz	73	0	0	0	0	0	0
94 proof	1 fl oz	76	0	0	0	0	0	0
GINGER (ground)	1 tbsp	19	0	0	2	4	1	0
GINGER ROOT (fresh)	1 tsp	2	0	0	0	0	0	0
GINKGO NUTS								
Canned	1 oz	31	0	0	87	6	3	1
Dried	1 oz	99	1	0	4	21	0	3
Fresh	1 oz	52	0	0	2	11	0	1
GOAT MILK	1 cup	168	10	7	122	11	0	9
GOOSE								
Eggs, fresh	1 egg	266	19	5	199	2	0	20
Fat	1 tbsp	115	13	4	0	0	0	0
Meat & skin, roasted, chopped	1 cup	427	31	10	98	0	0	35
Meat only, roasted	1/2 goose	1407	75	27	449	0	0	171
GOOSEBERRIES								
Canned in light syrup	1 cup	184	1	0	5	47	6	2
Fresh	1 cup	66	1	0	2	15	7	1

ITEM DESCRIPTION	Serving Size	Calories	Total Fat (g)	Saturated Fat (g)	Sodium (mg)	Carbohydrates (g)	Fiber (g)	Protein (g)
GRANOLA (homemade)	1 cup	597	29	5	30	65	11	18
GRANOLA BARS								
Coconut, chocolate coated	1 oz bar	151	9	6	43	16	2	1
Fruit filled, nonfat	1 oz bar	97	0	0	5	22	2	2
Hard, almond	1 oz bar	140	7	4	73	18	1	2
Hard, chocolate chip	1 oz bar	124	5	3	98	20	1	2
Hard, peanut	1 oz bar	136	6	1	79	18	1	3
Hard, peanut butter	1 oz bar	137	7	1	80	18	1	3
Hard, plain	1 oz bar	132	6	1	82	18	2	3
Oats, fruits & nut	1 oz bar	113	2	0	71	22	2	2
Soft, chocolate chip	1 oz bar	117	5	2	50	20	1	2
Soft, chocolate chip, graham & marshmallow	1 oz bar	120	4	3	88	20	1	2
Soft, chocolate chip, milk chocolate coated	1 oz bar	130	7	4	56	18	1	2
Soft, nut & raisin	1 oz bar	127	6	3	71	18	2	2
Soft, peanut butter	1 oz bar	119	4	1	115	18	1	3
Soft, peanut butter & chocolate chip	1 oz bar	121	6	2	92	17	1	3
Soft, peanut butter, milk chocolate coated	1 oz bar	144	9	5	55	15	1	3
Soft, plain	1 oz bar	124	5	2	78	19	1	2
Soft, raisin	1 oz bar	125	5	3	79	19	1	2
GRAPE DRINK (canned)	8 fl oz	152	0	0	40	39	0	0
GRAPE JUICE								
Canned or bottled	8 fl oz	152	0	0	13	37	0	1
Frozen concentrate, prepared w/ water	1 cup	128	0	0	5	32	0	0
Unsweetened	1 cup	152	0	0	13	37	1	1
GRAPE LEAVES								
Canned	1 leaf	3	0	0	114	0	0	0
Fresh	1 leaf	3	0	0	1	0	0	0
GRAPEFRUIT								
Pink & red, California & Arizona, fresh	1/2 fruit	46	0	0	1	12	0	1

ITEM DESCRIPTION	Serving Size	Calories	Total Fat (g)	Saturated Fat (g)	Sodium (mg)	Carbohydrates (g)	Fiber (g)	Protein (g)
ink & red, Florida, fresh	1/2 fruit	37	0	0	0	9	1	1
Sections, canned in juice	1 cup	92	0	0	17	23	1	2
Sections, canned in light syrup	1 cup	152	0	0	5	39	1	1
Sections, canned in water	1 cup	88	0	0	5	22	1	1
White, California, fresh	1/2 fruit	44	0	0	0	11	0	1
White, Florida, fresh	1/2 fruit	38	0	0	0	10	0	1
GRAPEFRUIT JUICE								
Pink	1 cup	96	0	0	2	23	0	1
White	1 cup	96	0	0	2	23	0	1
White, canned, sweetened	1 cup	115	0	0	5	28	0	1
White, canned, unsweetened	1 cup	94	0	0	2	22	0	1
White, frozen concentrate, unsweetened, prepared w/ water	1 cup	101	0	0	2	24	0	1
GRAPES								
American type	1 cup	62	0	0	2	16	1	1
Canned in heavy syrup	1 cup	195	0	0	13	50	2	1
Canned in water	1 cup	98	0	0	15	25	2	1
European red or green	1 cup	104	0	0	3	27	1	1
GRAPESEED OIL	1 tbsp	120	14	1	0	0	0	0
GRAVY								
Au jus, canned	1/4 cup	10	0	0	30	1	0	1
Au jus, dry	1 tsp	9	0	0	348	1	0	0
Beef, canned	1/4 cup	31	1	1	326	3	0	2
Brown, dry	1 tbsp	22	1	0	291	4	0	1
Campbell's Au Jus Gravy	1/4 cup	5	0	0	230	0	0	1
Campbell's Beef Gravy	1/4 cup	25	1	1	270	3	0	1
Campbell's Brown Gravy, w/ onions	1/4 cup	25	1	0	330	4	0	0
Campbell's Chicken Gravy	1/4 cup	40	3	1	260	3	0	0
Campbell's Country Style Cream Gravy	1/4 cup	45	3	1	190	3	0	1
Campbell's Country Style Sausage Gravy	1/4 cup	70	6	2	270	3	0	2
Campbell's Golden Pork Gravy	1/4 cup	45	3	2	310	3	0	1
Campbell's Mushroom Gravy	1/4 cup	20	1	0	280	3	0	0

ITEM DESCRIPTION	Serving Size	Calories	Total Fat (g)	Saturated Fat (g)	Sodium (mg)	Carbohydrates (g)	Fiber (g)	Protein (g)
Campbell's Turkey Gravy	1/4 cup	25	1	0	270	3	0	1
Chicken, canned	1/4 cup	47	3	1	343	3	0	1
Chicken, dry	1 tbsp	30	1	0	332	5	0	1
Franco-American Slow Roast Beef Gravy	1/4 cup	25	1	1	310	3	0	1
Franco-American Slow Roast Chick Gravy	1/4 cup	20	1	0	240	3	0	1
Franco-American Slow Roast Turkey Gravy	1/4 cup	25	1	0	320	4	0	1
Heinz Home Style Beef Gravy	1/4 cup	22	1	0	335	4	0	1
Meat or poultry, low sodium, prepared	1/4 cup	31	1	1	11	4	0	2
Mushroom, canned	1/4 cup	50	3	0	570	5	0	1
Pork, dry, powder	1 serv	25	1	0	359	4	0	1
Turkey, canned	1/4 cup	30	1	0	343	3	0	2
Turkey, dry	1 serv	26	1	0	307	5	0	1
GREAT NORTHERN BEANS								
Boiled	1 cup	209	1	0	4	37	12	15
Canned	1 cup	299	1	0	10	55	13	19
Fresh	1 cup	620	2	1	26	114	37	40
GREEN BEANS								
Canned, drained	1 cup	27	0	0	354	6	3	2
Fresh, cooked w/o salt	1 cup	44	0	0	1	10	4	2
GRENADINE SYRUP	1 tbsp	54	0	0	5	13	0	0
GRITS								
Quaker Instant Grits, cheddar cheese flavor, prepared w/ water	1 packet	102	2	0	508	20	1	2
Quaker Instant Grits, country bacon flavor, prepared w/ water	1 packet	97	0	0	413	21	1	3
Quaker Instant Grits, plain, prepared w/ water	1 cup	167	0	0	514	37	2	4
White, reg & quick, cooked w/ water	1 cup	143	0	0	5	31	1	3
Yellow, reg & quick, cooked w/ water	1 cup	143	0	0	5	31	1	3
GROUND CHERRIES (fresh)	1 cup	74	1	0	0	16	0	3

ITEM DESCRIPTION	Serving Size	Calories	Total Fat (g)	Saturated Fat (g)	Sodium (mg)	Carbohydrates (g)	Fiber (g)	Protein (g)
GROUPER (cooked in dry heat)	3 oz	100	1	0	45	0	0	21
GUANABANA NECTAR (canned)	1 cup	148	0	0	20	37	0	0
GUAVA NECTAR (canned)	1 cup	143	0	0	18	37	3	0
GUAVAS								
Fresh	1 fruit	37	1	0	1	8	3	1
Sauce, cooked	1 cup	86	0	0	10	23	9	1
Strawberry, fresh	1 fruit	4	0	0	2	1	0	0
GUM								
Bubble, Bazooka	1 pc	15	0	0	0	4	0	0
Chewing gum	1 stick	7	0	0	0	2	0	0
Chewing gum, sugarless	1 pc	5	0	0	0	2	0	0
HADDOCK								
Cooked in dry heat	3 oz	95	1	0	74	0	0	21
Smoked, boneless	1 oz	33	0	0	216	0	0	7
HALIBUT								
Atlantic & Pacific, cooked in dry heat	3 oz	119	3	0	59	0	0	23
Greenland, cooked in dry heat	3 oz	203	15	3	88	0	0	16
HAM								
Boneless, ex lean (approx 5% fat), roasted	3 oz	123	5	2	1023	1	0	18
Boneless, reg (approx 11% fat), roasted	3 oz	151	8	3	1275	0	0	19
Carl Buddig Smoked Slices	2 oz	93	5	2	787	1	0	11
Chopped, canned	1 oz	68	5	2	387	0	0	5
Chopped, from fresh	1 oz	50	3	1	372	1	0	5
Ex lean & reg, canned, roasted	3 oz	142	7	2	908	0	0	18
Ex lean (approx 4% fat), canned, roasted	3 oz	116	4	1	965	0	0	18
Ex lean, slices	1 slice, oval	29	1	0	286	0	0	5
Honey-smoked	2 oz	69	1	1	510	4	0	10
Hormel Cure 81	1 serv	89	3	1	872	0	0	15
Loaf or roll, w/ cheese	1 slice	67	5	2	302	1	0	4
Minced	1 oz	75	6	2	353	1	0	5
Oscar Mayer Ham, 96% fat free	1 slice	22	1	0	258	0	0	3

ITEM DESCRIPTION	Serving Size	Calories	Total Fat (g)	Saturated Fat (g)	Sodium (mg)	Carbohydrates (g)	Fiber (g)	Protein (g)
Oscar Mayer Ham & Cheese Loaf	1 serv	66	5	2	327	1	0	4
Oscar Mayer Ham, boiled	1 slice	22	1	0	283	0	0	3
Oscar Mayer Ham, chopped	1 slice	50	3	1	350	1	0	5
Oscar Mayer Ham, honey	1 slice	23	1	0	262	1	0	4
Oscar Mayer Ham, smoked	1 slice	21	1	0	255	0	0	3
Reg (approx 11% fat)	1 slice	46	2	1	365	1	0	5
Reg (approx 13% fat), canned, roasted	3 oz	142	13	4	800	0	0	17
Salad spread	1 tbsp	32	2	1	137	2	0	1
Spread, w/ cheese	1 tbsp	37	3	1	180	0	0	2
Whole, lean & fat, roasted	3 oz	207	14	5	1009	0	0	18
HAZELNUT OIL	1 tbsp	120	14	1	0	0	0	0
HAZELNUTS OR FILBERTS								
Blanched	1 oz	178	17	1	0	5	3	4
Dry roasted, w/o salt	1 oz	183	18	1	0	5	3	4
Oscar Mayer	1 serv	52	4	1	300	0	0	4
Raw	1 oz	178	17	1	0	5	3	4
HEARTS OF PALM (canned)	1 cup	41	1	0	622	7	4	4
HEAVY CREAM	1 tbsp	52	6	3	6	0	0	0
HERRING								
Atlantic, cooked in dry heat	3 oz	173	10	2	98	0	0	20
Atlantic, kippered, boneless	1 oz	62	4	1	260	0	0	7
Atlantic, pickled, boneless	1 oz	74	5	1	247	3	0	4
Pacific, cooked in dry heat	3 oz	213	15	4	81	0	0	18
HERRING OIL	1 tbsp	123	14	3	0	0	0	0
HICKORY NUTS (dried)	1 cup	788	77	8	1	22	8	15
HOISIN SAUCE	1 tbsp	35	1	0	258	7	0	1
HOMINY								
Canned, white	1 cup	119	1	0	346	24	4	2
Canned, yellow	1 cup	115	1	0	336	23	4	2
Quaker Hominy, white, quick, dry	1/4 cup	128	1	0	1	29	2	3
Quaker Hominy, white, reg, dry	1/4 cup	142	1	0	1	32	2	4
Quaker Hominy, yellow, quick, dry	1/4 cup	125	1	0	1	29	2	3

ITEM DESCRIPTION	Serving Size	Calories	Total Fat (g)	Saturated Fat (g)	Sodium (mg)	Carbohydrates (g)	Fiber (g)	Protein (g)
HONEY	1 tbsp	64	0	0	1	17	0	0
HONEYDEW (fresh, diced)	1 cup	61	0	0	31	15	1	1
HONEY LOAF (pork & beef)	1 slice	35	1	0	370	3	0	3
HORSERADISH (prepared)	1 tbsp	7	0	0	47	2	1	0
HUBBARD SQUASH								
Baked, cubed	1 cup	102	1	0	16	22	0	5
Boiled, mashed	1 cup	71	1	0	12	15	7	3
Fresh, cubed	1 cup	46	1	0	8	10	0	2
HUMMUS								
Commercial	1 tbsp	25	1	0	57	2	1	1
Homemade	1 tbsp	27	1	0	36	3	1	1
HUSH PUPPIES	1 cup	512	21	3	1015	70	4	12
ICE CREAM								
Bar, chocolate or caramel covered, w/ nuts	1 bar	171	11	7	50	17	0	2
Ben & Jerry's Half Baked	1/2 cup	270	13	8	85	33	1	4
Ben & Jerry's Phish Food	1/2 cup	270	12	9	80	37	1	4
Blue Bunny Premium Chocolate	1/2 cup	150	70	4.5	45	16	0	4
Blue Bunny Reduced Fat Vanilla	1/2 cup	110	5	3	65	16	2	3
Breyers Ice Cream, 98% fat free, chocolate	1/2 cup	92	1	1	51	21	4	3
Breyers Ice Cream, 98% fat free, vanilla	1/2 cup	93	1	1	50	21	4	2
Breyers Ice Cream, all natural, light, chocolate	1/2 cup	137	5	3	51	20	1	4
Breyers Ice Cream, all natural, light, mint chocolate chip	1/2 cup	133	5	3	46	19	0	3
Breyers Ice Cream, all natural, light, vanilla	1/2 cup	110	3	2	48	17	0	3
Breyers Ice Cream, all natural, light, vanilla, chocolate & strawberry	1/2 cup	109	3	2	47	18	0	3
Breyers Ice Cream, no sugar added, butter pecan	1/2 cup	122	7	3	112	14	1	3
Breyers Ice Cream, no sugar added, chocolate caramel	1/2 cup	107	4	3	55	18	1	3

ITEM DESCRIPTION	Serving Size	Calories	Total Fat (g)	Saturated Fat (g)	Sodium (mg)	Carbohydrates (g)	Fiber (g)	Protein (g)
Breyers Ice Cream, no sugar added, vanilla	1/2 cup	99	4	3	46	15	0	3
Breyers Ice Cream, no sugar added, vanilla, chocolate & strawberry	1/2 cup	97	4	3	46	15	1	3
Chocolate	1/2 cup	143	7	4	50	19	1	3
Chocolate, light	1 serv	137	5	3	48	17	1	3
Chocolate, light, no sugar added	1/2 cup	109	4	3	54	18	1	3
Chocolate, low carb	1/2 cup	127	8	5	50	10	3	3
Chocolate, rich	1/2 cup	189	13	8	42	15	1	3
Edy's Grand Chocolate	1/2 cup	150	8	4.5	35	17	1	3
Edy's Grand Vanilla	1/2 cup	140	8	4	35	15	0	2
Edy's Slow Churned Chocolate	1/2 cup	100	4	2	30	15	0	3
Edy's Slow Churned Vanilla	1/2 cup	100	3.5	2	45	15	0	3
French vanilla, soft serve	1/2 cup	191	11	6	52	19	1	4
Haagen-Dazs Chocolate	1/2 cup	270	18	11	60	22	1	5
Haagen-Dazs Vanilla Bean	1/2 cup	290	18	11	75	26	0	5
Healthy Choice, praline & caramel	1/2 cup	121	2	1	63	23	1	3
Klondike Slim-a-Bear, chocolate cone	1 cone	177	3	1	126	36	3	3
Klondike Slim-a-Bear, chocolate sandwich	1 sandwich	135	2	1	120	28	3	4
Klondike Slim-a-Bear, fudge bar, 98% fat free, no sugar added	3.5 oz bar	92	1	1	89	22	4	3
Klondike Slim-a-Bear, mint sandwich	1 sandwich	134	1	0	122	28	3	4
Klondike Slim-a-Bear, vanilla cone	1 cone	175	3	1	126	35	3	3
Klondike Slim-a-Bear, vanilla sandwich	1 sandwich	135	1	0	122	28	3	4
Turkey Hill Chocolate	1/2 cup	150	7	4.5	45	19	1	2
Turkey Hill Chocolate Peanut Butter Cup	1/2 cup	180	11	4.5	75	18	1	3
Turkey Hill Cookies 'n Cream	1/2 cup	150	8	4.5	60	19	0	2
Turkey Hill Original Vanilla	1/2 cup	140	7	4.5	45	16	0	2
Vanilla	1/2 cup	137	7.2	4	53	16	0.5	2
Vanilla, light	1/2 cup	125	4	2	56	20	0	4

ITEM DESCRIPTION	Serving Size	Calories	Total Fat (g)	Saturated Fat (g)	Sodium (mg)	Carbohydrates (g)	Fiber (g)	Protein (g)
Vanilla, light, no sugar added	1/2 cup	105	5	3	65	15	1	3
Vanilla, rich	1/2 cup	266	17	11	65	24	0	4
ICE CREAM CONES								
Cake or wafer	1 cone	17	0	0	6	3	0	0
Sugar	1 cone	40	0	0	32	8	0	1
ICE POPS								
Creamsicle Pops, no sugar added	1 pop	25	0	0	18	6	0	1
Creamsicle Pops, sugar free	1 pop	20	1	1	2	5	3	1
Fudgesicle Bars, fat free	1 pop	65	0	0	48	14	1	3
Fudgesicle Pops, no sugar added	1 serv	88	1	0	86	19	1	3
Popsicle Scribblers	1.2 oz pop	27	0	0	4	7	0	0
Popsicles, sugar free, orange, cherry & grape	1-3/4 oz pop	12	0	0	6	3	0	0
Regular	1-3/4 oz pop	41	0	0	4	10	0	0
Sweetened w/ low calorie sweetener	1-3/4 oz pop	13	0	0	6	3	0	0
ICED TEA, BRAND NAME								
Arizona Iced Tea, w/ lemon	8 fl oz	89	0	0	9	22	0	0
Lipton Brisk Iced Tea, w/ lemon	8 fl oz	86	0	0	51	22	0	0
Nestle Cool Nestea Iced Tea w/ lemon	8 fl oz	88	0	0	51	22	0	0
Snapple Lemon Iced Tea	8 fl oz	80	0	0	5	21	0	0
ICES								
Frozen fruit & juice bars	3 oz bar	80	0	0	4	19	1	1
Italian, restaurant prepared	1/2 cup	61	0	0	5	16	0	0
Lime	1/2 cup	127	0	0	22	32	0	0
Pineapple-coconut	1/2 cup	112	3	2	35	24	1	0
JACKFRUIT								
Canned in syrup	1 cup	164	0	0	20	43	2	1
Fresh, slices	1 cup	155	0	0	5	40	3	2
JAMS & PRESERVES								
Apricot	1 tbsp	48	0	0	8	13	0	0
Dietetic, any flavor	1 tbsp	18	0	0	0	8	0	0
Flavors other than apricot	1 tbsp	56	0	0	6	14	0	0

ITEM DESCRIPTION	Serving Size	Calories	Total Fat (g)	Saturated Fat (g)	Sodium (mg)	Carbohydrates (g)	Fiber (g)	Protein (g)
JAVA PLUM (Jambolan), fresh	3 fruit	5	0	0	1	1	0	0
JELLIES								
Jellies	1 tbsp	56	0	0	6	15	0	0
Red sugar, homemade	1 tbsp	34	0	0	0	9	0	0
JELLYFISH (dried, salted)	1 cup	21	1	0	5620	0	0	3
JICAMA (fresh, slices)	1 cup	46	0	0	5	11	6	1
JUICE DRINKS, BRAND NAME								
Juicy Juice Apple Juice	8 oz	110	0	0	20	28	0	n/a
Langers Cranberry Juice Cocktail	8 oz	140	0	0	10	35	0	0
Minute Maid® Mixed Berry	10 oz	150	0	0	25	36	0	0
Minute Maid® Pineapple Orange	8 oz	120	0	0	15	29	0	1
Northland Cranberry Juice	8 oz	130	0	0	35	33	0	0
Northland Pure Pomegranate	8 oz	140	0	0	25	34	0	0
Tropicana Berry Punch	8 oz	120	0	0	10	31	0	0
Tropicana Tropical Punch	8 oz	130	0	0	10	33	0	0
V8 Splash, berry blend	8 oz	70	0	0	51	18	0	0
V8 Splash, fruit medley	8 oz	80	0	0	51	19	0	0
V8 Splash, tropical blend	8 oz	70	0	0	51	18	0	0
V8 Splash Smoothies, strawberry banana	8 oz	91	0	0	71	20	0	3
V8 Splash Smoothies, tropical colada	8 oz	101	0	0	49	21	1	3
V8 Vegetable Juice, 100% vegetable juice	8 oz	51	0	0	481	10	2	2
V8 Vegetable Juice, low sodium	8 oz	51	0	0	141	10	2	2
V8 Vegetable Juice, spicy hot V8	8 oz	49	0	0	620	10	2	2
V8 V- Fusion Juices, acai berry	8 oz	111	0	0	69	27	0	0
V8 V- Fusion Juices, peach mango	8 oz	121	0	0	69	28	0	1
V8 V- Fusion Juices, strawberry banana	8 oz	121	0	0	69	29	0	1
JUTE								
Potherb, boiled	1 cup	32	0	0	10	6	2	3
Potherb, fresh	1 cup	10	0	0	2	2	0	1

ITEM DESCRIPTION	Serving Size	Calories	Total Fat (g)	Saturated Fat (g)	Sodium (mg)	Carbohydrates (g)	Fiber (g)	Protein (g)
KALE								
Boiled, chopped	1 cup	36	1	0	30	7	3	2
Fresh, chopped	1 cup	34	0	0	29	7	1	2
Frozen, boiled, chopped	1 cup	39	1	0	20	7	3	4
Scotch, boiled, chopped	1 cup	36	1	0	58	7	2	2
Scotch, fresh, chopped	1 cup	28	0	0	47	6	1	2
KAMUT (cooked)	1 cup	251	2	0	0	52	0	11
KANPYO (dried gourd strips)	1 strip	16	0	0	1	4	0	1
KETCHUP								
Reg sodium	1 tbsp	15	0	0	167	4	0	0
Low sodium	1 tbsp	15	0	0	3	4	0	0
KIDNEY BEANS								
California red, boiled	1 cup	219	0	0	7	40	17	16
California red, fresh	1 cup	607	0	0	20	110	46	45
Liquid from stewed kidney beans	1 cup	113	8	3	5	7	0	4
Red, boiled	1 cup	225	1	0	4	40	13	15
Red, canned	1 cup	215	1	0	660	40	14	13
Red, fresh	1 cup	620	2	0	22	113	28	41
Royal red, boiled	1 cup	218	0	0	9	39	17	17
Royal red, fresh	1 cup	605	1	0	24	107	46	47
Sprouted, fresh	1 cup	53	1	0	11	8	0	8
KIWI FRUIT (fresh, w/o skin)	1 fruit	56	0	0	3	13	3	1
KOHLRABI								
Boiled, slices	1 cup	48	0	0	35	11	2	3
Fresh	1 cup	36	0	0	27	8	5	2
KUMQUATS (fresh)	1 fruit	13	0	0	2	3	1	0
LAMB								
Australian, composite of retail cuts, 1/8" fat, cooked	3 oz	218	14	7	65	0	0	21
Australian, composite of retail cuts, lean, 1/8" fat, cooked	3 oz	218	8	3	68	0	0	23
Australian, foreshank, 1/8" fat, braised	3 oz	218	4	2	85	0	0	23
Australian, leg, center slice, bone in, 1/8" fat, broiled	3 oz	183	10	5	55	0	0	22

ITEM DESCRIPTION	Serving Size	Calories	Total Fat (g)	Saturated Fat (g)	Sodium (mg)	Carbohydrates (g)	Fiber (g)	Protein (g)
Australian, leg, shank half, 1/8" fat, roasted	3 oz	196	12	5	57	0	0	21
Australian, leg, sirloin chops, boneless, 1/8" fat, broiled	3 oz	200	12	5	54	0	0	22
Australian, leg, sirloin half, boneless, 1/8" fat, roasted	3 oz	239	16	8	66	0	0	21
Australian, leg, whole shank & sirloin, 1/8" fat, roasted	3 oz	207	13	6	60	0	0	21
Australian, loin, 1/8" fat, broiled	3 oz	186	10	5	66	0	0	22
Australian, rib, 1/8" fat, roasted	3 oz	235	17	8	65	0	0	19
Australian, shoulder, arm, 1/8" fat, braised	3 oz	264	17	8	62	0	0	25
Australian, shoulder, blade, 1/8" fat, broiled	3 oz	247	19	9	75	0	0	18
Australian, shoulder, whole arm & blade, 1/8" fat, cooked	3 oz	252	18	9	72	0	0	20
Domestic, composite of retail cuts, 1/4" fat, USDA Choice, cooked	3 oz	250	18	8	61	0	0	21
Domestic, composite of retail cuts, 1/8" fat, USDA Choice, cooked	3 oz	230	15	6	61	0	0	22
Domestic, cubed for stew, leg & shoulder, 1/4" fat, braised	3 oz	190	7	3	60	0	0	29
Domestic, cubed for stew, leg & shoulder, 1/4" fat, broiled	3 oz	158	6	2	65	0	0	24
Domestic, foreshank, 1/4" fat, USDA Choice, braised	3 oz	207	11	5	61	0	0	24
Domestic, foreshank, 1/8" fat, braised	3 oz	207	11	5	61	0	0	24
Domestic, leg, shank half, 1/4" fat, USDA Choice, roasted	3 oz	191	11	4	55	0	0	22
Domestic, leg, shank half, 1/8" fat, USDA Choice, roasted	3 oz	184	10	4	55	0	0	23
Domestic, leg, sirloin half, 1/4" fat, USDA Choice, roasted	3 oz	248	18	7	58	0	0	21
Domestic, leg, sirloin half, 1/8" fat, USDA Choice, roasted	3 oz	241	17	7	58	0	0	21
Domestic, leg, whole shank & sirloin, 1/4" fat, USDA Choice, roasted	3 oz	219	14	6	56	0	0	22

ITEM DESCRIPTION	Serving Size	Calories	Total Fat (g)	Saturated Fat (g)	Sodium (mg)	Carbohydrates (g)	Fiber (g)	Protein (g)
Domestic, leg, whole shank & sirloin, 1/8" fat, USDA Choice, roasted	3 oz	206	12	5	57	0	0	22
Domestic, loin, 1/4" fat, USDA Choice, broiled	3 oz	269	20	8	65	0	0	21
Domestic, loin, 1/4" fat, USDA Choice, roasted	3 oz	263	20	9	54	0	0	19
Domestic, loin, 1/8" fat, USDA Choice, broiled	3 oz	252	18	7	66	0	0	22
Domestic, loin, 1/8" fat, USDA Choice, roasted	3 oz	246	18	8	54	0	0	20
Domestic, rib, 1/4" fat, USDA Choice, broiled	3 oz	307	25	11	65	0	0	19
Domestic, rib, 1/4" fat, USDA Choice, roasted	3 oz	305	25	11	62	0	0	18
Domestic, rib, 1/8" fat, USDA Choice, broiled	3 oz	289	23	10	65	0	0	20
Domestic, rib, 1/8" fat, USDA Choice, roasted	3 oz	290	23	10	63	0	0	19
Domestic, shoulder, arm, 1/4" fat, USDA Choice, braised	3 oz	294	20	8	61	0	0	26
Domestic, shoulder, arm, 1/4" fat, USDA Choice, broiled	3 oz	239	17	7	65	0	0	21
Domestic, shoulder, arm, 1/8" fat, USDA Choice, roasted	3 oz	237	17	7	55	0	0	19
Domestic, shoulder, arm, 1/8" fat, broiled	3 oz	229	15	7	66	0	0	21
Domestic, shoulder, arm, 1/8" fat, USDA Choice, braised	3 oz	286	19	8	61	0	0	26
Domestic, shoulder, arm, 1/8" fat, USDA Choice, roasted	3 oz	227	16	7	55	0	0	19
Domestic, shoulder, blade, 1/4" fat, USDA Choice, braised	3 oz	293	21	9	64	0	0	24
Domestic, shoulder, blade, 1/4" fat, USDA Choice, broiled	3 oz	236	17	7	70	0	0	20
Domestic, shoulder, blade, 1/4" fat, USDA Choice, roasted	3 oz	239	18	7	56	0	0	19
Domestic, shoulder, blade, 1/8" fat, USDA Choice, braised	3 oz	288	20	8	64	0	0	25

ITEM DESCRIPTION	Serving Size	Calories	Total Fat (g)	Saturated Fat (g)	Sodium (mg)	Carbohydrates (g)	Fiber (g)	Protein (g)
Domestic, shoulder, blade, 1/8" fat, USDA Choice, broiled	3 oz	227	16	6	71	0	0	20
Domestic, shoulder, blade, 1/8" fat, USDA Choice, roasted	3 oz	230	16	7	57	0	0	19
Domestic, shoulder, whole arm & blade, 1/4" fat, USDA Choice, braised	3 oz	292	21	9	64	0	0	24
Domestic, shoulder, whole arm & blade, 1/4" fat, USDA Choice, broiled	3 oz	236	16	7	66	0	0	21
Domestic, shoulder, whole arm & blade, 1/4" fat, USDA Choice, roasted	3 oz	235	17	7	56	0	0	19
Domestic, shoulder, whole arm & blade, 1/8" fat, USDA Choice, braised	3 oz	287	20	8	63	0	0	25
Domestic, shoulder, whole arm & blade, 1/8" fat, USDA Choice, broiled	3 oz	228	16	6	70	0	0	20
Domestic, shoulder, whole arm & blade, 1/8" fat, USDA Choice, roasted	3 oz	229	16	7	56	0	0	19
Ground, broiled	3 oz	241	17	7	69	0	0	21
Quarters, boiled, chopped	1 cup	58	1	0	52	9	4	6
LARD	1 tbsp	115	13	5	0	0	0	0
LASAGNA (vegetable, frozen, baked)	1 cup	314	14	5	796	32	4	16
LEEKS								
Boiled	1 leek	38	0	0	12	9	1	1
Freeze-dried	1 tbsp	1	0	0	0	0	0	0
Fresh	1 leek	54	0	0	18	13	2	1
LEMONADE								
Frozen concentrate, pink, prepared w/ water	8 fl oz	99	0	0	10	26	0	0
Frozen concentrate, yellow, prepared w/ water	8 fl oz	99	0	0	10	26	0	0
Lemonade-flavor drink, powder, prepared w/ water	8 fl oz	66	0	0	33	17	0	0
Powder, low calorie, w/ aspartame, prepared w/ water	8 fl oz	7	0	0	10	2	0	0
Powder, prepared w/ water	8 fl oz	98	0	0	8	26	0	0
LEMON GRASS (citronella, fresh)	1 tbsp	5	0	0	0	1	0	0

ITEM DESCRIPTION	Serving Size	Calories	Total Fat (g)	Saturated Fat (g)	Sodium (mg)	Carbohydrates (g)	Fiber (g)	Protein (g)
LEMON JUICE								
Canned or bottled	2 tbsp	6	0	0	6	2	0	0
Fresh	2 tbsp	8	0	0	0	3	0	0
Frozen, unsweetened	2 tbsp	7	0	0	0	2	0	0
LEMONS								
Fresh, sections	1 cup	61	1	0	4	20	6	2
Fresh, whole	1 fruit	22	0	0	3	12	5	1
Peel, fresh	1 tbsp	3	0	0	0	1	1	0
LENTILS								
Boiled	1 cup	230	1	0	4	40	16	18
Sprouted, fresh	1 cup	82	0	0	8	17	0	7
LETTUCE								
Bibb, shredded	1 cup	7	0	0	3	1	1	1
Boston, shredded	1 cup	7	0	0	3	1	1	1
Cos, shredded	1 cup	8	0	0	4	2	1	1
Green leaf, shredded	1 cup	5	0	0	10	1	0	0
Iceberg, shredded	1 cup	10	0	0	7	2	1	1
Red leaf, shredded	1 cup	4	0	0	7	1	0	0
Romaine, shredded	1 cup	8	0	0	4	2	1	1
LIGHT CREAM (whipped)	1 cup	350	37	23	41	4	0	3
LIMA BEANS								
Boiled	1/2 cup	105	0	0	14	20	5	6
Boiled, baby	1/2 cup	115	0	0	3	21	7	7
Boiled, large	1/2 cup	108	0	0	2	20	7	7
Canned, no salt	1/2 cup	88	0	0	5	17	5	5
Canned, w/ salt	1/2 cup	88	0	0	312	17	5	5
Fresh	1/2 cup	88	1	0	6	16	4	5
Fresh, baby	1/2 cup	338	1	0	13	63	21	21
Fresh, large	1/2 cup	301	1	0	16	56	17	19
Frozen, boiled, baby	1/2 cup	94	0	0	26	18	5	6
LIMEADE (frozen concentrate, prepared w/ water)	8 fl oz	128	0	0	7	34	0	0
LIME JUICE								
Canned or bottled,								

ITEM DESCRIPTION	Serving Size	Calories	Total Fat (g)	Saturated Fat (g)	Sodium (mg)	Carbohydrates (g)	Fiber (g)	Protein (g)
unsweetened	1 fl oz	6	0	0	5	2	0	0
Fresh	1 fl oz	8	0	0	1	3	0	0
LIMES fresh (2" dia)	1 fruit	20	0	0	1	7	2	0
LING (cooked in dry heat)	3 oz	94	1	0	147	0	0	21
LINGCOD (cooked in dry heat)	3 oz	93	1	0	65	0	0	19
LITCHIS								
Dried	1 fruit	7	0	0	0	2	0	0
Fresh	1 fruit	6	0	0	0	2	0	0
LIVERWURST SPREAD	1/4 cup	168	14	5	385	3	1	7
LOBSTER								
Northern, cooked in moist heat	3 oz	83	1	0	323	1	0	17
Spiny, cooked in moist heat	3 oz	122	2	0	193	3	0	22
LOGANBERRIES (frozen)	1 cup	81	0	0	1	19	8	2
LOQUATS (fresh)	1 lg	9	0	0	0	2	0	0
LOTUS ROOT								
Boiled	1/2 cup	40	0	0	27	10	2	1
Fresh (9 1/2" long)	1 root	85	0	0	46	20	6	3
MACADAMIA NUTS								
Dry roasted	1 cup	948	100	16	5	18	11	10
Dry roasted, w/ salt	1 cup	945	100	16	350	17	11	10
Fresh	1 cup	962	102	16	7	19	12	11
MACE (ground)	1 tbsp	25	2	1	4	3	1	0
MACKEREL								
Atlantic, cooked in dry heat	3 oz	223	15	4	71	0	0	20
Jack, canned, drained	1 cup	296	12	4	720	0	0	44
King, cooked in dry heat	3 oz	114	2	0	173	0	0	22
Pacific & Jack, cooked in dry heat	3 oz	171	9	2	94	0	0	22
Salted, cooked	1 cup	415	34	10	6052	0	0	25
Spanish, cooked in dry heat	3 oz	134	5	2	56	0	0	20
MALABAR SPINACH (cooked)	1 bunch	4	0	0	9	0	0	0
MALT (beverage)	1 cup	88	0	0	31	19	0	0
MALTED DRINK MIX								
Chocolate, powder, prepared w/ whole milk	8 fl oz	225	9	5	159	30	1	9

ITEM DESCRIPTION	Serving Size	Calories	Total Fat (g)	Saturated Fat (g)	Sodium (mg)	Carbohydrates (g)	Fiber (g)	Protein (g)
powder, prepared w/ whole milk	8 fl oz	233	10	5	209	27	0	10
MALT SYRUP	1 tbsp	76	0	0	8	17	0	1
MANGO								
Nectar, canned	1 cup	128	0	0	13	33	1	0
fresh	1 fruit	135	1	0	4	35	4	1
MANGOSTEEN								
canned in syrup, drained)	1 cup	143	1	0	14	35	4	1
MAPLE SYRUP	1 tbsp	52	0	0	2	13	0	0
MARGARINE								
40% fat	1 tbsp	26	3	0	110	0	0	0
40% fat, no salt	1 tbsp	22	3	0	0	0	0	0
48% fat , tub	1 tbsp	59	7	1	90	0	0	0
60% fat, stick	1 tbsp	77	9	2	112	0	0	0
60% fat, stick, no salt	1 tbsp	75	8	2	0	0	0	0
60% fat, stick, tub, bottle	1 tbsp	75	8	1	112	0	0	0
60% fat, tub or bottle, unsalted	1 tbsp	75	8	2	4	0	0	0
70% fat, soybean & part hydrogenated soybean oil, stick	1 tbsp	87	10	2	98	0	0	0
80% fat, composite, stick, unsalted	1 tbsp	102	11	2	0	0	0	0
80% fat, composite, stick, w/ salt	1 tbsp	100	11	2	132	0	0	0
80% fat, composite, tub, unsalted	1 tbsp	101	11	2	4	0	0	0
80% fat, composite, tub, w/ salt	1 tbsp	101	11	2	93	0	0	0
80% fat, corn & soybean oils, stick	1 tbsp	100	11	2	92	0	0	0
Fat free, tub	1 tbsp	7	0	0	85	1	0	0
Hard, soybean oils	1 tbsp	101	11	2	133	0	0	0
Hard, sunflower, soybean & cottonseed oils	1 tbsp	101	11	2	133	0	0	0
Liquid, soybean & cottonseed oils	1 tbsp	102	11	2	111	0	0	0
Margarine-butter blend, soybean oil & butter	1 tbsp	101	11	2	89	0	0	0
No salt	1 tbsp	101	11	2	0	0	0	0
Salted	1 tbsp	101	11	2	133	0	0	0

ITEM DESCRIPTION	Serving Size	Calories	Total Fat (g)	Saturated Fat (g)	Sodium (mg)	Carbohydrates (g)	Fiber (g)	Protein (g)
MARGARINE SUBSTITUTE								
Benecol Light Spread	1 tbsp	50	5	1	94	1	0	0
Smart Balance Light Buttery Spread	1 tbsp	47	5	1	81	0	0	0
Smart Balance Omega Plus Spread	1 tbsp	85	9	3	102	0	0	0
Smart Balance Regular Buttery Spread	1 tbsp	85	9	3	90	0	0	0
Spread, 37% fat, unspecified oils	1 tbsp	51	6	1	88	0	0	1
Spread, 40% fat, reduced calorie, made w/ yogurt, salted	1 tbsp	46	5	1	88	0	0	0
Spread, 40% fat, reduced calorie, stick, salted	1 tbsp	50	6	1	139	0	0	0
Spread, 60% fat, vegetable oil, tub	1 tbsp	75	8	2	110	0	0	0
Spread, 67-70% fat, vegetable oil, tub	1 tbsp	85	10	2	75	0	0	0
Spread, 70% fat, liquid, salted	1 tbsp	87	10	1	139	0	0	0
Spread, fat free, liquid, salted	1 tbsp	6	0	0	125	0	0	0
Spread, made w/ yogurt, stick, salted	1 tbsp	88	10	2	83	0	0	0
Spread, stick or tub, sweetened	1 tbsp	75	7	1	76	2	0	0
MARINARA SAUCE	1/2 cup	111	3	1	535	18	3	2
Low sodium	1/2 cup	111	3	1	38	18	3	2
MARJORAM (dried)	1 tbsp	5	0	0	1	1	1	0
MARSHMALLOWS	1 reg	23	0	0	6	6	0	0
Marshmallow topping	1 oz	91	0	0	23	22	0	0
MAYONNAISE								
Cholesterol free	1 tbsp	103	12	2	73	0	0	0
Diet or reduced calorie, cholesterol free	1 tbsp	49	5	1	107	1	0	0
Diet, cholesterol free	1 tbsp	57	5	1	105	4	0	0
Hellmann's Canola	1 tbsp	90	10	1	90	0	0	0
Hellmann's Olive Oil	1 tbsp	100	11	1	85	0	0	.2
Kraft Mayo, fat free	1 tbsp	11	0	0	120	2	0	0
Kraft Mayo, light	1 tbsp	50	5	1	120	1	0	0
Light	1 tbsp	49	5	1	101	1	0	0
Low calorie	1 tbsp	38	3	0	100	3	0	0

ITEM DESCRIPTION	Serving Size	Calories	Total Fat (g)	Saturated Fat (g)	Sodium (mg)	Carbohydrates (g)	Fiber (g)	Protein (g)
low sodium, low calorie or diet	1 tbsp	32	3	0	15	2	0	0
reg, w/ salt	1 tbsp	59	5	1	107	4	0	0
soybean & safflower oil, w/ salt	1 tbsp	99	11	1	78	0	0	0
soybean oil, w/o salt	1 tbsp	99	11	2	4	0	0	0
soybean oil, w/ salt	1 tbsp	99	11	2	78	0	0	0
MAYONNAISE SUBSTITUTE								
fat free	1 tbsp	13	0	0	126	2	0	0
imitation, milk cream	1 tbsp	15	1	0	76	2	0	0
imitation, soybean	1 tbsp	35	3	0	75	2	0	0
imitation, soybean, no cholesterol	1 tbsp	68	7	1	50	2	0	0
Kraft Miracle Whip Free, nonfat	1 tbsp	13	0	0	126	2	0	0
Kraft Miracle Whip, light	1 tbsp	37	3	0	131	2	0	0
Made w/ tofu	1 tbsp	48	5	0	116	0	0	1
MENHADEN								
fish oil	1 tbsp	123	14	4	0	0	0	0
fish oil, fully hydrogenated	1 tbsp	113	13	12	0	0	0	0
MILK								
Canned, condensed, sweetened	1 cup	982	27	17	389	166	0	24
Canned, evaporated	1 cup	338	19	12	267	25	0	17
Canned, evaporated, nonfat	1 cup	200	1	0	294	29	0	19
Dry, nonfat, instant	1 cup	243	0	0	373	35	0	24
Dry, nonfat, reg	1 cup	434	1	1	642	62	0	43
Dry, whole	1 cup	635	34	21	475	49	0	34
imitation, non-soy	1 cup	112	5	1	134	13	0	4
Low fat, 1% milkfat	1 cup	102	2	2	107	12	0	8
Low sodium	1 cup	149	8	5	7	11	0	8
Nonfat, calcium fortified, fat free or skim	1 cup	86	0	0	127	12	0	8
Reduced fat, 2% milkfat	1 cup	122	5	3	100	11	0	8
Whole, 3.25% milkfat	1 cup	146	8	5	98	11	0	8
MILKFISH (cooked in dry heat)	3 oz	162	7	0	78	0	0	22
MILK SHAKES								
Thick, chocolate	8 fl oz	270	6	4	252	48	1	7
Thick, vanilla	8 fl oz	254	7	4	216	40	0	9

ITEM DESCRIPTION	Serving Size	Calories	Total Fat (g)	Saturated Fat (g)	Sodium (mg)	Carbohydrates (g)	Fiber (g)	Protein (g)
MILLET								
Millet, cooked	1 cup	207	2	0	3	41	2	6
Millet, puffed	1 cup	74	1	0	1	17	1	3
Millet, fresh	1 cup	756	8	1	10	146	17	22
MISO	1 cup	547	17	3	10252	73	15	32
MIXED FRUIT								
Peaches, cherries, raspberries, grapes, & boysenberries, frozen, sweetened	10 oz pkg	278	1	0	9	69	5	4
Peaches, pears, & pineapple, canned in heavy syrup	1 cup	184	0	0	10	48	3	1
Prunes, apricots, & pears, dried	11 oz pkg	712	1	0	53	188	23	7
MIXED NUTS								
Dry roasted, w/ peanuts, w/o salt	1 cup	814	70	9	16	35	12	24
Dry roasted, w/ peanuts, w/ salt	1 cup	814	70	9	917	35	12	24
Oil roasted, w/o peanuts, w/o salt	1 cup	886	81	13	16	32	8	22
Oil roasted, w/ peanuts, w/o salt	1 cup	876	80	12	16	30	14	24
Oil roasted, w/o peanuts, w/ salt	1 cup	886	81	13	441	32	8	22
Oil roasted, w/ peanuts, w/ salt	1 cup	876	80	12	595	30	13	24
MIXED VEGETABLES								
Canned	1 cup	88	1	0	549	17	9	3
Canned, drained	1 cup	80	0	0	243	15	5	4
Canned, no salt	1 cup	67	0	0	47	13	6	3
Frozen, boiled	10 oz pkg	179	0	0	96	36	12	8
MOCHA MIX (w/ whitener & low calorie sweetener)	1 tsp, dry	16	1	1	32	5	0	1
MOLASSES	1 tbsp	58	0	0	7	15	0	0
MOLE SAUCE (dry mix, prepared)	1 cup	1513	110	0	3085	111	27	20
MONKFISH (cooked in dry heat)	3 oz	82	2	0	20	0	0	16
MORTADELLA (beef, pork)	1 slice	47	4	1	187	0	0	2
MOTH BEANS								
Boiled	1 cup	207	1	0	18	37	0	14
Fresh	1 cup	672	3	1	59	121	0	45

EM DESCRIPTION	Serving Size	Calories	Total Fat (g)	Saturated Fat (g)	Sodium (mg)	Carbohydrates (g)	Fiber (g)	Protein (g)
OUSSE (homemade, chocolate)	1/2 cup	454	32	18	77	32	1	8
UFFINS								
etty Crocker Wild Blueberry Muffin, om mix	1 serv	128	2	0	186	26	0	2
ueberry, commercial (2.75" dia)	1	259	13	2	208	33	1	3
ueberry, commercial, low fat	1	181	3	1	224	36	3	3
ueberry, homemade, ade w/ 2% milk	1	162	6	1	251	23	0	4
ueberry, toaster type	1	103	3	0	158	18	1	2
orn, commercial, small	1	201	6	1	344	34	2	4
orn, homemade, made w/ 2% milk, mall	1	180	7	1	333	25	0	4
orn, toaster type	1	114	4	1	142	19	1	2
usteaz Almond Poppyseed Muffin, om mix	1 serv	167	4	1	236	30	1	2
at bran, small	1	178	5	1	259	32	3	5
ain, homemade, made w/ 2% milk	1	169	7	1	266	24	2	4
heat bran, toaster type w/ raisins	1	106	3	0	178	19	3	2
ULBERRIES (fresh)	10 fruit	6	0	0	2	1	0	0
ULLET (striped, cooked in dry heat)	3 oz	128	4	1	60	0	0	21
ULTIGRAIN CHIPS								
unChips Multigrain Snack, ench onion	1 oz	141	6	1	132	19	2	2
unChips Multigrain Snack, arvest cheddar	1 oz	139	6	1	153	18	2	2
unChips Multigrain Snack, original	1 oz	139	6	1	93	19	2	2
UNG BEANS								
oiled	1 cup	212	1	0	4	39	15	14
resh	1 cup	718	2	1	31	130	34	49
prouted, boiled	1 cup	26	0	0	12	5	1	3
prouted, canned	1 cup	15	0	0	175	3	1	2
prouted, fresh	1 cup	31	0	0	6	6	2	3
prouted, stir-fried	1 cup	62	0	0	11	13	2	5
USHROOMS								
oiled	1 cup, pcs	44	1	0	3	8	3	3

ITEM DESCRIPTION	Serving Size	Calories	Total Fat (g)	Saturated Fat (g)	Sodium (mg)	Carbohydrates (g)	Fiber (g)	Protein (g)
Brown, Italian, or cremini, fresh, slices	1 cup	19	0	0	4	3	0	2
Canned	1 cup	39	0	0	663	8	4	3
Cloud ears, dried	1 cup	80	0	0	10	20	20	3
Enoki, fresh	1 lg	2	0	0	0	0	0	0
Maitake, fresh, diced	1 cup	26	0	0	1	5	2	1
Oyster, fresh	1 large	64	1	0	27	10	3	5
Portabella, grilled, slices	1 cup	42	1	0	12	6	3	5
Portabella, fresh, diced	1 cup	22	0	0	5	4	1	2
Shiitake	1 cup, pcs	81	0	0	6	21	3	2
Shiitake, dried	1 mushroom	11	0	0	0	3	0	0
Shiitake, stir-fried, slices	1 cup	47	0	0	5	7	4	3
Straw, canned	1 cup	58	1	0	699	8	5	7
White, fresh	1 cup, pcs	15	0	0	4	2	1	2
White, stir-fried, slices	1 cup	28	0	0	13	4	2	4
MUSSELS								
Blue, cooked in moist heat	3 oz	146	4	1	314	6	0	20
Blue, fresh	1 med	14	0	0	46	1	0	2
MUSTARD (yellow, prepared)	1 tsp	3	0	0	57	0	0	0
MUSTARD GREENS								
Boiled, chopped	1 cup	21	0	0	22	3	3	3
Fresh, chopped	1 cup	15	0	0	14	3	2	2
Frozen, boiled, chopped	1 cup	28	0	0	38	5	4	3
MUSTARD OIL	1 tbsp	124	14	2	0	0	0	0
MUSTARD SEED (yellow)	1 tbsp	53	3	0	1	4	2	3
MUSTARD SPINACH								
Boiled, chopped	1 cup	29	0	0	25	5	4	3
Fresh, chopped	1 cup	33	0	0	32	6	4	3
NATTO	1 cup	371	19	3	12	25	9	31
NAVY BEANS								
Boiled	1 cup	255	1	0	0	47	19	15
Canned	1 cup	296	1	0	1174	54	13	20
Fresh	1 cup	701	3	0	10	126	51	46
Fresh, sprouted	1 cup	70	1	0	14	14	0	6
NECTARINES (fresh, whole)	1 sml	57	0	0	0	14	2	1

ITEM DESCRIPTION	Serving Size	Calories	Total Fat (g)	Saturated Fat (g)	Sodium (mg)	Carbohydrates (g)	Fiber (g)	Protein (g)
NOODLES								
Cellophane, dehydrated	1 cup	491	0	0	14	121	1	0
Chinese restaurant noodles, flat, crunchy	1 cup	234	14	2	170	23	0	5
Chow mein	1 cup	237	14	2	198	26	2	4
Egg	1 cup	221	3	1	8	40	2	7
Egg, w/ salt	1 cup	221	3	0	264	40	2	7
Long rice & mung bean, dehydrated	1 cup	491	0	0	14	121	1	0
Rice	1 cup	192	0	0	33	44	2	2
Soba	1 cup	113	0	0	68	24	0	6
Somen	1 cup	231	0	0	283	48	0	7
Spinach egg	1 cup	211	3	1	19	39	4	8
NUTMEG								
Ground	1 tbsp	37	3	2	1	3	1	0
Butter oil	1 tbsp	120	14	12	0	0	0	0
NUTRITIONAL SUPPLEMENT (Ensure Plus, liquid nutrition)	1 cup	355	11	2	239	50	0	13
NUTS IN SYRUP TOPPING	2 tbsp	184	9	1	17	24	1	2
OAT BRAN								
Cooked	1 cup	88	2	0	2	25	6	7
Fresh	1 cup	231	7	1	4	62	14	16
OAT OIL	1 tbsp	120	14	3	0	0	0	0
OCEAN PERCH (Atlantic, cooked in dry heat)	3 oz	103	2	0	82	0	0	20
OCTOPUS (cooked in moist heat)	3 oz	139	2	0	391	4	0	25
OILS (corn, peanut, & olive)	1 tbsp	124	14	2	0	0	0	0
OKRA								
Boiled, slices	1/2 cup	18	0	0	5	4	2	1
Fresh	1 cup	31	0	0	8	7	3	2
Frozen, boiled, slices	1/2 cup	26	0	0	3	5	3	2
OLIVE LOAF								
Pork	1 slice	66	5	2	416	3	0	3
Oscar Mayer, chicken, pork, & turkey	1 serv	74	6	2	369	2	0	3
OLIVE OIL (salad or cooking)	1 tbsp	119	14	2	0	0	0	0

ITEM DESCRIPTION	Serving Size	Calories	Total Fat (g)	Saturated Fat (g)	Sodium (mg)	Carbohydrates (g)	Fiber (g)	Protein (g)
OLIVES								
Pickled, canned or bottled	1 olive	4	0	0	42	0	0	0
Ripe, canned, jumbo to colossal	1 jumbo	7	1	0	75	0	0	0
Ripe, canned, small to extra large	1 lg	5	0	0	38	0	0	0
ONION POWDER	1 tbsp	24	0	0	4	6	0	1
ONION RINGS (Breaded, heated in oven) (3-4" dia)	10 rings	289	19	6	266	27	1	4
ONIONS								
Boiled	1 cup	92	0	0	6	21	3	3
Canned, chopped	1 cup	43	0	0	831	9	3	2
Dehydrated flakes	1/4 cup	49	0	0	3	12	1	1
Fresh, chopped	1 cup	64	0	0	6	15	3	2
Frozen, chopped, boiled	1/2 cup	29	0	0	13	7	2	1
Frozen, whole, boiled	1 cup	59	0	0	17	14	3	1
Sweet, fresh	1 onion	106	0	0	26	25	3	3
Yellow, sauteed, chopped	1 cup	115	9	0	10	7	2	1
Young green	1 stalk	3	0	0	0	1	0	0
ORANGE & APRICOT JUICE DRINK (canned)	8 fl oz	128	0	0	5	32	0	1
ORANGE DRINK								
Breakfast drink	8 fl oz	108	0	0	5	27	1	0
Breakfast drink, frozen concentrate w/ juice & pulp, prepared w/ water	8 fl oz	112	0	0	25	28	0	0
Breakfast drink, powder, prepared w/ water	6 fl oz	100	0	0	10	26	0	0
Canned	8 fl oz	122	0	0	7	31	0	0
Orange juice drink	8 fl oz	134	0	0	5	33	0	0
ORANGE-GRAPEFRUIT JUICE (canned, unsweetened)	1 cup	106	0	0	7	25	0	1
ORANGE JUICE								
California, chilled, including juice from concentrate	1 cup	110	1	0	2	25	0	2
Canned, unsweetened	1 cup	117	0	0	10	27	1	2
Fresh	1 cup	112	1	0	2	26	1	2

ITEM DESCRIPTION	Serving Size	Calories	Total Fat (g)	Saturated Fat (g)	Sodium (mg)	Carbohydrates (g)	Fiber (g)	Protein (g)
Frozen concentrate, unsweetened, prepared w/ water	1 cup	112	0	0	2	27	1	2
ORANGE MARMALADE	1 tbsp	49	0	0	11	13	0	0
ORANGE ROUGHY (cooked in dry heat)	3 oz	89	1	0	59	0	0	19
ORANGES								
Fresh, all varieties (2-5/8" dia)	1 fruit	62	0	0	0	15	3	1
Fresh, California, Valencia (2-5/8" dia)	1 fruit	59	0	0	0	14	3	1
Fresh, Florida (2-5/8" dia)	1 fruit	65	0	0	0	16	3	1
Fresh, navel (2-7/8" dia)	1 fruit	69	0	0	1	18	3	1
Peel only, fresh	1 tbsp	6	0	0	0	2	1	0
ORANGE-STRAWBERRY-BANANA JUICE	1 cup	117	0	0	9	29	1	1
OREGANO (dried, ground)	1 tsp	6	0	0	0	1	0	0
OYSTERS								
Eastern, breaded & fried	3 oz	167	11	3	354	10	0	7
Eastern, canned, drained	1 cup	112	4	1	181	6	0	11
Eastern, farmed, cooked in dry heat	3 oz	67	2	1	139	6	0	6
Eastern, farmed, fresh	3 oz	50	1	0	151	5	0	4
Eastern, wild, cooked in dry heat	3 oz	61	2	0	207	4	0	7
Eastern, wild, cooked in moist heat	3 oz	116	4	1	359	7	0	12
Eastern, wild, fresh	3 oz	116	2	1	179	3	0	6
Pacific, cooked in moist heat	3 oz	139	4	1	180	8	0	16
Pacific, fresh	3 oz	69	2	0	90	4	0	8
OYSTER SAUCE	1 tbsp	9	0	0	492	2	0	0
OYSTER STEW (Campbell's Red & White, condensed)	1/2 cup	79	6	4	910	5	0	2
PALM KERNEL OIL	1 tbsp	117	14	11	0	0	0	0
PALM OIL	1 tbsp	120	14	7	0	0	0	0
PAM COOKING SPRAY	1 spray	2	0	0	0	0	0	0
PANCAKES								
Blueberry, homemade (4" dia)	1	84	4	1	157	11	0	2
Buttermilk, homemade (4" dia)	1	86	4	1	198	11	0	3
Kellogg's Eggo Buttermilk Pancakes	1	90	3	1	205	15	0	2
Plain, dry mix, complete, prepared (4" dia)	1	74	1	0	239	14	1	2

ITEM DESCRIPTION	Serving Size	Calories	Total Fat (g)	Saturated Fat (g)	Sodium (mg)	Carbohydrates (g)	Fiber (g)	Protein (g)
Plain, dry mix, plus egg (4" dia)	1	83	3	1	192	11	1	3
Plain, frozen	1	92	2	0	207	16	1	2
Plain, frozen, microwavable	1	91	2	0	215	17	1	2
Plain, homemade (4" dia)	1	86	4	0	167	11	0	2
Whole wheat, dry mix, plus egg (4" dia)	1	92	3	1	252	13	1	4
PANCAKE SYRUP								
Cane, 15% maple	1 tbsp	56	0	0	21	14	0	0
Corn, refiner & sugar	1 tbsp	64	0	0	14	17	0	0
Reduced calorie	1 tbsp	25	0	0	27	7	0	0
Regular	1 tbsp	47	0	0	16	12	0	0
With 2% maple	1 tbsp	53	0	0	12	14	0	0
With butter	1 tbsp	59	0	0	20	15	0	0
PAPAYA								
Nectar, canned	1 cup	142	0	0	12	36	2	0
Fresh, cubed	1 cup	55	0	0	4	14	3	1
PAPRIKA	1 tbsp	20	1	0	2	4	3	1
PARSLEY								
Dried	1 tbsp	4	0	0	7	1	1	0
Freeze-dried	1 tbsp	1	0	0	2	0	0	0
Fresh	1 tbsp	1	0	0	2	0	0	0
PARSNIPS								
Boiled, slices	1 cup	111	0	0	16	27	6	2
Fresh, slices	1 cup	100	0	0	13	24	7	2
PASSION FRUIT								
Purple, fresh	1 fruit	17	0	0	5	4	2	0
Juice, purple, fresh	1 cup	126	0	0	15	34	1	1
Juice, yellow, fresh	1 cup	148	0	0	15	36	1	2
PASTA								
Corn	1 cup	176	1	0	0	39	7	4
Fresh, refrigerated, plain	2 oz	75	1	0	3	14	0	3
Fresh, refrigerated, spinach	2 oz	74	1	0	3	14	0	3
Homemade, made w/ egg	2 oz	74	1	0	47	13	0	3
Homemade, made w/o egg	2 oz	71	1	0	42	14	0	2

ITEM DESCRIPTION	Serving Size	Calories	Total Fat (g)	Saturated Fat (g)	Sodium (mg)	Carbohydrates (g)	Fiber (g)	Protein (g)
Macaroni, elbows	1 cup	221	1	0	1	43	3	8
Macaroni, protein fortified, small shells	1 cup	189	0	0	6	36	0	9
Macaroni, vegetable, spirals	1 cup	172	0	0	8	36	6	6
Macaroni, whole wheat, elbows	1 cup	174	1	0	4	37	4	7
Spaghetti, cooked	1 cup	221	1	0	1	43	3	8
Spaghetti, protein fortified, cooked	1 cup	230	0	0	7	44	2	11
Spaghetti, spinach, cooked	1 cup	182	1	0	20	37	0	6
Spaghetti, whole wheat, cooked	1 cup	174	1	0	4	37	6	7
Tortellini, w/ cheese filling	3/4 cup	249	6	3	279	38	2	11
Vermicelli, made from soy	1 cup	463	0	0	6	115	6	0
PASTA ENTRÉE								
Chef Boyardee Beefaroni, canned	1 cup	236	7	3	959	35	1	8
Chef Boyardee Beef Ravioli, tomato & meat sauce	1 cup	224	7	3	910	33	1	8
Chef Boyardee Mini Beef Ravioli, tomato & meat sauce	1 cup	232	8	3	935	31	3	8
Chef Boyardee Spaghetti & Meatballs, tomato sauce, canned	1 serv	257	10	4	925	31	4	11
Healthy Choice Beef Macaroni, frozen	1 serv	211	2	1	444	33	5	14
Hodgson Mill Whole Wheat Macaroni & Cheese, mix	1 serv	263	3	1	428	48	5	10
Kraft Macaroni & Cheese, mix	1 serv	259	3	1	561	48	2	11
Lean Cuisine Angel Hair Pomodoro	1	250	5	2	620	42	4	8
Lipton Alfredo Egg Noodles, creamy sauce, mix	1 cup	389	11	4	1646	58	0	14
Macaroni & cheese, canned	1 serv	200	6	2	1027	28	1	8
Pasta w/ sliced franks in tomato sauce, canned	1 serv	262	12	4	1215	30	2	9
Spaghettios A to Z's	1 serv	176	1	0	879	36	3	6
Spaghettios A to Z's, w/ meatballs	1 serv	257	9	4	990	33	3	11
Spaghettios Original	1 serv	179	0	0	630	37	3	6
Spaghettios Raviolios, beef ravioli, meat sauce	1 serv	267	8	4	1091	38	4	11
Spaghettios, w/ meatballs	1 serv	239	8	4	660	32	4	11

ITEM DESCRIPTION	Serving Size	Calories	Total Fat (g)	Saturated Fat (g)	Sodium (mg)	Carbohydrates (g)	Fiber (g)	Protein (g)
Spaghettios, w/ sliced franks	1 serv	234	10	5	930	27	5	9
Spaghetti, w/ meatballs, canned	1 cup	273	13	5	1035	28	0	11
Spaghetti w/ meat sauce, frozen	1 serv	255	3	1	473	43	5	14
Stouffer's Fettuccini Alfredo	1 serv	610	34	9	1030	57	5	18
Stouffer's Lasagna Bake w/ Meat Sauce	1 serv	350	10	4	960	49	5	17
Velveeta Shells and Cheese	4 oz	360	12	4	940	49	2	13
PASTRAMI								
Beef, 98% fat free	1 slice	9	0	0	96	0	0	2
Carl Buddig Smoked Beef, chopped, pressed	2 oz	80	4	2	602	1	0	11
PÂTÉ								
Chicken liver, canned	1 tbsp	26	2	1	50	1	0	2
Foie gras, goose liver, canned, smoked	1 tbsp	60	6	2	91	1	0	1
Liver, canned	1 tbsp	41	4	1	91	0	0	2
Truffle flavor	2 oz	183	16	6	452	4	0	6
PEACH NECTAR (canned)	1 cup	134	0	0	17	35	2	1
PEACHES								
Canned in ex heavy syrup, slices	1 cup	252	0	0	21	68	3	1
Canned in ex light syrup, slices	1 cup	104	0	0	12	27	3	1
Canned in heavy syrup	1 cup	194	0	0	16	52	3	1
Canned in heavy syrup, drained	1 cup	171	0	0	13	44	5	1
Canned in juice	1 cup	110	0	0	10	29	3	2
Canned in light syrup, slices	1 cup	136	0	0	13	37	3	1
Canned in water, slices	1 cup	59	0	0	7	15	3	1
Dehydrated, stewed	1 cup	322	1	0	10	83	0	5
Dehydrated, uncooked	1 cup	377	1	0	12	96	0	6
Dried, stewed, w/o sugar	1 cup	199	1	0	5	51	7	3
Dried, stewed, w/ sugar	1 cup	278	1	0	5	72	7	3
Dried, uncooked, halves	1 cup	382	1	0	11	98	13	6
Fresh (2-1/2" dia)	1 fruit	51	0	0	0	12	2	1
Frozen, slices, sweetened, thawed	1 cup	235	0	0	15	60	5	2
Spiced, canned in heavy syrup	1 cup	182	0	0	10	49	3	1

ITEM DESCRIPTION	Serving Size	Calories	Total Fat (g)	Saturated Fat (g)	Sodium (mg)	Carbohydrates (g)	Fiber (g)	Protein (g)
PEANUT BUTTER								
Chunky, w/o salt	2 tbsp	188	16	3	5	7	3	8
Chunky, w/ salt	2 tbsp	188	16	3	156	7	3	8
Creamy	2 tbsp	201	18	3	117	6	2	8
Reduced sodium	2 tbsp	202	16	2	65	7	2	8
Smooth, w/o salt	2 tbsp	188	16	3	5	6	2	8
Smooth, w/ salt	2 tbsp	188	16	3	147	6	2	8
PEANUT FLOUR								
Defatted	1 cup	196	0	0	108	21	10	31
Low fat	1 cup	257	13	2	1	19	10	20
PEANUT OIL	1 tbsp	124	14	2	0	0	0	0
PEANUTS								
All types, boiled, w/ salt	1 oz	290	6	1	213	6	3	4
All types, dry roasted, w/o salt	1 oz	166	14	2	2	6	3	4
All types, dry roasted, w/ salt	1 oz	166	14	2	230	6	2	7
All types, fresh	1 cup	828	72	10	26	24	12	38
All types, oil roasted, w/o salt, chopped	1 cup	773	66	9	8	25	9	35
All types, oil roasted, w/ salt, chopped	1 cup	863	76	13	461	22	14	40
Spanish, fresh	1 cup	832	72	11	32	23	14	38
Spanish, oil roasted, w/o salt	1 cup	851	72	11	9	26	13	41
Spanish, oil roasted, w/ salt	1 cup	851	72	11	637	26	13	41
Valencia, fresh	1 cup	832	69	11	1	31	13	37
Valencia, oil roasted, w/o salt	1 cup	848	74	11	9	23	13	39
Valencia, oil roasted, w/ salt	1 cup	848	74	11	1112	23	13	39
Virginia, fresh	1 cup	822	71	9	15	24	12	37
Virginia, oil roasted, w/o salt	1 cup	827	70	9	9	28	13	37
Virginia, oil roasted, w/ salt	1 cup	827	70	9	619	28	13	37
PEANUT SPREAD (reduced sugar)	2 tbsp	202	17	3	139	4	2	8
PEAR NECTAR (canned)	1 cup	150	0	0	10	39	2	0
PEARS								
Asian, fresh (2 1/2" dia)	1 fruit	51	0	0	0	13	4	1
Canned in ex heavy syrup, halves	1 cup	258	0	0	13	67	4	1
Canned in ex light syrup, halves	1 cup	116	0	0	5	30	4	1

ITEM DESCRIPTION	Serving Size	Calories	Total Fat (g)	Saturated Fat (g)	Sodium (mg)	Carbohydrates (g)	Fiber (g)	Protein (g)
Canned in heavy syrup	1 cup	197	0	0	13	51	4	1
Canned in heavy syrup, drained	1 cup	149	0	0	10	38	5	0
Canned in juice, halves	1 cup	124	0	0	10	32	4	1
Canned in light syrup, halves	1 cup	143	0	0	13	38	4	0
Canned in water, halves	1 cup	71	0	0	5	19	4	0
Dried, stewed, w/o sugar, halves	1 cup	324	1	0	8	86	16	2
Dried, stewed, w/ sugar, halves	1 cup	392	1	0	8	104	16	2
Dried, uncooked, halves	1 cup	472	1	0	11	125	14	3
Fresh, whole	1 sml	86	0	0	1	23	5	1
PEAS								
Boiled	1/2 cup	34	0	0	3	6	2	3
Frozen, boiled	1/2 cup	34	0	0	4	7	2	3
Green, boiled	1/2 cup	67	0	0	2	13	4	4
Green, canned, seasoned	1/2 cup	57	0	0	290	11	2	4
Green, canned, w/o salt	1/2 cup	66	0	0	11	12	4	4
Green, canned, w/o salt, drained	1/2 cup	59	0	0	2	11	3	4
Green, canned, w/ salt	1/2 cup	60	1	0	255	10	4	4
Green, fresh	1/2 cup	59	0	0	4	10	4	4
Green, frozen, boiled	1/2 cup	62	0	0	58	11	4	4
PEAS & CARROTS								
Canned, w/o salt	1/2 cup	48	0	0	5	11	4	3
Canned, w/ salt	1/2 cup	48	0	0	332	11	3	3
Frozen, boiled	1/2 cup	38	0	0	54	8	2	2
PEAS & ONIONS								
Canned	1/2 cup	31	0	0	265	5	1	2
Frozen, boiled	1/2 cup	40	0	0	33	8	2	2
PECANS								
Chopped	1 cup	753	78	7	0	15	11	10
Dry roasted, w/o salt	1 oz	201	21	2	0	4	3	3
Dry roasted, w/ salt	1 oz	201	21	2	109	4	3	3
Oil roasted, w/o salt	1 cup	786	83	8	1	14	10	10
Oil roasted, w/ salt	1 cup	787	83	8	432	14	10	10
PECTIN (unsweetened, dry mix)	1-3/4 oz pkg	162	0	0	100	45	4	0
PEPEAO (dried)	1 cup	72	0	0	17	19	0	1

ITEM DESCRIPTION	Serving Size	Calories	Total Fat (g)	Saturated Fat (g)	Sodium (mg)	Carbohydrates (g)	Fiber (g)	Protein (g)
PEPPER								
Black	1 tbsp	16	0	0	3	4	2	1
Red or cayenne	1 tbsp	17	1	0	2	3	1	1
White	1 tbsp	21	0	0	0	5	2	1
PEPPER SAUCE								
Hot sauce	1 tsp	1	0	0	124	0	0	0
Hot chili, green, canned	1 tbsp	3	0	0	4	1	0	0
Hot chili, red, canned	1 tbsp	3	0	0	4	1	0	0
PEPPERED LOAF (pork & beef)	1 slice	42	2	1	432	1	0	5
PEPPERMINT (fresh)	2 tbsp	2	0	0	1	0	0	0
PEPPERONI (pork, beef)	1 oz	138	12	4	463	0	0	6
PEPPERS								
Ancho, dried	1 pepper	48	1	0	7	9	4	2
Banana, fresh (4" long)	1 pepper	9	0	0	4	2	1	1
Hot chili, green, canned, w/o seeds	1 pepper	15	0	0	856	4	1	1
Hot chili, green, fresh	1 pepper	18	0	0	3	4	1	1
Hot chili, red, canned, w/o seeds	1 pepper	15	0	0	856	4	1	1
Hot chili, red, fresh	1 pepper	18	0	0	4	4	1	1
Hot chili, sun-dried	1 pepper	3	0	0	1	1	0	0
Hungarian, fresh	1 pepper	8	0	0	0	2	0	0
Jalapeño, canned, chopped	1 cup	37	1	0	2273	6	4	1
Jalapeño, fresh, slices	1 cup	27	1	0	1	5	3	1
Pace Diced Green Chilies	2 tbsp	8	0	0	100	2	1	0
Pace Jalapeños Nacho Sliced Peppers	2 tbsp	4	0	0	300	1	1	0
Pasilla, dried	1 pepper	24	1	0	6	4	2	1
Serrano, fresh, chopped	1 cup	34	0	0	10	7	4	2
Sweet, green, boiled, chopped	1 cup	38	0	0	3	9	2	1
Sweet, green, canned, halves	1 cup	25	0	0	1917	5	2	1
Sweet, green, freeze-dried	1 tbsp	1	0	0	1	0	0	0
Sweet, green, fresh, chopped	1 cup	30	0	0	4	7	3	1
Sweet, red, boiled, strips	1 cup	38	0	0	3	9	2	1
Sweet, red, canned, halves	1 cup	25	0	0	1917	5	2	1
Sweet, red, freeze-dried	1 tbsp	1	0	0	1	0	0	0

ITEM DESCRIPTION	Serving Size	Calories	Total Fat (g)	Saturated Fat (g)	Sodium (mg)	Carbohydrates (g)	Fiber (g)	Protein (g)
Sweet, red, fresh, chopped	1 cup	46	0	0	6	9	3	1
Sweet, red, frozen, boiled, chopped	1 cup	22	0	0	5	4	0	1
Sweet, yellow, fresh	1 lg	50	0	0	4	12	2	2
PERCH (cooked in dry heat)	3 oz	99	1	0	67	0	0	21
PERSIMMONS								
Japanese, dried	1 fruit	93	0	0	1	25	5	0
Japanese, fresh	1 fruit	118	0	0	2	31	6	1
Native, fresh	1 fruit	32	0	0	0	8	0	0
PHEASANT (cooked, chopped)	1 cup	346	17	5	60	0	0	45
PHYLLO DOUGH	1 sheet	57	1	0	92	10	0	1
PICANTE SAUCE								
Pace Organic Picante Sauce	2 tbsp	8	0	0	220	2	1	0
Pace Picante Sauce	2 tbsp	8	0	0	250	2	1	0
PICKLE RELISH								
Hamburger	1 tbsp	19	0	0	164	5	1	0
Hot dog	1 tbsp	14	0	0	164	4	0	0
Sweet	1 tbsp	20	0	0	122	5	0	0
PICKLES								
Chowchow, sweet, w/ cauliflower, onion & mustard	1 cup	296	2	0	1291	65	4	4
Cucumber, dill, low sodium	1 med	12	0	0	12	3	1	0
Cucumber, dill or kosher dill (4" long)	1 pickle	16	0	0	1181	4	2	1
Cucumber, sour (4" long)	1 pickle	15	0	0	1631	3	2	0
Cucumber, sour, low sodium (4" long)	1 pickle	15	0	0	24	3	2	0
Cucumber, sweet, gherkin (3" long)	1 pickle	32	0	0	160	7	0	0
Cucumber, sweet, low sodium	1 med	43	0	0	6	12	0	0
PICO DE GALLO (Pace)	2 tbsp	10	0	0	150	3	0	0
PIE								
Apple, commercial (9" dia)	1/8 pie	296	14	5	332	43	2	2
Apple, homemade (9" dia)	1/8 pie	411	19	5	327	58	0	4
Banana cream, homemade (9" dia)	1/8 pie	387	20	5	346	47	1	6

ITEM DESCRIPTION	Serving Size	Calories	Total Fat (g)	Saturated Fat (g)	Sodium (mg)	Carbohydrates (g)	Fiber (g)	Protein (g)
Banana cream, prepared from no-bake mix (9" dia)	1/8 pie	231	12	6	267	29	1	3
Blueberry, commercial (9" dia)	1/8 pie	290	13	2	406	44	1	2
Blueberry, homemade (9" dia)	1/8 pie	360	17	4	272	49	0	4
Cherry, commercial (9" dia)	1/8 pie	325	14	3	308	50	1	3
Cherry, fried (5" x 3.75")	1 pie	404	21	3	479	55	3	4
Cherry, homemade (9" dia)	1/8 pie	486	22	5	344	69	0	5
Chocolate cream, commercial (8" dia)	1/6 pie	344	22	6	154	38	2	3
Chocolate mousse, prepared from no-bake mix (9" dia)	1/8 pie	247	15	8	437	28	0	3
Coconut cream, commercial (7" dia)	1/8 pie	143	8	3	122	18	1	1
Coconut cream, prepared from no-bake mix (9" dia)	1/8 pie	259	17	8	309	27	1	3
Coconut custard, commercial (8" dia)	1/6 pie	270	14	6	348	31	2	6
Dutch apple, commercial (9" dia)	1/8 pie	380	15	3	262	58	2	3
Egg custard, commercial (8" dia)	1/6 pie	220	12	2	252	22	2	6
Fruit, fried (5" x 3.75")	1 pie	404	21	3	479	55	3	4
Lemon, fried (5" x 3.75")	1 pie	404	21	3	479	55	3	4
Lemon meringue, commercial (8" dia)	1/6 pie	303	10	2	165	53	1	2
Lemon meringue, homemade (9" dia)	1/8 pie	362	16	4	307	50	0	5
Mince, homemade (9" dia)	1/8 pie	477	18	4	419	79	4	4
Peach (8" dia)	1/6 pie	261	12	2	316	38	1	2
Pecan, commercial	1 slice	541	22	4	319	79	3	6
Pecan, homemade (9" dia)	1/8 pie	503	27	5	320	64	0	6
Pumpkin, commercial	1 slice	323	13	3	310	46	2	5
Pumpkin, homemade (9" dia)	1/8 pie	316	14	5	349	41	0	7
Vanilla cream, homemade (9" dia)	1/8 pie	350	18	5	328	41	1	6
PIE CRUST								
Chocolate cookie, commercial	1/8 crust	110	5	1	114	15	1	1
Chocolate wafer, chilled, homemade (9" dia)	1/8 crust	142	9	2	188	15	0	1

ITEM DESCRIPTION	Serving Size	Calories	Total Fat (g)	Saturated Fat (g)	Sodium (mg)	Carbohydrates (g)	Fiber (g)	Protein (g)
Deep dish, frozen, baked	1/8 crust	132	8	2	99	13	1	2
Graham cracker, baked, homemade (9" dia)	1/8 crust	148	7	2	171	20	1	2
Graham cracker, chilled, homemade (9" dia)	1/8 crust	145	7	2	168	19	1	1
Graham cracker, commercial (9" dia)	1/8 crust	115	6	1	75	15	0	1
Nabisco Nilla Pie Crust	1 serv	144	8	1	63	18	1	1
Refrigerated, reg, baked	1/8 crust	125	7	3	117	14	0	1
Standard, baked, from mix (9" dia)	1/8 crust	100	6	2	146	10	0	1
Standard, baked, homemade (9" dia)	1/8 crust	121	8	2	125	11	0	1
Standard, frozen, enriched (9" dia)	1/8 crust	98	6	2	90	11	1	1
Standard, frozen, unenriched (9" dia)	1/8 crust	73	5	1	92	7	0	1
Vanilla wafer, chilled, homemade (9" dia)	1/8 crust	117	8	2	113	11	0	1
PIGEON PEAS								
Immature seeds, boiled	1 cup	170	2	0	8	30	9	9
Immature seeds, fresh	1 cup	209	3	1	8	37	8	11
Mature seeds, boiled	1 cup	203	1	0	8	39	11	11
Mature seeds, fresh	1 cup	703	3	1	35	129	31	44
PIKE								
Northern, cooked in dry heat	3 oz	96	1	0	42	0	0	21
Walleye, cooked in dry heat	3 oz	101	1	0	55	0	0	21
PILINUTS (dried)	1 cup	863	95	37	4	5	0	13
PIMENTO (canned)	1 tbsp	3	0	0	2	1	0	0
PIMIENTO LOAF								
Oscar Mayer Pickle Pimiento Loaf, chicken	1 serv	75	6	2	357	3	0	3
Pork & pickles	1 slice	86	6	2	496	3	1	4
PIÑA COLADA								
Canned	1 fl oz	77	2	2	23	9	0	0
Homemade	1 fl oz	55	1	1	2	7	0	0
PINEAPPLE								
Canned in ex heavy syrup, chunks	1 cup	216	0	0	3	56	2	1

ITEM DESCRIPTION	Serving Size	Calories	Total Fat (g)	Saturated Fat (g)	Sodium (mg)	Carbohydrates (g)	Fiber (g)	Protein (g)
anned in heavy syrup, chunks	1 cup	198	0	0	3	51	2	1
anned in juice, chunks	1 cup	149	0	0	2	39	2	1
anned in juice, drained, chunks	1 cup	109	0	0	2	28	2	1
anned in light syrup, chunks	1 cup	131	0	0	3	34	2	1
anned in water, chunks	1 cup	79	0	0	2	20	2	1
resh, ex sweet varieties, chunks	1 cup	84	0	0	2	22	2	1
resh, traditional varieties, chunks	1 cup	74	0	0	2	19	0	1
rozen, sweetened, chunks	1 cup	211	0	0	5	54	3	1
INEAPPLE & GRAPEFRUIT UICE DRINK (canned)	8 fl oz	118	0	0	35	29	0	1
INEAPPLE & ORANGE JUICE DRINK (canned)	8 fl oz	125	0	0	8	30	0	3
INEAPPLE JUICE								
rozen concentrate, unsweetened, repared w/ water	1 cup	130	0	0	3	32	1	1
nsweetened, canned	1 cup	133	0	0	5	32	1	1
INEAPPLE TOPPING	2 tbsp	106	0	0	18	28	0	0
INE NUTS (dried)	1 cup	909	92	7	3	18	5	18
INK BEANS								
oiled	1 cup	252	1	0	3	47	9	15
resh	1 cup	720	2	1	17	135	27	44
INTO BEANS								
oiled	1 cup	245	1	0	2	45	15	15
anned	1 cup	206	2	0	706	37	11	12
resh	1 cup	670	2	0	23	121	30	41
rozen, boiled	10 oz pkg	460	1	0	236	88	24	26
ISTACHIO NUTS								
ry roasted, w/o salt	1 cup	700	56	7	12	34	13	26
ry roasted, w/ salt	1 cup	696	56	7	496	33	13	26
resh	1 cup	682	54	7	1	34	13	25
ITA BREAD white (6-1/2" dia)	1 pita	165	1	0	322	33	1	5
ITANGA (Surinam cherry, fresh)	1 fruit	2	0	0	0	1	0	0
IZZA								
eleste Pizza for One, original	1	350	17	4	1090	39	2	9

ITEM DESCRIPTION	Serving Size	Calories	Total Fat (g)	Saturated Fat (g)	Sodium (mg)	Carbohydrates (g)	Fiber (g)	Protein (g)
DiGiorno, Personal Pepperoni	1	770	35	14	1430	83	6	30
DiGiorno, Personal Sausage	1	760	33	13	1300	85	5	30
DiGiorno, Personal Supreme	1	790	36	14	1460	85	6	31
Lean Cuisine, Four Cheese Pizza	1	350	6	2	600	55	3	20
Red Baron Singles, Meat-Trio	1	400	18	8	790	46	3	15
Red Baron Singles, Supreme	1	420	19	9	770	46	2	16
Stouffer's French Bread Pizza	1pc/2	360	15	6	530	43	4	14
Tony's Pizza for One, cheese	1	380	14	6	700	50	2	13
Tony's Pizza for One, pepperoni	1	410	18	9	840	48	2	15
PIZZA SAUCE (canned)	1/4 cup	34	1	0	117	5	1	1
PLANTAIN CHIPS	1 oz	158	10	3	111	16	1	0
PLANTAINS								
Cooked, mashed	1 cup	232	0	0	10	62	5	2
Fresh	1 med	218	1	0	7	57	4	2
PLUMS								
Canned in ex heavy syrup	1 cup	264	0	0	50	69	3	1
Canned in heavy syrup	1 cup	230	0	0	49	60	2	1
Canned in heavy syrup, drained	1 cup	163	0	0	35	42	3	1
Canned in juice	1 cup	146	0	0	3	38	2	1
Canned in light syrup	1 cup	159	0	0	50	41	2	1
Canned in water	1 cup	102	0	0	2	27	2	1
Fresh (2-1/8" dia)	1 fruit	30	0	0	0	8	1	0
PLUM SAUCE	1 tbsp	35	0	0	102	8	0	0
POI	1 cup	269	0	0	29	65	1	1
POKE								
Boiled	1 cup	33	1	0	30	5	2	4
Fresh	1 cup	37	1	0	37	6	3	4
POLLOCK (Atlantic, cooked in dry heat)	3 oz	100	1	0	94	0	0	21
POMEGRANATE JUICE (bottled)	1 cup	134	1	0	22	33	0	0
POMEGRANATES fresh (4" dia)	1 fruit	234	3	0	8	53	11	5
POMPANO (Florida, cooked in dry heat)	3 oz	179	10	4	65	0	0	20
POPCORN								
Air popped	2/3 cup	110	1	0	2	22	4	4

ITEM DESCRIPTION	Serving Size	Calories	Total Fat (g)	Saturated Fat (g)	Sodium (mg)	Carbohydrates (g)	Fiber (g)	Protein (g)
Caramel coated, fat free	2/3 cup	108	0	0	81	26	1	1
Caramel coated, w/o peanuts	2/3 cup	122	4	1	58	22	2	1
Caramel coated, w/ peanuts	2/3 cup	113	2	0	84	23	1	2
Cheese flavor	2/3 cup	149	9	2	252	15	3	3
Microwave, butter, w/ palm oil	2/3 cup	150	9	4	219	16	3	2
Microwave, butter, w/ partially hydrogenated oil	2/3 cup	149	8	2	219	16	3	2
Microwave, low fat, low sodium	2/3 cup	122	3	0	139	21	4	4
Oil popped	2/3 cup	142	12	2	300	13	2	2
Oil popped, low fat	2/3 cup	108	2	0	178	22	4	3
Oil popped, unsalted	2/3 cup	148	8	1	1	16	3	3
Unpopped kernels	1 oz	106	1	0	2	21	4	3
POPCORN CAKES	1 cake	38	0	0	29	8	0	1
POPOVERS (dry mix, enriched)	1 oz	105	1	0	257	20	0	3
POPPYSEEDS	1 tbsp	46	4	0	2	2	2	2
POPPYSEED OIL	1 tbsp	120	14	2	0	0	0	0
PORK								
Back ribs, roasted	3 oz	315	25	9	86	0	0	21
Canned	1/8 can	200	13	4	217	1	0	20
Composite of retail cuts, cooked	3 oz	315	15	5	53	0	0	23
Composite of retail cuts, lean, cooked	3 oz	315	8	3	50	0	0	25
Cured, bacon, broiled, pan fried or roasted	1 slice	43	3	1	185	0	0	3
Cured, bacon, broiled, pan fried or roasted, low sodium	1 slice	43	3	1	82	0	0	3
Cured, Canadian-style bacon, grilled	1 slice	43	2	1	363	0	0	6
Cured, feet, pickled	3 oz	315	9	3	476	0	0	10
Cured, shoulder, arm picnic, roasted	3 oz	315	18	7	911	0	0	17
Cured, shoulder, blade roll, roasted	3 oz	315	20	7	827	0	0	15
Ground, cooked	3 oz	315	18	7	62	0	0	22
Hormel Always Tender, center cut chops	1 serv	187	11	4	423	1	0	21
Hormel Always Tender, loin	1 serv	162	8	3	401	1	0	21
Hormel Always Tender, loin filets, lemon & garlic	1 serv	132	5	2	661	2	0	20

ITEM DESCRIPTION	Serving Size	Calories	Total Fat (g)	Saturated Fat (g)	Sodium (mg)	Carbohydrates (g)	Fiber (g)	Protein (g)
Hormel Always Tender, tenderloin, peppercorn	1 serv	123	4	1	665	2	0	19
Hormel Always Tender, tenderloin, teriyaki	1 serv	133	3	1	463	5	0	20
Leg, rump half, roasted	3 oz	214	12	4	53	0	0	25
Leg, shank half, roasted	3 oz	246	17	6	50	0	0	22
Leg, whole, roasted	3 oz	232	15	5	51	0	0	23
Loin, blade chops, braised	3 oz	275	22	8	47	0	0	19
Loin, blade chops, broiled	3 oz	272	21	8	60	0	0	19
Loin, blade chops, pan fried	3 oz	291	24	9	57	0	0	18
Loin, blade roast, roasted	3 oz	275	21	8	26	0	0	20
Loin, center loin chops, braised	3 oz	210	12	5	50	0	0	24
Loin, center loin chops, broiled	3 oz	178	9	3	47	0	0	22
Loin, center loin chops, pan fried	3 oz	235	14	5	68	0	0	25
Loin, center loin roast, roasted	3 oz	199	11	4	54	0	0	22
Loin, center rib chops, braised	3 oz	212	13	5	34	0	0	23
Loin, center rib chops, broiled	3 oz	189	11	4	47	0	0	21
Loin, center rib chops, pan fried	3 oz	225	14	5	42	0	0	22
Loin, center rib roast, roasted	3 oz	217	13	5	41	0	0	23
Loin, country-style ribs, braised	3 oz	232	15	5	49	0	0	23
Loin, country-style ribs, roasted	3 oz	279	22	8	44	0	0	20
Loin, sirloin chops, braised	3 oz	208	13	5	43	0	0	22
Loin, sirloin chops, broiled	3 oz	220	14	5	58	0	0	23
Loin, sirloin chops, lean, broiled	3 oz	164	6	2	48	0	0	26
Loin, sirloin roast, lean, roasted	3 oz	173	8	2	50	0	0	24
Loin, sirloin roast, roasted	3 oz	196	11	3	48	0	0	23
Loin, tenderloin, broiled	3 oz	171	7	2	54	0	0	25
Loin, tenderloin, roasted	3 oz	125	3	1	48	0	0	22
Loin, top loin chops, braised	3 oz	198	11	4	36	0	0	24
Loin, top loin chops, broiled	3 oz	167	8	3	37	0	0	23
Loin, top loin chops, pan fried	3 oz	218	13	5	47	0	0	25
Loin, top loin roast, roasted	3 oz	163	8	2	39	0	0	22
Oriental style, dehydrated	1 cup	135	14	5	151	0	0	3
Pickled pork hocks	100 grams	171	11	3	1050	0	0	19

ITEM DESCRIPTION	Serving Size	Calories	Total Fat (g)	Saturated Fat (g)	Sodium (mg)	Carbohydrates (g)	Fiber (g)	Protein (g)
Shoulder, arm picnic, braised	3 oz	280	20	7	75	0	0	24
Shoulder, arm picnic, roasted	3 oz	269	20	7	60	0	0	20
Shoulder, blade, Boston roast, roasted	3 oz	229	16	6	57	0	0	20
Shoulder, blade, Boston steak, broiled	3 oz	220	14	5	59	0	0	22
Shoulder, Boston butt, blade steak, braised	3 oz	315	15	6	49	0	0	21
Shoulder breast, broiled	1 pc	604	17	5	202	0	0	106
Shoulder, petite tender, broiled	1 pc	143	4	1	49	0	0	25
Spareribs, braised	3 oz	337	26	9	79	0	0	25
Spareribs, roasted	3 oz	315	26	8	77	0	0	18
Various meats & by-products, feet, simmered	3 oz	197	14	4	62	0	0	19
Various meats & by-products, liver, braised	3 oz	140	4	1	42	3	0	22
Various meats & by-products, tail, simmered	3 oz	337	30	11	21	0	0	14
PORK ENTRÉE								
Campbell's Pork & Beans	1 serv	138	1	1	439	25	7	6
Supper Bakes, Savory Pork Chops w/ Herb Stuffing	1 serv	153	1	0	780	31	2	5
PORK FAT (cooked)	1 oz	180	19	7	8	0	0	3
PORK SKINS								
BBQ flavor	1 oz	153	9	3	756	0	0	16
Plain	1 oz	154	9	3	521	0	0	17
POTATO CHIPS								
Baked, white, restructured	1 cup	159	6	1	312	24	2	2
BBQ	1 oz	139	9	2	213	15	1	2
Cheese	1 oz	141	8	2	225	16	2	2
Cheese, made from dried potatoes	1 oz	156	10	3	214	14	1	2
Fat free, salted	1 oz	107	0	0	182	24	2	3
Fat free, w/ Olestra	1 oz	78	0	0	157	18	2	2
Fat free, w/ Olestra, made from dried potatoes	1 oz	72	0	0	122	16	2	1
Light	1 oz	134	6	1	139	19	2	2
Light, made from dried potatoes	1 oz	142	7	2	117	18	1	1

ITEM DESCRIPTION	Serving Size	Calories	Total Fat (g)	Saturated Fat (g)	Sodium (mg)	Carbohydrates (g)	Fiber (g)	Protein (g)
Plain, made from dried potatoes	1 oz	158	11	3	110	15	1	1
Plain, salted	1 oz	155	11	3	149	14	1	2
Plain, unsalted	1 oz	152	10	3	2	15	1	2
Plain, w/ partially hydrogenated soybean oil, salted	1 oz	152	10	2	168	15	1	2
Plain, w/ partially hydrogenated soybean oil, unsalted	1 oz	152	10	2	2	15	1	2
Reduced fat, w/o salt	1 oz	138	6	1	2	19	2	2
Sour cream & onion	1 oz	151	10	3	177	15	1	2
Sour cream & onion, made from dried potatoes	1 oz	155	10	3	204	15	0	2
POTATO FLOUR	1 cup	571	1	0	88	133	9	11
POTATO PANCAKES (2.75" dia)	1	59	3	1	168	6	1	1
POTATOES								
Au gratin, dry mix, prepared w/ water, whole milk & butter	5.5 oz pkg	764	34	21	3609	106	7	19
Au gratin, homemade, w/ butter	1 cup	323	19	12	1061	28	4	12
Au gratin, homemade, w/ margarine	1 cup	323	19	9	1061	28	4	12
Baked (2-1/4" x 3-1/4")	1 potato	160	0	0	17	36	4	4
Baked, flesh only	1/2 cup	57	0	0	3	13	1	1
Baked, skin only	1 skin	115	0	0	12	27	5	2
Boiled, cooked in skin, flesh only	1/2 cup	68	0	0	3	16	1	1
Boiled, cooked in skin, skin only	1 skin	27	0	0	5	6	1	1
Boiled, cooked w/o skin (2-1/4" x 3-1/4")	1 potato	144	0	0	8	33	3	3
Canned	1 cup	132	0	0	651	30	4	4
Canned, drained	1 cup	108	0	0	394	24	4	3
Canned, drained, no salt	1 cup	112	0	0	9	24	4	3
French fried, cottage cut, frozen, oven heated w/o salt	10 fries	109	4	2	22	17	2	2
French fried, frozen, oven heated, w/o salt	10 fries	166	9	3	307	20	2	2
Hashed browns, frozen, plain, prepared	1 patty	63	3	1	10	8	1	1

ITEM DESCRIPTION	Serving Size	Calories	Total Fat (g)	Saturated Fat (g)	Sodium (mg)	Carbohydrates (g)	Fiber (g)	Protein (g)
Hashed browns, homemade	1 cup	413	20	3	534	55	5	5
Mashed, dehydrated, prepared w/ milk, water & margarine	1 cup	244	10	3	359	34	3	5
Mashed, dehydrated, prepared w/o milk & butter	1 cup	227	10	6	540	30	5	4
Mashed, homemade, whole milk added	1 cup	174	1	1	634	37	3	4
Mashed, homemade, whole milk & butter added	1 cup	237	9	4	666	35	3	4
Microwaved, cooked in skin (2-3/4" x 4-3/4")	1 potato	212	0	0	16	49	5	5
Microwaved, cooked in skin, flesh only	1/2 cup	78	0	0	5	18	1	2
Microwaved, cooked in skin, skin only	1 skin	77	0	0	9	17	3	3
O'Brien, homemade	1 cup	157	2	2	421	30	0	5
Puffs, frozen, oven heated	1 cup	243	11	2	614	36	3	3
Red, baked (2-1/4" x 3-1/4")	1 potato	154	0	0	21	34	3	4
Red, fresh (2-1/4" x 3-1/4")	1 potato	149	0	0	13	34	4	4
Russet, baked (2-1/4" x 3-1/4")	1 potato	168	0	0	24	37	4	5
Russet, fresh (2-1/4" x 3-1/4")	1 potato	168	0	0	11	38	3	5
Scalloped, homemade w/ butter or margarine	1 cup	216	9	6	821	26	5	7
Scalloped, mix, prepared w/ water, whole milk, & butter	5.5 oz pkg	764	35	22	2803	105	9	17
White, baked (2-1/4" x 3-1/4")	1 potato	130	0	0	10	29	3	3
White, fresh (2-1/4" x 3-1/4")	1 potato	147	0	0	13	33	5	4
POTATO SALAD (homemade)	1 cup	358	21	4	1322	28	3	7
POTATO STICKS	1/2 cup	94	6	2	45	10	1	1
POULTRY SEASONING	1 tbsp	14	0	0	1	3	1	0
POUT (cooked in dry heat)	3 oz	87	1	0	66	0	0	18
PRETZELS								
Hard, chocolate coated	1 oz	130	5	2	161	20	0	2
Hard, plain, salted	1 oz	108	1	0	486	22	1	3
Hard, plain, unsalted	1 oz	108	1	0	82	22	1	3
Hard, whole wheat	1 oz	103	1	0	58	23	2	3

ITEM DESCRIPTION	Serving Size	Calories	Total Fat (g)	Saturated Fat (g)	Sodium (mg)	Carbohydrates (g)	Fiber (g)	Protein (g)
Soft, salted	1 med	389	4	1	1615	80	2	9
Soft, unsalted	1 med	389	4	1	794	82	2	9
PRICKLY PEARS (fresh)	1 fruit	42	1	0	5	10	4	1
PRUNE JUICE (canned)	1 cup	182	0	0	10	45	3	2
PRUNES								
Canned in heavy syrup	1 cup	246	0	0	7	65	9	2
Dehydrated, stewed	1 cup	316	1	0	6	83	0	3
Dehydrated, uncooked	1 cup	447	1	0	7	118	0	5
Puree	2 tbsp	93	0	0	8	23	1	1
Stewed, w/ added sugar	1 cup	308	1	0	5	82	9	3
Stewed, w/o added sugar	1 cup	265	0	0	2	70	8	2
Uncooked	1 cup	417	1	0	3	111	12	4
PUDDINGS								
Chocolate, instant, prepared w/ whole milk	1/2 cup	163	5	3	417	28	1	5
Chocolate, reg, prepared w/ whole milk	1/2 cup	169	4	3	136	28	1	5
Chocolate, ready to eat	1/2 cup	153	5	1	164	25	0	2
Coconut cream, instant, prepared w/ 2% milk	1/2 cup	157	3	2	362	28	0	4
Coconut cream, instant, prepared w/ whole milk	1/2 cup	172	5	3	362	28	0	4
Coconut cream, reg, prepared w/ 2% milk	1/2 cup	146	4	3	228	25	0	4
Coconut cream, reg, prepared w/ whole milk	1/2 cup	160	5	4	227	25	0	4
Lemon, instant, prepared w/ whole milk	1/2 cup	169	4	3	392	30	0	4
Rice, ready to eat	1/2 cup	133	3	2	139	22	1	4
Tapioca, ready to eat	1/2 cup	143	4	1	160	24	0	2
Tapioca, ready to eat, fat free	1/2 cup	105	0	0	209	24	0	2
Vanilla, instant, prepared w/ whole milk	1/2 cup	162	4	2	406	28	0	4
Vanilla, ready to eat	1/2 cup	143	4	1	156	25	0	2
Vanilla, ready to eat, fat free	3-1/2 oz	88	0	0	189	20	0	2
Vanilla, reg, prepared w/ whole milk	1/2 cup	157	4	2	216	26	0	4

ITEM DESCRIPTION	Serving Size	Calories	Total Fat (g)	Saturated Fat (g)	Sodium (mg)	Carbohydrates (g)	Fiber (g)	Protein (g)
PUFF PASTRY								
Sheet, frozen, baked	1/6 sheet	228	16	2	104	19	1	3
Shell, frozen, baked	1 shell	223	15	2	101	18	1	3
PUMMELO (fresh)	1 fruit	231	0	0	6	59	6	5
PUMPKIN								
Boiled, mashed	1 cup	49	0	0	2	12	3	2
Canned, w/o salt	1 cup	83	1	0	12	20	7	3
Canned, w/ salt	1 cup	83	1	0	590	20	7	3
Fresh, cubed	1 cup	30	0	0	1	8	1	1
PUMPKIN FLOWERS								
Boiled	1 cup	20	0	0	8	4	1	1
Fresh	1 cup	5	0	0	2	1	0	0
PUMPKIN LEAVES								
Boiled	1 cup	15	0	0	6	2	2	2
Fresh	1 cup	7	0	0	4	1	0	1
PUMPKIN PIE MIX (canned)	1 cup	281	0	0	562	71	22	3
PUMPKIN PIE SPICE	1 tbsp	19	1	0	3	4	1	0
PUMPKIN SEEDS								
Dried	1 oz	151	13	2	5	5	1	7
Kernels, roasted, w/o salt	1 oz	146	12	2	5	4	1	9
Kernels, roasted, w/ salt	1 oz	146	12	2	161	4	1	9
Whole, roasted, w/o salt	1 oz	125	5	1	5	15	0	5
Whole, roasted, w/ salt	1 oz	125	5	1	161	15	0	5
PURSLANE								
Boiled	1 cup	21	0	0	51	4	0	2
Fresh	1 cup	7	0	0	19	1	0	1
QUAIL EGGS (fresh)	1 egg	14	1	0	13	0	0	1
QUINCES (fresh)	1 fruit	52	0	0	4	14	2	0
QUINOA (cooked)	1 cup	222	4	0	13	39	5	8
RABBIT (domestic, composite of cuts, stewed)	3 oz	167	7	2	40	0	0	25
RADICCHIO (fresh, shredded)	1 cup	9	0	0	9	2	0	1
RADISHES								
Fresh, slices	1 cup	19	0	0	45	4	2	1

ITEM DESCRIPTION	Serving Size	Calories	Total Fat (g)	Saturated Fat (g)	Sodium (mg)	Carbohydrates (g)	Fiber (g)	Protein (g)
Hawaiian style, pickled	1 cup	42	0	0	1184	8	3	2
Oriental, boiled, slices	1 cup	25	0	0	19	5	2	1
Oriental, dried	1 cup	314	1	0	322	74	0	9
Oriental, fresh (7" long)	1 radish	61	0	0	71	14	5	2
White icicle, fresh, slices	1 cup	14	0	0	16	3	1	1
RADISH SEEDS (fresh)	1 cup	16	1	0	2	1	0	1
RAISINS								
Golden, seedless	1 cup	498	1	0	20	131	7	6
Purple, seedless	1 cup	493	1	0	18	131	6	5
RAMBUTAN (canned in syrup)	1 cup	123	0	0	16	31	1	1
RASPBERRIES								
Fresh	1 cup	64	1	0	1	15	8	1
Red, canned in heavy syrup	1 cup	233	0	0	8	60	8	2
Red, frozen, sweetened	1 cup	258	0	0	2	65	11	2
REFRIED BEANS								
Canned, fat free	1 cup	182	1	0	1012	31	11	12
Canned, frijoles rojos volteados	1 cup	336	16	2	874	36	11	12
Canned, traditional	1 cup	217	3	1	1069	36	12	13
Canned, vegetarian	1 cup	201	2	0	1041	33	11	13
Pace Salsa Refried Beans	1/2 cup	72	0	0	590	14	4	4
Pace Spicy Jalapeño Refried Beans	1/2 cup	76	0	0	590	14	5	5
Pace Traditional Refried Beans	1/2 cup	80	0	0	690	13	5	5
RHUBARB								
Fresh, diced	1 cup	26	0	0	5	6	2	1
Frozen, cooked, w/ sugar	1 cup	278	0	0	2	75	5	1
RICE								
Brown, long grain, cooked	1 cup	216	2	0	10	45	4	5
Brown, medium grain, cooked	1 cup	218	2	0	2	46	4	5
Brown rice flour	1 cup	574	4	1	13	121	7	11
White, from Chinese restaurant, steamed	1 cup	199	0	0	7	45	1	4
White, glutinous	1 cup	169	0	0	9	37	2	4
White, long grain	1 cup	205	0	0	2	45	1	4
White, long grain, instant	1 cup	193	1	0	7	41	1	4
White, long grain, parboiled	1 cup	194	1	0	3	41	1	5

ITEM DESCRIPTION	Serving Size	Calories	Total Fat (g)	Saturated Fat (g)	Sodium (mg)	Carbohydrates (g)	Fiber (g)	Protein (g)
White, medium grain	1 cup	242	0	0	0	53	1	4
White, short grain	1 cup	242	0	0	0	53	0	4
White, w/ pasta	1 cup	246	6	1	1147	43	5	5
White rice flour	1 cup	578	2	1	0	127	4	9
Wild, cooked	1 cup	166	1	0	5	35	3	7
RICE BRAN (crude)	1 cup	373	25	5	6	59	25	16
RICE BRAN OIL	1 tbsp	120	14	3	0	0	0	0
RICE CAKES								
Brown rice, buckwheat	1 cake	34	0	0	10	7	0	1
Brown rice, buckwheat, unsalted	1 cake	34	0	0	0	7	0	1
Brown rice, corn	1 cake	35	0	0	26	7	0	1
Brown rice, multigrain	1 cake	35	0	0	23	7	0	1
Brown rice, multigrain, unsalted	1 cake	35	0	0	0	7	0	1
Brown rice, plain	1 cake	35	0	0	29	7	0	1
Brown rice, plain, unsalted	1 cake	35	0	0	2	7	0	1
Brown rice, rye	1 cake	35	0	0	10	7	0	1
Brown rice, sesame seed	1 cake	35	0	0	20	7	0	1
Brown rice, sesame seed, unsalted	1 cake	35	0	0	0	7	0	1
ROAST BEEF HASH (Hormel, canned)	1 cup	385	24	10	793	23	4	21
ROCKFISH (Pacific, cooked in dry heat)	3 oz	103	2	0	65	0	0	20
ROE (cooked in dry heat)	3 oz	173	7	2	99	2	0	24
ROLLS								
Dinner, egg (2-1/2" dia)	1 roll	107	2	1	191	18	1	3
Dinner, oat bran	1 roll	78	2	0	136	13	1	3
Dinner, plain, commercial (2" sq)	1 roll	78	2	0	134	13	1	3
Dinner, plain, homemade, made w/ 2% milk (2-1/2" dia)	1 roll	111	3	1	145	19	1	3
Dinner, rye (2-3/8" dia)	1 roll	80	1	0	250	15	1	3
Dinner, wheat	1 roll	76	2	0	95	13	1	2
French	1 roll	105	2	0	231	19	1	3
Hamburger or hot dog, mixed grain	1 roll	113	3	1	197	19	2	4
Hamburger or hot dog, plain	1 roll	120	2	0	206	21	1	4
Hamburger or hot dog, reduced calorie	1 roll	84	1	0	190	18	3	4
Kaiser (3-1/2" dia)	1 roll	167	2	0	310	30	1	6

ITEM DESCRIPTION	Serving Size	Calories	Total Fat (g)	Saturated Fat (g)	Sodium (mg)	Carbohydrates (g)	Fiber (g)	Protein (g)
Pillsbury Cinnamon Rolls, w/ icing	1 serv	145	5	2	340	23	1	2
Pumpernickel (2-1/2" dia)	1 roll	100	1	0	205	19	2	4
Sweet, cinnamon, commercial w/raisins (2-3/4" dia)	1 roll	223	10	2	230	31	1	4
Sweet, cinnamon, refrigerated dough w/ frosting	1 roll	109	4	1	250	17	0	2
Sweet, w/ cheese	1 roll	238	12	4	236	29	1	5
Wonder Hamburger Rolls	1 roll	117	2	0	256	22	1	3
ROSEMARY								
Fresh	1 tbsp	2	0	0	0	0	0	0
Dried	1 tbsp	11	1	0	2	2	1	0
ROUGHY (orange, cooked in dry heat)	3 oz	89	1	0	59	0	0	19
ROWAL (fresh)	1/2 cup	127	2	0	5	27	7	3
RUM								
80 proof	1 fl oz	64	0	0	0	0	0	0
86 proof	1 fl oz	70	0	0	0	0	0	0
90 proof	1 fl oz	73	0	0	0	0	0	0
94 proof	1 fl oz	76	0	0	0	0	0	0
RUTABAGAS								
Boiled, cubed	1 cup	66	0	0	34	15	3	2
Fresh	1 large	278	2	0	154	63	19	9
RYE FLOUR								
Dark	1 cup	415	3	0	1	88	29	18
Light	1 cup	374	1	0	2	82	15	9
Medium	1 cup	361	2	0	3	79	15	10
SABLEFISH								
Cooked in dry heat	3 oz	212	17	3	61	0	0	15
Smoked	1 oz	73	6	1	209	0	0	5
SAFFLOWER								
Oil, linoleic, over 70%	1 tbsp	120	14	1	0	0	0	0
Oil, oleic, over 70%	1 tbsp	120	14	1	0	0	0	0
Seed meal, defatted	1 oz	97	1	0	1	14	0	10
Seeds, dried	1 oz	147	11	1	1	10	0	5
SAFFRON	1 tbsp	7	0	0	3	1	0	0

ITEM DESCRIPTION	Serving Size	Calories	Total Fat (g)	Saturated Fat (g)	Sodium (mg)	Carbohydrates (g)	Fiber (g)	Protein (g)
SAGE (ground)	1 tbsp	6	0	0	0	1	1	0
SAKE	1 fl oz	39	0	0	1	1	0	0
SALAD DRESSINGS								
1000 Island, commercial	1 tbsp	59	6	1	138	2	0	0
1000 Island, fat free	1 tbsp	21	0	0	117	5	1	0
1000 Island, reduced fat	1 tbsp	29	2	0	125	4	0	0
Bacon & tomato	1 tbsp	49	5	1	163	0	0	0
Blue or Roquefort cheese, commercial	1 tbsp	71	8	1	140	1	0	0
Blue or Roquefort cheese, fat free	1 tbsp	20	0	0	138	4	0	0
Blue or Roquefort cheese, low calorie	1 tbsp	15	1	0	180	0	0	1
Blue or Roquefort cheese, reduced calorie	1 tbsp	14	0	0	258	2	0	0
Buttermilk, light	1 tbsp	30	2	0	136	3	0	0
Caesar	1 tbsp	80	9	1	158	0	0	0
Caesar, low calorie	1 tbsp	16	1	0	162	3	0	0
Creamy, w/ sour cream or buttermilk & oil, reduced calorie	1 tbsp	24	2	0	153	1	0	0
Creamy, w/ sour cream or buttermilk & oil, reduced calorie, cholesterol free	1 tbsp	21	1	0	140	2	0	0
Creamy, w/ sour cream or buttermilk & oil, reduced calorie, fat free	1 tbsp	18	0	0	170	3	0	0
French, commercial	1 tbsp	73	7	1	134	2	0	0
French, commercial, w/o salt	1 tbsp	69	7	1	0	2	0	0
French, fat free	1 tbsp	21	0	0	126	5	0	0
French, homemade	1 tbsp	88	10	2	92	0	0	0
French, reduced calorie	1 tbsp	32	2	0	160	4	0	0
French, reduced fat	1 tbsp	36	2	0	126	5	0	0
French, reduced fat, w/o salt	1 tbsp	37	2	0	5	5	0	0
Green goddess	1 tbsp	64	7	1	130	1	0	0
Honey mustard, reduced calorie	1 tbsp	31	2	0	135	4	0	0
Italian, commercial	1 tbsp	43	4	1	243	2	0	0
Italian, commercial, w/o salt	1 tbsp	43	4	1	4	2	0	0
Italian, fat free	1 tbsp	7	0	0	158	1	0	0
Italian, reduced calorie	1 tbsp	28	3	0	199	1	0	0

ITEM DESCRIPTION	Serving Size	Calories	Total Fat (g)	Saturated Fat (g)	Sodium (mg)	Carbohydrates (g)	Fiber (g)	Protein (g)
Italian, reduced fat	1 tbsp	11	1	0	205	1	0	0
Italian, reduced fat, w/o salt	1 tbsp	11	1	0	4	1	0	0
Ken's Steak House Caesar Dressing & Marinade	2 tbsp	170	18	2.5	430	1	0	0
Ken's Steak House Italian Dressing & Marinade	2 tbsp	150	16	2.5	450	1	0	0
Ken's Steak House Ranch Dressing	2 tbsp	140	15	2	310	2	0	0
Ken's Steak House Red Wine Vinegar & Olive Oil	2 tbsp	120	12	1.5	360	2	0	0
Kraft Free Fat Free Italian Dressing	1 tbsp	10	0	0	215	2	0	0
Kraft Free Fat Free Ranch Dressing	1 tbsp	24	0	0	177	5	0	0
Kraft Light Done Right! Italian Dressing	1 tbsp	26	2	0	114	1	0	0
Kraft Light Done Right! Ranch Dressing	1 tbsp	38	3	0	151	2	0	0
Kraft Ranch Dressing	1 tbsp	74	8	1	144	1	0	0
Kraft Zesty Italian Dressing	1 tbsp	54	6	1	253	1	0	0
Newman's Own Balsamic Vinaigrette	2 tbsp	90	9	1	350	3	0	0
Newman's Own Caesar Dressing	2 tbsp	150	16	1.5	420	1	0	1
Newman's Own Family Recipe Italian Dressing	2 tbsp	120	13	1	400	1	0	1
Newman's Own Ranch Dressing	2 tbsp	150	16	2.5	310	2	0	0
Peppercorn, commercial	1 tbsp	76	8	1	143	0	0	0
Ranch, commercial	1 tbsp	73	8	1	122	1	0	0
Ranch, fat free	1 tbsp	17	0	0	106	4	0	0
Ranch, reduced fat	1 tbsp	29	2	0	136	3	0	0
Russian	1 tbsp	53	4	0	149	5	0	0
Russian, low calorie	1 tbsp	23	1	0	139	4	0	0
Sesame seed	1 tbsp	66	7	1	150	1	0	0
Spray, assorted flavors	~10 sprays	13	1	0	88	1	0	0
Sweet & sour	1 tbsp	2	0	0	33	1	0	0
Vinegar & oil, homemade	1 tbsp	72	8	1	0	0	0	0
SALAMI								
Beef & pork, cooked	3 slices	124	10	3	535	1	0	8
Beef & pork, less sodium	3.5 oz	396	31	11	623	15	0	15

ITEM DESCRIPTION	Serving Size	Calories	Total Fat (g)	Saturated Fat (g)	Sodium (mg)	Carbohydrates (g)	Fiber (g)	Protein (g)
Beef, cooked	1 slice	68	6	3	296	0	0	3
Dry or hard, pork	3 slices	122	10	4	678	0	0	7
Dry or hard, pork & beef	3 slices	104	8	3	543	1	0	6
Italian pork	1 oz	119	10	4	529	0	0	6
Oscar Mayer Salami, beer	1 slice	52	4	1	283	0	0	3
Oscar Mayer Salami Cotto, beef	1 slice	47	4	2	301	0	0	3
Oscar Mayer Salami Cotto, beef, pork & chicken	1 slice	56	5	2	252	1	0	3
Oscar Mayer Salami, Genoa	1 slice	35	3	1	164	0	0	2
Oscar Mayer Salami, hard	1 slice	33	3	1	178	0	0	2
SALMON								
Atlantic, farmed, cooked in dry heat	3 oz	175	11	2	52	0	0	19
Atlantic, wild, cooked in dry heat	3 oz	155	7	1	48	0	0	22
Chinook, cooked in dry heat	3 oz	196	11	3	51	0	0	22
Chinook, smoked	1 oz	33	1	0	222	0	0	5
Chinook, smoked, lox	1 oz	33	1	0	567	0	0	5
Chum, canned	3 oz	175	5	1	414	0	0	18
Chum, canned, w/o salt	3 oz	175	5	1	64	0	0	18
Chum, cooked in dry heat	3 oz	131	4	1	54	0	0	22
Coho, farmed, cooked in dry heat	3 oz	151	7	2	44	0	0	21
Coho, wild, cooked in dry heat	3 oz	118	4	1	49	0	0	20
Coho, wild, cooked in moist heat	3 oz	156	6	1	45	0	0	23
Pink, canned	3 oz	118	5	1	471	0	0	17
Pink, canned, w/o salt	3 oz	118	5	1	64	0	0	17
Pink, cooked in dry heat	3 oz	127	4	1	73	0	0	22
Sockeye, canned	3 oz	141	6	1	306	0	0	20
Sockeye, canned, w/o salt	3 oz	130	6	1	64	0	0	17
Sockeye, cooked in dry heat	3 oz	184	9	2	56	0	0	23
SALMON OIL	1 tbsp	123	14	3	0	0	0	0
SALSA								
Pace Chipotle Chunky Salsa	2 tbsp	8	0	0	230	2	1	0
Pace Cilantro Chunky Salsa	2 tbsp	8	0	0	270	2	1	0
Pace Lime & Garlic Chunky Salsa	2 tbsp	12	0	0	210	3	1	0
Pace Salsa Verde	2 tbsp	15	0	0	230	2	0	0

ITEM DESCRIPTION	Serving Size	Calories	Total Fat (g)	Saturated Fat (g)	Sodium (mg)	Carbohydrates (g)	Fiber (g)	Protein (g)
Pace Tequila Lime Salsa	2 tbsp	15	0	0	190	3	0	0
Pace Thick & Chunky Salsa	2 tbsp	8	0	0	230	2	1	0
Pace Triple Pepper Salsa	2 tbsp	15	0	0	190	3	1	1
Ready to serve	2 tbsp	9	0	0	192	2	1	0
SALSIFY								
Boiled, slices	1 cup	92	0	0	22	21	4	4
Fresh, slices	1 cup	109	0	0	27	25	4	4
SALT (table)	1 tbsp	0	0	0	6976	0	0	0
SANDWICH SPREAD								
Meatless	1 tbsp	22	1	0	94	1	1	1
Oscar Mayer Sandwich Spread, pork, chicken, beef	1 serv	71	5	2	246	5	0	2
Pork & beef	1 tbsp	35	3	1	152	2	0	1
Poultry salad	1 tbsp	26	2	0	49	1	0	2
SARDINE OIL	1 tbsp	123	14	4	0	0	0	0
SARDINES								
Atlantic, canned in oil	1 cup	310	17	2	752	0	0	37
Pacific, canned in tomato sauce	1 cup	166	9	2	368	1	0	19
SAUERKRAUT								
Canned	1 cup	27	0	0	939	6	4	1
Canned, low sodium	1 cup	31	0	0	437	6	4	1
SAUSAGE								
Beerwurst, beer salami, pork & beef	2 oz	155	13	5	410	2	1	8
Beerwurst, pork (4" dia x 1/8" thick)	1 slice	55	4	1	285	0	0	3
Berliner, pork, beef	1 slice	53	4	1	298	1	0	4
Blood	1 slice	95	9	3	170	0	0	4
Bratwurst, beef & pork, smoked	2.3 oz	196	17	4	560	1	0	8
Bratwurst, chicken, cooked	3 oz	148	9	0	60	0	0	16
Bratwurst, pork, beef & turkey, light, smoked	2.3 oz	123	9	0	648	1	0	10
Bratwurst, pork, cooked	1 link	283	25	8	719	2	0	12
Bratwurst, veal, cooked	2.96 oz	286	27	13	50	0	0	12
Chicken & beef, smoked	1 cup, pcs	408	33	10	1408	0	0	26
Chorizo, pork & beef (4" link)	1 link	273	23	9	741	1	0	14

ITEM DESCRIPTION	Serving Size	Calories	Total Fat (g)	Saturated Fat (g)	Sodium (mg)	Carbohydrates (g)	Fiber (g)	Protein (g)
Honey roll, beef (4" dia x 1/8" thick)	1 slice	42	2	1	304	1	0	4
Italian, pork, cooked (1/4 lb link)	1 link	286	23	8	1002	4	0	16
Italian, sweet links	3 oz link	125	7	3	479	2	0	14
Kielbasa, pork & beef, nonfat dry milk	1 link	232	20	7	678	2	0	9
Kielbasa, turkey & beef, smoked	2 oz	127	10	3	672	2	0	7
Knockwurst, pork & beef	1 link	221	20	7	670	2	0	8
Liverwurst, pork (2-1/2" dia x 1/4" thick)	1 slice	59	5	2	155	0	0	3
Oscar Mayer Braunschweiger Liver Sausage, slices	1 slice	93	8	3	325	1	0	4
Oscar Mayer Braunschweiger Liver Sausage, tube	1 serv	191	17	6	626	1	0	8
Oscar Mayer Pork Sausage Links	1 link	82	7	3	201	0	0	4
Oscar Mayer Smokie Links	1 link	130	12	4	433	1	0	5
Oscar Mayer Smokies, beef	1 link	127	11	5	416	1	0	5
Oscar Mayer Smokies, cheese	1 link	130	12	4	450	1	0	6
Oscar Mayer Smokies Sausage Little, cheese, pork & turkey	1 link	28	3	1	93	0	0	1
Oscar Mayer Smokies Sausage Little, pork & turkey	1 link	27	2	1	92	0	0	1
Oscar Mayer Summer Sausage, beef thuringer	1 slice	71	6	3	328	0	0	3
Oscar Mayer Summer Sausage, thuringer	1 slice	70	6	2	329	0	0	3
Polish, beef & chicken, hot	5 pcs	142	11	4	847	2	0	10
Polish, beef & pork, smoked	2.7 oz	229	20	7	644	2	0	9
Polish, pork (10" long x 1-1/4" dia)	1 link	740	65	23	1989	4	0	32
Pork & beef, patty	1 patty	107	10	3	217	1	0	4
Pork & turkey, patty	1 patty	77	6	2	220	0	0	6
Pork sausage rice links, brown & serve	2 links	183	17	3	310	1	0	6
Smoked link, pork (4" long x 1-1/8" dia)	1 link	209	19	6	562	0	0	8
Smoked link, pork & beef	1 oz	320	29	10	911	2	0	12
Smoked link, pork & beef, w/ flour & nonfat dry milk (4" long x 1-1/8" dia)	1 link	182	15	5	865	3	0	10

ITEM DESCRIPTION	Serving Size	Calories	Total Fat (g)	Saturated Fat (g)	Sodium (mg)	Carbohydrates (g)	Fiber (g)	Protein (g)
Smoked link, pork & beef, w/ nonfat dry milk (4" long x 1-1/8" dia)	1 link	213	19	7	798	1	0	9
Turkey, pork, & beef, reduced fat, smoked	1 cup	353	25	9	1407	4	0	27
Vienna, canned, chicken, beef & pork (2" long x 7/8" dia)	1 link	37	3	1	155	0	0	2
SAUSAGE BISCUITS (Jimmy Dean, frozen)	1 sandwich	192	14	4	441	12	1	5
SAUSAGE SUBSTITUTE								
Meatless	1 link	64	5	1	222	2	1	5
Morningstar Farms Sausage Style Recipe Crumbles, frozen	2/3 cup	90	2	0	445	8	1	10
Morningstar Farms Veggie Sausage Links, frozen	1 link	72	3	0	302	3	2	9
Morningstar Farms Veggie Sausage Patties, frozen	1 patty	80	3	0	255	3	2	10
Worthington Low Fat Veja-Links, canned	1 link	38	1	0	190	1	0	5
Worthington Prosage Links, frozen	2 links	64	2	0	369	2	1	9
Worthington Saucettes, canned	1 link	83	6	0	202	2	1	6
Worthington Veja-Links, canned	1 link	48	3	0	164	1	1	5
SAVORY (ground)	1 tbsp	12	0	0	1	3	2	0
SCALLIONS (fresh, chopped)	1 tbsp	2	0	0	1	0	0	0
SCALLOPS (breaded & fried)	6 pcs	386	19	5	919	38	0	16
SCALLOP SQUASH								
Boiled, mashed	1 cup	38	0	0	2	8	5	2
Fresh, slices	1 cup	23	0	0	1	5	0	2
SCALLOPS SUBSTITUTE (imitation, made from surimi)	3 oz	84	0	0	676	9	0	11
SCUP (cooked in dry heat)	3 oz	115	3	0	46	0	0	21
SEA BASS (cooked in dry heat)	3 oz	105	2	1	74	0	0	20
SEA TROUT (cooked in dry heat)	3 oz	113	4	1	63	0	0	18
SEAWEED								
Agar, fresh	2 tbsp	3	0	0	1	1	0	0
Irish moss, fresh	2 tbsp	5	0	0	7	1	0	0

ITEM DESCRIPTION	Serving Size	Calories	Total Fat (g)	Saturated Fat (g)	Sodium (mg)	Carbohydrates (g)	Fiber (g)	Protein (g)
Kelp, fresh	2 tbsp	4	0	0	23	1	0	0
Laver, fresh	2 tbsp	4	0	0	5	1	0	1
Spirulina, dried	1 tbsp	20	1	0	73	2	0	4
Wakame, fresh	2 tbsp	4	0	0	87	1	0	0
SEMOLINA	1 cup	601	2	0	2	122	7	21
SESAME BUTTER								
High fat	1 oz	149	11	1	12	8	0	9
Low fat	1 oz	94	0	0	11	10	0	14
Part defatted	1 oz	108	3	0	12	10	0	11
Paste	1 tbsp	94	8	1	2	4	1	3
Tahini	1 tbsp	89	8	1	5	3	1	3
Tahini, from fresh & ground kernels	1 tbsp	86	7	1	11	4	1	3
Tahini, from roasted & toasted kernels	1 tbsp	89	8	1	17	3	1	3
Tahini, from unroasted kernels	1 tbsp	85	8	1	0	3	1	3
SESAME MEAL (part defatted)	1 oz	161	14	2	11	7	0	5
SESAME OIL	1 tbsp	120	14	2	0	0	0	0
SESAME SEEDS								
Kernels, dried	1 tbsp	50	5	1	4	1	1	2
Kernels, toasted, w/o salt	1 tbsp	45	4	1	3	2	1	1
Kernels, toasted, w/ salt	1 tbsp	45	4	1	47	2	1	1
Whole, dried	1 tbsp	52	5	1	1	2	1	2
Whole, roasted & toasted	1 tbsp	51	4	1	1	2	1	2
SESAME STICKS								
Wheat based, salted	1 oz	153	10	2	422	13	1	3
Wheat based, unsalted	1 oz	153	10	2	8	13	0	3
SESBANIA FLOWER								
Fresh	1 cup	5	0	0	3	1	0	0
Steamed	1 cup	23	0	0	11	5	0	1
SHAD (American, cooked in dry heat)	3 oz	214	15	0	55	0	0	18
SHAKES								
Fast food, chocolate	12 fl oz	358	10	7	274	58	5	10
Fast food, strawberry	12 fl oz	319	8	5	234	53	1	10
Fast food, vanilla	12 fl oz	370	16	10	202	49	2	8

ITEM DESCRIPTION	Serving Size	Calories	Total Fat (g)	Saturated Fat (g)	Sodium (mg)	Carbohydrates (g)	Fiber (g)	Protein (g)
SHALLOTS								
Freeze-dried	1 tbsp	3	0	0	1	1	0	0
Fresh, chopped	1 tbsp	7	0	0	1	2	0	0
SHARK (cooked, battered & fried)	3 oz	194	12	3	104	5	0	16
SHEANUT OIL	1 tbsp	120	14	6	0	0	0	0
SHELLIE BEANS (canned)	1 cup	74	0	0	818	15	8	4
SHERBET (orange)	1/2 cup	107	1	1	34	23	1	1
SHORTENING								
Baking, soybean, palm & cottonseed, hydrogenated	1 tbsp	113	13	4	0	0	0	0
Cakes & frostings, soybean, hydrogenated	1 tbsp	113	13	3	0	0	0	0
Confectionery, coconut or palm oil, hydrogenated	1 tbsp	113	13	12	0	0	0	0
Confectionery, fractionated palm	1 tbsp	120	14	9	0	0	0	0
Frying, heavy, beef tallow & cottonseed	1 tbsp	115	13	6	0	0	0	0
Frying, heavy, palm, hydrogenated	1 tbsp	113	13	6	0	0	0	0
Frying, heavy, soybean, hydrogenated	1 tbsp	113	13	3	0	0	0	0
Frying, soybean & cottonseed, hydrogenated	1 tbsp	113	13	2	0	0	0	0
Household, lard & vegetable oil	1 tbsp	115	13	5	0	0	0	0
Household, soybean & cottonseed, hydrogenated	1 tbsp	113	13	3	0	0	0	0
Household, soybean & palm, hydrogenated	1 tbsp	113	13	3	0	0	0	0
Household, vegetable	1 tbsp	113	13	3	1	0	0	0
Soybean & cottonseed, hydrogenated	1 tbsp	113	13	3	0	0	0	0
SHRIMP								
Breaded & fried	3 oz	206	10	2	292	10	0	18
Canned	3 oz	85	1	0	660	0	0	17
Cooked in moist heat	3 oz	84	1	0	190	0	0	18
Imitation, made from surimi	3 oz	86	1	0	599	8	0	11
SMELT (rainbow, cooked in dry heat)	3 oz	105	3	0	65	0	0	19

ITEM DESCRIPTION

	Serving Size	Calories	Total Fat (g)	Saturated Fat (g)	Sodium (mg)	Carbohydrates (g)	Fiber (g)	Protein (g)
SNACK BARS								
Cocoavia Chocolate Almond Snack Bar	1 bar	76	3	1	57	11	1	2
Cocoavia Chocolate Blueberry Snack Bar	1 bar	72	2	1	57	13	1	1
Corn flake crust, w/ fruit	1 oz bar	107	2	0	47	21	1	1
Crisped rice bar, chocolate chip	1 oz bar	113	4	1	78	20	1	1
Fiber One Oats & Caramel	1 bar	140	4	2	105	30	9	2
Fiber One Oats & Chocolate	1 bar	140	4	2	95	29	9	2
Fiber One Oats & Peanut Butter	1 bar	150	5	2	105	28	9	3
Kudos Whole Grain Bar, chocolate chip	1 bar	118	4	1	69	20	1	1
Kudos Whole Grain Bar, M&M's milk chocolate	1 bar	100	3	2	82	18	1	1
Kudos Whole Grain Bar, peanut butter	1 bar	130	6	3	75	18	1	2
Nature Valley Crunchy Granola Bars, Cinnamon	2	180	6	.5	170	29	2	4
Nature Valley Crunchy Granola Bars, Oats 'n Honey	2	190	6	.5	160	29	2	4
Nature Valley Crunchy Granola Bars, Peanut Butter	2	190	7	1	180	28	2	5
Power Bar, chocolate	1 bar	247	2	1	99	47	4	10
Quaker Chewy Granola Bars, Chocolate Chip	1	100	3	1.5	75	18	1	1
Quaker Chewy Granola Bars, Peanut Butter Chocolate Chip	1	100	3	1	95	17	1	2
Quaker Chewy Granola Bars, SMores	1	100	2	.5	80	19	1	1
Snickers Marathon Chewy Chocolate Peanut Bar	1 bar	218	7	3	254	26	1	13
Snickers Marathon Double Chocolate Nut Bar	1 bar	151	4	2	147	23	5	10
Snickers Marathon Energy Bar	1 bar	170	5	2	169	22	3	10
Snickers Marathon Honey Nut Oat Bar	1 bar	166	3	2	140	24	5	10
Snickers Marathon Multi-Grain Bar	1 bar	223	7	3	230	30	2	10
Snickers Marathon Protein Perfect Bar, caramel nut	1 bar	322	8	4	180	42	8	20

ITEM DESCRIPTION	Serving Size	Calories	Total Fat (g)	Saturated Fat (g)	Sodium (mg)	Carbohydrates (g)	Fiber (g)	Protein (g)
SNACK CAKES								
Crème filled, chocolate w/ frosting	1 cake	200	8	2	194	30	2	2
Crème filled, sponge	1 cake	157	5	2	168	27	0	1
SNAP BEANS								
Canned, all styles, seasoned	1/2 cup	18	0	0	425	4	2	1
Green, boiled	1 cup	44	0	0	1	10	4	2
Green, canned	1 cup	36	0	0	409	7	4	2
Green, canned, no salt	1 cup	36	0	0	34	8	4	2
Green, fresh	1 cup	34	0	0	7	8	4	2
Green, frozen, all styles, microwaved	1 cup	44	0	0	3	8	4	2
Green, frozen, boiled	1 cup	38	0	0	1	9	4	2
Yellow, boiled	1 cup	44	0	0	4	10	4	2
Yellow, canned	1 cup	36	0	0	622	8	4	2
Yellow, canned, no salt	1 cup	36	0	0	34	8	4	2
Yellow, fresh	1 cup	34	0	0	7	8	4	2
Yellow, frozen, boiled	1 cup	38	0	0	12	9	4	2
SNAPPER (cooked in dry heat)	3 oz	109	1	0	48	0	0	22
SODA								
Chocolate flavored	1 fl oz	13	0	0	27	3	0	0
Club soda	16 fl oz	0	0	0	100	0	0	0
Cola	16 fl oz	201	0	0	20	52	0	0
Cola or pepper, w/ aspartame, w/o caffeine	16 fl oz	5	0	0	19	1	0	1
Cola or pepper, w/ saccharine, w/ caffeine	16 fl oz	0	0	0	76	0	0	0
Cola, reduced sugar, w/ sweeteners	8 fl oz	71	0	0	14	18	0	0
Cream soda	16 fl oz	252	0	0	59	66	0	0
Ginger ale	16 fl oz	166	0	0	34	43	0	0
Grape	16 fl oz	213	0	0	74	56	0	0
Lemon-lime	16 fl oz	202	0	0	49	51	0	0
Orange	16 fl oz	238	0	0	60	61	0	0
Pepper	16 fl oz	201	0	0	49	51	0	0
Root beer	16 fl oz	202	0	0	64	52	0	0

ITEM DESCRIPTION	Serving Size	Calories	Total Fat (g)	Saturated Fat (g)	Sodium (mg)	Carbohydrates (g)	Fiber (g)	Protein (g)
Other than cola or pepper, low calorie	16 fl oz	0	0	0	28	0	0	0
Other than cola or pepper, low calorie, w/ aspartame	16 fl oz	0	0	0	28	0	0	0
Other than cola or pepper, low calorie, w/ saccharine	16 fl oz	0	0	0	76	0	0	0
SOFRITO SAUCE (homemade)	1/2 cup	244	19	0	1179	6	2	13
SORGHUM	1 cup	651	6	1	12	143	12	22
SORGHUM SYRUP	1 tbsp	61	0	0	2	16	0	0
SOUP								
Bean w/ bacon, mix, prepared w/ water	1 cup	106	2	1	928	16	9	5
Bean w/ frankfurters, canned, prepared w/ water	1 cup	188	7	2	1092	22	0	10
Bean w/ ham, canned, chunky, ready to serve	1 cup	231	9	3	972	27	11	13
Bean w/ pork, canned, prepared w/ water	1 cup	168	6	1	928	22	8	8
Beef & mushroom, canned, prepared w/ water	1 cup	73	3	1	942	6	0	6
Beef & mushroom, low sodium, chunky	1 cup	173	6	4	63	24	1	11
Beef, chunky, canned, ready to serve	1 cup	162	3	1	880	25	2	10
Beef noodle, canned, prepared w/ water	1 cup	83	3	1	930	9	1	5
Beef stroganoff, canned, chunky, ready to serve	1 cup	235	11	6	1044	22	1	12
Beef w/ country vegetable, chunky, canned, ready to serve	1 pkg	334	7	3	1978	46	0	22
Black bean, canned, prepared w/ water	1 cup	114	2	0	1203	19	8	6
Cheese, canned, prepared w/ milk	1 cup	231	15	9	1019	16	1	9
Cheese, canned, prepared w/ water	1 cup	156	10	7	958	11	1	5
Chicken, chunky, canned, ready to serve	1 cup	174	6	2	867	17	2	12
Chicken corn chowder, chunky, ready to serve	1 pkg	534	34	9	1612	40	5	17

ITEM DESCRIPTION	Serving Size	Calories	Total Fat (g)	Saturated Fat (g)	Sodium (mg)	Carbohydrates (g)	Fiber (g)	Protein (g)
Chicken gumbo, canned, prepared w/ water	1 cup	56	1	0	954	8	2	3
Chicken mushroom, canned, prepared w/ water	1 cup	132	9	2	942	9	0	4
Chicken mushroom chowder, chunky, ready to serve	1 pkg	431	24	6	1827	38	8	16
Chicken noodle, canned, prepared w/ water	1 cup	62	2	1	657	7	1	3
Chicken noodle, chunky, canned, ready to serve	1 cup	91	2	1	840	10	1	8
Chicken noodle, low sodium, canned, prepared w/ water	1 cup	62	2	1	429	7	1	3
Chicken noodle, mix, prepared w/ water	1 cup	56	1	0	561	9	0	2
Chicken rice, canned, chunky, ready to serve	1 cup	127	3	1	888	13	1	12
Chicken rice, mix, prepared w/ water	1 cup	58	1	0	931	9	1	2
Chicken vegetable, canned, prepared w/ water	1 cup	77	3	1	972	9	4	4
Chicken vegetable, chunky, canned, ready to serve	1 cup	166	5	1	833	19	0	12
Chicken vegetable, chunky, reduced fat, reduced sodium, ready to serve	1 pkg	182	2	1	872	29	0	12
Chicken w/ dumplings, canned, prepared w/ water	1 cup	96	6	1	860	6	1	6
Chicken w/ rice, canned, prepared w/ water	1 cup	58	2	0	812	7	1	4
Chili beef, canned, prepared w/ water	1 cup	149	3	2	1013	24	3	7
Clam chowder, Manhattan style, canned, chunky, ready to serve	1 cup	134	3	2	1001	19	3	7
Clam chowder, Manhattan style, canned, prepared w/ water	1 cup	75	2	0	563	12	2	2
Clam chowder, New England, canned, prepared w/ 2% milk	1 cup	154	5	2	902	19	1	8
Clam chowder, New England, canned, prepared w/ water	1 cup	87	3	1	853	13	1	4

ITEM DESCRIPTION	Serving Size	Calories	Total Fat (g)	Saturated Fat (g)	Sodium (mg)	Carbohydrates (g)	Fiber (g)	Protein (g)
Consomme, w/ gelatin, mix, prepared w/ water	1 cup	17	0	0	3299	2	0	2
Crab, canned, ready to serve	1 cup	76	2	0	1235	10	1	5
Cream of asparagus, canned, prepared w/ milk	1 cup	161	8	3	1042	16	1	6
Cream of asparagus, canned, prepared w/ water	1 cup	85	4	1	981	11	1	2
Cream of celery, canned, prepared w/ milk	1 cup	164	10	4	1009	15	1	6
Cream of celery, canned, prepared w/ water	1 cup	90	6	1	949	9	1	2
Cream of chicken, canned, prepared w/ milk	1 cup	191	11	5	1047	15	0	7
Cream of chicken, canned, prepared w/ water	1 cup	117	7	2	986	9	0	3
Cream of chicken, mix, prepared w/ water	1 cup	107	5	3	1185	13	0	2
Cream of mushroom, canned, prepared w/ 2% milk	1 cup	169	10	3	837	14	0	6
Cream of mushroom, canned, prepared w/ water	1 cup	104	7	2	789	8	0	2
Cream of mushroom, low sodium, ready to serve	1 cup	129	9	2	49	11	1	2
Cream of onion, canned, prepared w/ milk	1 cup	186	9	4	1004	18	1	7
Cream of onion, canned, prepared w/ water	1 cup	107	5	1	927	13	1	3
Cream of potato, canned, prepared w/ milk	1 cup	149	6	4	1061	17	1	6
Cream of potato, canned, prepared w/ water	1 cup	73	2	1	1000	11	1	2
Cream of shrimp, canned, prepared w/ water	1 cup	88	5	3	954	8	0	3
Egg drop, Chinese restaurant	1 cup	65	1	0	892	10	0	3
Escarole, canned, ready to serve	1 cup	27	2	1	3864	2	0	2
Gazpacho, canned, ready to serve	1 cup	46	0	0	739	4	1	7
Green pea, canned, prepared w/ milk	1 cup	239	7	4	970	32	3	13

ITEM DESCRIPTION	Serving Size	Calories	Total Fat (g)	Saturated Fat (g)	Sodium (mg)	Carbohydrates (g)	Fiber (g)	Protein (g)
Green pea, canned, prepared w/ water	1 cup	161	3	1	891	26	5	8
Hot & sour, Chinese restaurant	1 cup	91	3	1	876	10	0	6
Lentil, w/ ham, canned, ready to serve	1 cup	139	3	1	1319	20	0	9
Minestrone, canned, prepared w/ water	1 cup	82	3	1	911	11	1	4
Minestrone, chunky, canned, ready to serve	1 cup	127	3	1	864	21	6	5
Mushroom barley, canned, prepared w/ water	1 cup	73	2	0	891	12	1	2
Mushroom w/ beef stock, canned, prepared w/ water	1 cup	85	4	2	969	9	1	3
Mushroom, mix, prepared w/ water	1 cup	83	5	1	1020	11	1	2
Onion, canned, prepared w/ water	1 cup	56	2	0	1028	8	1	4
Onion, mix, prepared w/ water	1 cup	28	0	0	796	6	1	1
Oxtail, mix, prepared w/ water	1 cup	68	2	1	1159	9	0	3
Oyster stew, canned, prepared w/ milk	1 cup	135	8	5	1041	10	0	6
Oyster stew, canned, prepared w/ water	1 cup	58	4	3	981	4	0	2
Pea, low sodium, prepared w/ water	1 cup	161	3	1	26	26	5	8
Pepperpot, canned, prepared w/ water	1 cup	100	5	2	948	9	1	6
Potato ham chowder, chunky, ready to serve	1 pkg	431	28	9	1962	30	3	15
Ramen noodle, beef	1 pkg	371	13	7	1702	54	2	9
Ramen noodle, chicken	1 pkg	371	13	6	1760	54	2	9
Scotch broth, canned, prepared w/ water	1 cup	80	3	1	1000	9	1	5
Shark fin, restaurant prepared	1 cup	99	4	1	1082	8	0	7
Sirloin burger w/ vegetable, ready to serve	1 pkg	415	20	7	1946	37	12	23
Split pea, canned, reduced sodium, prepared w/ water	1 cup	180	2	1	420	30	5	10
Split pea, w/ ham, canned, prepared w/ water	1 cup	190	4	2	1007	28	2	10

ITEM DESCRIPTION	Serving Size	Calories	Total Fat (g)	Saturated Fat (g)	Sodium (mg)	Carbohydrates (g)	Fiber (g)	Protein (g)
Split pea, w/ ham, chunky, canned, ready to serve	1 cup	185	4	2	965	27	4	11
Split pea, w/ ham, chunky, reduced fat, reduced sodium, ready to serve	1 pkg	410	6	2	1849	61	0	28
Stockpot, canned, prepared w/ water	1 cup	99	4	1	1047	11	0	5
Tomato beef w/ noodle, canned, prepared w/ water	1 cup	137	4	2	895	21	2	4
Tomato bisque, canned, prepared w/ milk	1 cup	198	7	3	1109	29	1	6
Tomato bisque, canned, prepared w/ water	1 cup	124	3	1	1047	24	1	2
Tomato, canned, prepared w/ 2% milk	1 cup	139	3	2	723	22	2	6
Tomato, canned, prepared w/ water	1 cup	74	1	0	675	16	2	2
Tomato, low sodium, prepared w/ water	1 cup	74	1	0	60	16	2	2
Tomato, mix, prepared w/ water	1 cup	101	2	1	943	19	1	2
Tomato rice, canned, prepared w/ water	1 cup	116	3	0	788	21	2	2
Tomato vegetable, mix, prepared w/ water	1 cup	54	1	0	323	10	1	2
Turkey, chunky, canned, ready to serve	1 cup	135	4	1	923	14	0	10
Turkey noodle, canned, prepared w/ water	1 cup	68	2	1	815	9	1	4
Turkey vegetable, canned, prepared w/ water	1 cup	72	3	1	906	9	1	3
Vegetable beef, canned, prepared w/ water	1 cup	76	2	1	773	10	2	5
Vegetable beef, microwavable	1 pkg	128	2	1	1098	10	4	18
Vegetable beef, mix, prepared w/ water	1 cup	53	1	1	789	8	1	3
Vegetable, chunky, canned, ready to serve	1 cup	125	4	1	880	19	1	4
Vegetable, condensed, low sodium, prepared w/ water	1 cup	83	1	0	491	15	3	3

ITEM DESCRIPTION	Serving Size	Calories	Total Fat (g)	Saturated Fat (g)	Sodium (mg)	Carbohydrates (g)	Fiber (g)	Protein (g)
Vegetable w/ beef broth, canned, prepared w/ water	1 cup	80	2	0	800	13	2	3
Vegetable w/ chicken, canned, prepared w/ water, low sodium	1 cup	166	5	1	84	21	1	12
Vegetarian vegetable, canned, prepared w/ water	1 cup	67	2	0	815	12	1	2
Wonton, Chinese restaurant	1 cup	71	1	0	905	12	0	5
SOUP, BRAND NAME								
Campbell's Chunky, baked potato w/ cheddar & bacon bits	1 cup	159	6	1	870	23	2	4
Campbell's Chunky, beef rib roast w/ potatoes & herbs	1 cup	108	1	1	889	17	3	8
Campbell's Chunky, beef w/ country vegetable	1 cup	147	3	1	889	21	4	10
Campbell's Chunky, beef w/ white & wild rice	1 cup	159	3	1	990	24	3	8
Campbell's Chunky, chicken & dumplings	1 cup	181	7	2	889	19	4	9
Campbell's Chunky, chicken, broccoli, cheese, & potato	1 cup	201	11	4	909	14	1	7
Campbell's Chunky, chicken corn chowder	1 cup	194	9	1	850	20	3	8
Campbell's Chunky, classic chicken noodle	1 cup	115	3	1	889	15	2	8
Campbell's Chunky, fajita chicken w/ rice & beans	1 cup	142	1	0	850	23	4	9
Campbell's Chunky, grilled chicken sausage gumbo	1 cup	140	3	1	850	21	3	8
Campbell's Chunky, grilled chicken, vegetable, & pasta	1 cup	100	2	1	880	15	2	8
Campbell's Chunky, grilled sirloin steak, hearty vegetable	1 cup	125	2	1	889	19	4	8
Campbell's Chunky, Healthy Request, chicken noodle	1 cup	120	3	1	480	15	1	7
Campbell's Chunky, Healthy Request, vegetable	1 cup	118	0	0	480	24	4	4
Campbell's Chunky, hearty bean & ham	1 cup	181	2	1	779	30	8	11

ITEM DESCRIPTION	Serving Size	Calories	Total Fat (g)	Saturated Fat (g)	Sodium (mg)	Carbohydrates (g)	Fiber (g)	Protein (g)
Campbell's Chunky, hearty chicken w/ vegetable	1 cup	93	1	1	789	13	2	7
Campbell's Chunky, herb roasted chicken, potatoes, garlic	1 cup	113	1	1	870	17	3	8
Campbell's Chunky, Manhattan clam chowder	1 cup	127	4	1	831	19	3	5
Campbell's Chunky, New England clam chowder	1 cup	211	9	1	889	25	5	7
Campbell's Chunky, old fashioned potato & ham chowder	1 cup	191	11	4	801	17	2	6
Campbell's Chunky, old fashioned vegetable beef	1 cup	130	3	1	889	18	4	9
Campbell's Chunky, roadhouse beef bean chili	1 cup	233	8	4	870	25	8	15
Campbell's Chunky, Salisbury steak w/ mushrooms & onions	1 cup	152	5	2	889	19	5	9
Campbell's Chunky, savory chicken w/ white & wild rice	1 cup	118	2	1	811	18	2	7
Campbell's Chunky, savory pot roast	1 cup	118	1	1	880	18	3	8
Campbell's Chunky, savory vegetable	1 cup	108	1	1	769	22	4	3
Campbell's Chunky, slow roasted beef w/ mushrooms	1 cup	118	1	1	831	18	3	8
Campbell's Chunky, split pea & ham	1 cup	169	3	1	779	27	4	12
Campbell's Chunky, steak & potato	1 cup	130	2	1	921	18	2	10
Campbell's Healthy Request, chicken w/ rice, condensed	1/2 cup	73	2	1	480	9	1	2
Campbell's Healthy Request, cream of celery, condensed	1/2 cup	67	2	0	480	12	1	1
Campbell's Healthy Request, cream of chicken, condensed	1/2 cup	81	3	1	460	12	1	2
Campbell's Healthy Request, cream of mushroom, condensed	1/2 cup	69	2	1	470	10	1	2
Campbell's Healthy Request, homestyle chicken noodle, condensed	1/2 cup	60	2	1	480	8	1	3

ITEM DESCRIPTION	Serving Size	Calories	Total Fat (g)	Saturated Fat (g)	Sodium (mg)	Carbohydrates (g)	Fiber (g)	Protein (g)
Campbell's Healthy Request, minestrone, condensed	1/2 cup	80	1	0	460	15	3	3
Campbell's Healthy Request, tomato, condensed	1/2 cup	91	2	1	470	17	1	2
Campbell's Healthy Request, vegetable, condensed	1/2 cup	100	1	0	480	19	3	4
Campbell's Red & White, 25% less sodium, chicken noodle, condensed	1/2 cup	60	2	1	660	8	1	3
Campbell's Red & White, 25% less sodium, cream of mushroom, condensed	1/2 cup	110	8	1	650	9	2	1
Campbell's Red & White, 25% less sodium, tomato, condensed	1/2 cup	91	0	0	529	20	1	2
Campbell's Red & White, 98% fat free, broccoli cheese, condensed	1/2 cup	71	2	1	790	12	1	3
Campbell's Red & White, 98% fat free, cream of broccoli, condensed	1/2 cup	69	2	1	701	10	2	2
Campbell's Red & White, 98% fat free, cream of celery, condensed	1/2 cup	60	3	1	580	8	1	1
Campbell's Red & White, 98% fat free, cream of chicken, condensed	1/2 cup	69	3	1	590	10	1	2
Campbell's Red & White, 98% fat free, cream of mushroom, condensed	1/2 cup	69	3	1	630	9	1	2
Campbell's Red & White, bean w/ bacon, condensed	1/2 cup	170	4	2	860	25	8	8
Campbell's Red & White, beef consomme, condensed	1/2 cup	20	0	0	810	1	0	4
Campbell's Red & White, beef noodle, condensed	1/2 cup	71	2	1	820	8	1	4
Campbell's Red & White, beef w/ vegetable & barley, condensed	1/2 cup	89	2	1	890	15	3	5
Campbell's Red & White, beefy mushroom, condensed	1/2 cup	50	2	1	890	6	0	3
Campbell's Red & White, broccoli cheese, condensed	1/2 cup	100	5	2	820	12	0	2
Campbell's Red & White, cheddar cheese, condensed	1/2 cup	110	5	2	890	12	1	2

ITEM DESCRIPTION	Serving Size	Calories	Total Fat (g)	Saturated Fat (g)	Sodium (mg)	Carbohydrates (g)	Fiber (g)	Protein (g)
Campbell's Red & White, chicken alphabet, condensed	1/2 cup	71	2	1	660	11	1	4
Campbell's Red & White, chicken & dumplings, condensed	1/2 cup	71	2	1	760	10	1	3
Campbell's Red & White, chicken & stars, condensed	1/2 cup	71	2	1	640	10	1	3
Campbell's Red & White, chicken gumbo, condensed	1/2 cup	60	1	1	869	10	1	2
Campbell's Red & White, chicken noodle, condensed	1/2 cup	60	2	1	890	8	1	3
Campbell's Red & White, chicken noodle, Noodleo's, condensed	1/2 cup	79	2	1	620	12	1	4
Campbell's Red & White, chicken vegetable, condensed	1/2 cup	79	1	1	890	15	2	3
Campbell's Red & White, chicken w/ rice, condensed	1/2 cup	71	2	1	820	13	1	2
Campbell's Red & White, chicken wonton, condensed	1/2 cup	60	1	1	869	8	0	4
Campbell's Red & White, cream of asparagus, condensed	1/2 cup	110	7	2	830	9	3	2
Campbell's Red & White, cream of broccoli, condensed	1/2 cup	91	4	1	750	12	1	2
Campbell's Red & White, cream of celery, condensed	1/2 cup	91	6	1	861	9	3	1
Campbell's Red & White, cream of chicken, condensed	1/2 cup	120	8	3	870	10	2	3
Campbell's Red & White, cream of chicken w/ herbs, condensed	1/2 cup	81	4	1	810	9	2	2
Campbell's Red & White, cream of mushroom, condensed	1/2 cup	100	6	2	870	9	2	1
Campbell's Red & White, cream of mushroom w/ roasted garlic, condensed	1/2 cup	69	3	1	711	11	2	2
Campbell's Red & White, cream of onion, condensed	1/2 cup	100	6	2	800	10	3	1
Campbell's Red & White, cream of potato, condensed	1/2 cup	91	2	1	800	15	2	2

ITEM DESCRIPTION	Serving Size	Calories	Total Fat (g)	Saturated Fat (g)	Sodium (mg)	Carbohydrates (g)	Fiber (g)	Protein (g)
Campbell's Red & White, cream of shrimp, condensed	1/2 cup	91	5	1	861	8	1	2
Campbell's Red & White, creamy chicken noodle, condensed	1/2 cup	120	7	2	870	11	4	4
Campbell's Red & White, curly noodle, condensed	1/2 cup	79	2	0	630	11	1	4
Campbell's Red & White, double noodle in chicken broth, condensed	1/2 cup	100	2	1	620	17	2	4
Campbell's Red & White, fiesta nacho cheese, condensed	1/2 cup	120	8	3	790	10	1	3
Campbell's Red & White, French onion, condensed	1/2 cup	45	2	1	900	6	1	2
Campbell's Red & White, golden mushroom, condensed	1/2 cup	81	4	1	890	10	1	2
Campbell's Red & White, green pea, condensed	1/2 cup	180	3	1	870	28	4	9
Campbell's Red & White, homestyle chicken noodle, condensed	1/2 cup	71	2	1	706	8	1	4
Campbell's Red & White, Italian style wedding, condensed	1/2 cup	89	2	1	810	12	3	4
Campbell's Red & White, lentil, condensed	1/2 cup	140	1	1	800	24	6	9
Campbell's Red & White, Manhattan clam chowder, condensed	1/2 cup	71	1	1	879	12	2	2
Campbell's Red & White, mega noodle, condensed	1/2 cup	89	2	1	600	14	2	4
Campbell's Red & White, minestrone, condensed	1/2 cup	89	1	1	960	17	3	4
Campbell's Red & White, New England clam chowder, condensed	1/2 cup	89	2	1	879	13	1	4
Campbell's Red & White, old fashioned tomato rice, condensed	1/2 cup	110	2	1	770	23	1	1
Campbell's Red & White, pepper pot, condensed	1/2 cup	89	4	1	980	9	1	5
Campbell's Red & White, Southwest-style chicken vegetable, condensed	1/2 cup	110	1	1	830	21	4	5

ITEM DESCRIPTION	Serving Size	Calories	Total Fat (g)	Saturated Fat (g)	Sodium (mg)	Carbohydrates (g)	Fiber (g)	Protein (g)
Campbell's Red & White, split pea w/ ham & bacon, condensed	1/2 cup	180	3	2	850	27	5	10
Campbell's Red & White, tomato bisque, condensed	1/2 cup	130	4	1	879	23	1	2
Campbell's Red & White, tomato, condensed	1/2 cup	91	0	0	711	20	1	2
Campbell's Red & White, vegetable beef, condensed	1/2 cup	79	1	1	890	15	3	5
Campbell's Red & White, vegetable, condensed	1/2 cup	100	1	1	890	20	3	4
Campbell's Select, 98% fat free, New England clam chowder	1 cup	105	2	0	870	16	3	6
Campbell's Select, chicken w/ egg noodles	1 cup	100	3	1	480	13	2	7
Campbell's Select, Italian-style wedding	1 cup	110	3	1	789	15	2	7
Campbell's Select, Mexican style chicken tortilla	1 cup	127	3	1	921	18	3	8
Campbell's Select, minestrone	1 cup	96	0	0	899	19	4	4
Campbell's Select, savory chicken & long grain rice	1 cup	93	0	0	970	15	1	7
Campbell's Soup at Hand, chicken & stars	1 serv	64	1	1	891	10	2	3
Campbell's Soup at Hand, chicken w/ mini noodles	1 serv	79	2	1	979	11	2	4
Campbell's Soup at Hand, cream of broccoli	1 serv	143	7	2	891	17	7	3
Campbell's Soup at Hand, creamy chicken	1 serv	131	9	2	891	13	4	4
Campbell's Soup at Hand, creamy tomato	1 serv	189	4	1	939	34	4	4
Campbell's Soup at Hand, New England clam chowder	1 serv	122	6	1	891	13	4	4
Campbell's Soup at Hand, vegetable beef	1 serv	61	1	1	930	10	1	3
Healthy Choice, bean & ham	1 cup	180	2.5	1	480	28	6	11
Healthy Choice, beef pot roast	1 cup	110	.5	0	470	19	3	7
Healthy Choice, chicken & rice, canned	1 cup	89	1	0	434	14	2	6

ITEM DESCRIPTION	Serving Size	Calories	Total Fat (g)	Saturated Fat (g)	Sodium (mg)	Carbohydrates (g)	Fiber (g)	Protein (g)
Healthy Choice, chicken noodle, canned	1 cup	100	2	1	474	13	2	9
Healthy Choice, country vegetable	1 cup	90	.5	0	480	18	4	4
Healthy Choice, garden vegetable, canned	1 cup	125	1	0	480	25	5	5
Healthy Choice, Italian-style wedding	1 cup	120	2.5	1	430	16	3	9
Healthy Choice, split pea & ham	1 cup	160	2.5	1	470	27	6	12
Healthy Choice, vegetable beef	1 cup	130	1.5	0	420	21	4	9
Progresso Beef Pot Roast	1 cup	120	2	.5	690	16	2	8
Progresso Chicken Noodle	1 cup	100	2.5	.5	690	12	1	7
Progresso Chicken & Wild Rice	1 cup	100	1.5	.5	650	15	1	6
Progresso Creamy Mushroom	1 cup	120	8	2	890	9	1	2
Progresso Lentil	1 cup	160	2	.5	810	30	5	9
Progresso Minestrone	1 cup	100	2	.5	690	20	4	4
Progresso New England Clam Chowder	1 cup	180	8	2	860	22	2	5
Progresso Tomato Basil	1 cup	150	3	.5	680	29	2	3
Progresso Vegetable	1 cup	80	0	0	660	15	3	5
SOUR CREAM								
Cultured	1 tbsp	23	2	1	10	0	0	0
Imitation, cultured	2 tbsp	60	6	5	29	2	0	1
Kraft Breakstone's, fat free	2 tbsp	29	0	0	23	5	0	2
Kraft Breakstone's, reduced fat	2 tbsp	47	4	2	18	2	0	1
Reduced fat, cultured	1 tbsp	20	2	1	6	1	0	0
SOYBEAN OIL								
Hydrogenated, w/ cottonseed	1 tbsp	120	14	2	0	0	0	0
Lecithin	1 tbsp	104	14	2	0	0	0	0
Partially hydrogenated	1 tbsp	120	14	2	0	0	0	0
Regular	1 tbsp	120	14	2	0	0	0	0
SOYBEANS								
Boiled	1 cup	298	15	2	2	17	10	29
Curd cheese	1 cup	340	18	3	45	16	0	28
Dry roasted	1 cup	776	37	5	3	56	14	68
Fresh	1 cup	830	37	5	4	56	17	68
Green, boiled	1 cup	254	12	1	25	20	8	22
Green, fresh	1 cup	376	17	2	38	28	11	33

ITEM DESCRIPTION	Serving Size	Calories	Total Fat (g)	Saturated Fat (g)	Sodium (mg)	Carbohydrates (g)	Fiber (g)	Protein (g)
Roasted	1 cup	810	44	6	7	58	30	61
Sprouted, fresh	1 cup	85	5	1	10	7	1	9
Sprouted, steamed	1 cup	76	4	1	9	6	1	8
Sprouted, steamed, w/ salt	1 cup	76	4	1	231	6	1	8
SOY CHIPS (or crisps, salted)	1 oz	107	2	0	239	15	1	8
SOY CREAMER								
Silk French Vanilla Creamer	1 tbsp	20	1	0	10	3	0	0
Silk Hazelnut Creamer	1 tbsp	20	1	0	10	3	0	0
Silk Original Creamer	1 tbsp	15	1	0	10	1	0	0
SOY FLOUR								
Defatted	1 cup	346	1	0	21	40	18	49
Defatted, crude protein, stirred	1 cup	372	9	1	9	31	16	50
Full fat, fresh, crude protein, stirred	1 cup	369	18	3	11	27	8	32
Full fat, fresh, stirred	1 cup	366	17	3	11	30	8	29
Full fat, roasted, crude protein, stirred	1 cup	373	19	3	10	26	8	32
Full fat, roasted, stirred	1 cup	375	19	3	10	29	8	30
Low fat, crude protein, stirred	1 cup	325	6	1	16	30	9	45
Low fat, stirred	1 cup	330	8	1	8	31	14	40
SOY MEAL (defatted, fresh)	1 cup	414	3	0	4	49	0	55
SOYMILK								
All flavors, enhanced	1 cup	109	5	1	122	8	1	7
All flavors, lowfat	1 cup	100	2	0	90	18	2	4
All flavors, nonfat	1 cup	66	0	0	139	10	1	6
All flavors, unsweetened	1 cup	80	4	1	90	4	1	7
Chocolate	1 cup	153	4	1	129	24	1	5
Chocolate & other flavors, light	1 cup	114	2	0	112	20	2	5
Original & vanilla	1 cup	104	4	0	114	12	1	6
Original & vanilla, light	1 cup	73	2	0	117	9	1	6
Original & vanilla, light, unsweetened	1 cup	83	2	0	153	9	2	6
Silk, chai	1 cup	129	4	1	100	19	0	6
Silk, chocolate	1 cup	141	4	1	100	23	2	5
Silk, coffee	1 cup	151	4	1	100	25	0	5
Silk, light, chocolate	1 cup	119	2	0	100	22	2	5

ITEM DESCRIPTION	Serving Size	Calories	Total Fat (g)	Saturated Fat (g)	Sodium (mg)	Carbohydrates (g)	Fiber (g)	Protein (g)
Silk, light, plain	1 cup	70	2	0	119	8	1	6
Silk, light, vanilla	1 cup	80	2	0	95	10	1	6
Silk, mocha	1 cup	141	4	1	100	22	0	5
Silk, nog	1/2 cup	90	2	0	74	15	0	3
Silk, plain	1 cup	100	4	1	119	8	1	7
Silk Plus Fiber	1 cup	100	4	1	95	14	5	6
Silk Plus, for bone health	1 cup	100	4	1	95	11	2	6
Silk Plus Omega-3 DHA	1 cup	109	5	1	119	8	1	7
Silk, unsweetened	1 cup	80	4	1	85	4	1	7
Silk, vanilla	1 cup	100	4	1	95	10	1	6
Silk, very vanilla	1 cup	129	4	1	141	19	1	6
Vitasoy, light, vanilla	1 cup	73	2	0	119	10	0	4
Vitasoy Organic Classic Original Soymilk	1 cup	114	4	1	160	11	1	8
Vitasoy Organic Creamy Original Soymilk	1 cup	107	4	0	160	11	1	7
SOY PROTEIN								
Concentrate, acid wash	1 oz	94	0	0	255	9	2	16
Concentrate, alcohol extraction	1 oz	94	0	0	1	9	2	16
Isolate	1 oz	96	1	0	285	2	2	23
Isolate, potassium type	1 oz	92	0	0	14	3	2	23
SOY SAUCE								
Made from hydrolyzed vegetable protein	1 tbsp	7	0	0	1024	1	0	0
Made from soy & wheat (shoyu)	1 tbsp	8	0	0	902	1	0	1
Made from soy & wheat (shoyu), low sodium	1 tbsp	8	0	0	533	1	0	1
Made from soy (tamari)	1 tbsp	11	0	0	1005	1	0	2
SOY YOGURT								
Silk, banana strawberry	1 container	150	2	0	26	29	1	4
Silk, black cherry	1 container	150	2	0	20	29	1	4
Silk, blueberry	1 container	150	2	0	26	29	1	4
Silk, key lime	1 container	150	2	0	26	30	1	4
Silk, peach	1 container	160	2	0	26	32	1	4

ITEM DESCRIPTION	Serving Size	Calories	Total Fat (g)	Saturated Fat (g)	Sodium (mg)	Carbohydrates (g)	Fiber (g)	Protein (g)
...ilk, plain	1 container	150	4	0	30	22	1	6
...ilk, raspberry	1 container	150	2	0	26	30	1	4
...ilk, strawberry	1 container	160	2	0	26	31	1	4
...ilk, vanilla, family size	1 container	179	4	0	30	31	1	6
...ilk, vanilla, single serving	1 container	150	3	0	20	25	1	5
SPAGHETTI SAUCE								
...marinara, ready to serve)	1 cup	224	7	2	1054	35	7	5
SPAGHETTI SQUASH								
...oiled or baked	1 cup	42	0	0	28	10	2	1
...resh, cubed	1 cup	31	1	0	17	7	0	1
SPAM								
...ormel luncheon meat, pork & chicken, canned, light	2 oz	107	8	3	578	1	0	9
...ormel luncheon meat, pork w/ ham, canned	2 oz	174	15	6	767	2	0	7
SPEARMINT								
...ried	1 tbsp	5	0	0	6	1	0	0
...resh	2 tbsp	5	0	0	3	1	1	0
SPELT (cooked)	1 cup	246	2	0	10	51	8	11
SPICES								
...regano, dried	1 tsp	3	0	0	0	1	0	0
...arragon, dried	1 tsp	2	0	0	0	0	0	0
...hyme, dried	1 tsp	3	0	0	1	1	0	0
SPINACH								
...oiled	1 cup	41	0	0	126	7	4	5
...anned	1 cup	44	1	0	746	7	4	5
...anned, drained	1 cup	49	1	0	58	7	5	6
...anned, no salt	1 cup	44	1	0	176	7	5	5
...resh	1 cup	7	0	0	24	1	1	1
...rozen, chopped or leaf	1 cup	45	1	0	115	7	5	6
...rozen, chopped or leaf, boiled	10 oz pkg	75	2	0	213	11	8	9
...ew Zealand, boiled, chopped	1 cup	22	0	0	193	4	0	2
...ew Zealand, fresh, chopped	1 cup	8	0	0	73	1	0	1
SPINACH SOUFFLÉ	1 cup	233	18	8	770	8	1	11

ITEM DESCRIPTION	Serving Size	Calories	Total Fat (g)	Saturated Fat (g)	Sodium (mg)	Carbohydrates (g)	Fiber (g)	Protein (g)
SPLIT PEAS								
Boiled	1 cup	231	1	0	4	41	16	16
Fresh	1 cup	672	2	0	30	119	50	48
SPORTS DRINKS								
Fluid replacement, electrolyte solution	8 fl oz	25	0	0	252	6	0	0
Fruit flavored, low calorie	8 fl oz	26	0	0	84	7	0	0
Gatorade, Frost	8 fl oz	50	0	0	110	14	0	0
Gatorade, Fruit Punch	8 fl oz	25	0	0	110	7	0	0
Gatorade, Orange	8 fl oz	50	0	0	110	14	0	0
Powerade, Fruit Punch	8 fl oz	50	0	0	100	14	0	0
Powerade, Lemon Lime	8 fl oz	50	0	0	100	14	0	0
Powerade, Mountain Berry Blast	8 fl oz	50	0	0	100	14	0	0
Propel Fitness Water, fruit flavored	8 fl oz	12	0	0	31	3	0	0
SPOT (cooked in dry heat)	3 oz	134	5	2	31	0	0	20
SPRING ONIONS (fresh, chopped)	1 tbsp	2	0	0	1	0	0	0
SQUID (fried)	3 oz	149	6	2	260	7	0	15
STRAWBERRIES								
Canned in heavy syrup	1 cup	234	1	0	10	60	4	1
Fresh, halved	1 cup	49	0	0	2	12	3	1
Frozen, sweetened, whole	1 cup	199	0	0	3	54	5	1
Frozen, sweetened, slices	1 cup	245	0	0	8	66	5	1
Frozen, unsweetened	1 cup	77	0	0	4	20	5	1
STRAWBERRY-FLAVOR DRINK								
(mix, powder, prepared w/ whole milk)	8 fl oz	234	8	5	128	33	0	8
STRAWBERRY TOPPING	2 tbsp	107	0	0	9	28	0	0
STRIPED BASS (cooked in dry heat)	3 oz	105	3	1	75	0	0	19
STUFFING								
Brownberry, sage & onion mix	1 serv	261	3	1	1126	49	4	9
Stove Top, chicken flavor, prepared	1/2 cup	107	1	0	429	20	1	4
STURGEON								
Cooked in dry heat	3 oz	115	4	1	59	0	0	18
Smoked	1 oz	49	1	0	210	0	0	9

ITEM DESCRIPTION	Serving Size	Calories	Total Fat (g)	Saturated Fat (g)	Sodium (mg)	Carbohydrates (g)	Fiber (g)	Protein (g)
SUCCOTASH								
Boiled	1 cup	221	2	0	33	47	9	10
Canned, w/ cream style corn	1 cup	205	1	0	652	47	8	7
Canned, w/ whole kernel corn	1 cup	161	1	0	564	36	7	7
Frozen, boiled	1 cup	158	2	0	76	34	7	7
SUCKER (white, cooked in dry heat)	3 oz	101	3	0	43	0	0	18
SUGAR								
Brown	1 cup	836	0	0	62	216	0	0
Granulated	1 tsp	16	0	0	0	4	0	0
Maple	1 tsp	11	0	0	0	3	0	0
Powdered, sifted	1 cup	389	0	0	1	100	0	0
Powdered, unsifted	1 cup	467	0	0	1	120	0	0
SUMMER SQUASH								
All varieties, boiled, slices	1 cup	36	1	0	2	8	3	2
All varieties, fresh, slices	1 cup	18	0	0	2	4	1	1
SUNFISH (pumpkin seed, cooked in dry heat)	3 oz	97	1	0	88	0	0	21
SUNFLOWER OIL								
High oleic, 70% & over	1 tbsp	124	14	1	0	0	0	0
Linoleic, 65%	1 tbsp	120	14	1	0	0	0	0
Linoleic, hydrogenated	1 tbsp	120	14	2	0	0	0	0
Linoleic, less than 60%	1 tbsp	120	14	1	0	0	0	0
SUNFLOWER SEED BUTTER								
w/o salt	1 tbsp	93	8	1	0	4	0	3
w/ salt	1 tbsp	93	8	1	83	4	0	3
SUNFLOWER SEED FLOUR (part defatted)	1 cup	209	1	0	2	23	3	31
SUNFLOWER SEEDS								
Dry roasted, w/ salt	1 cup	745	64	7	525	31	12	25
Oil roasted, w/o salt	1 cup	799	69	10	4	31	14	27
Oil roasted, w/ salt	1 cup	799	69	10	554	31	14	27
Toasted, w/o salt	1 cup	829	76	8	4	28	15	23
Toasted, w/ salt	1 cup	829	76	8	821	28	15	23
SURIMI	3 oz	84	1	0	122	6	0	13

ITEM DESCRIPTION	Serving Size	Calories	Total Fat (g)	Saturated Fat (g)	Sodium (mg)	Carbohydrates (g)	Fiber (g)	Protein (g)
SWAMP CABBAGE								
Boiled, chopped	1 cup	20	0	0	120	4	2	2
Fresh, chopped	1 cup	11	0	0	63	2	1	1
SWEETENERS								
Aspartame, Equal	1 tsp	13	0	0	0	3	0	0
Fructose, dry, powder	1 tsp	15	0	0	1	4	0	0
Saccharine	1 pckt	4	0	0	4	1	0	0
Sucralose, Splenda	1 pckt	3	0	0	0	1	0	0
SWEET POTATO CHIPS	1 oz	141	7	1	10	18	1	1
SWEET POTATOES								
Canned in syrup	1 cup	203	0	0	100	48	6	2
Canned in syrup, drained	1 cup	212	1	0	76	50	6	3
Canned, mashed	1 cup	258	1	0	191	59	4	5
Canned, vacuum packed, mashed	1 cup	232	1	0	135	54	5	4
Cooked, baked in skin (5" long x 2" dia)	1 potato	103	0	0	41	24	4	2
Cooked, boiled, w/o skin, mashed	1 cup	249	0	0	89	58	8	4
Cooked, candied, homemade (2-1/1" x 2" dia)	1 pc	151	3	1	74	29	3	1
Fresh, cubed	1 cup	114	0	0	73	27	4	2
Frozen, baked, cubed	1 cup	176	0	0	14	41	3	3
Leaves, fresh, chopped	1 cup	12	0	0	3	2	1	1
Leaves, steamed	1 cup	22	0	0	8	5	1	1
SWISS CHARD								
Boiled, chopped	1 cup	35	0	0	313	7	4	3
Fresh	1 cup	7	0	0	77	1	1	1
SWORDFISH (cooked in dry heat)	3 oz	132	4	1	98	0	0	22
TABASCO SAUCE	1 tsp	1	0	0	30	0	0	0
TACO SAUCE								
Pace Green	2 tbsp	4	0	0	100	1	0	0
Pace Red	1 tbsp	8	0	0	130	2	0	0
TACO SEASONING MIX (Pace)	2 tbsp	10	0	0	428	3	1	0
TACO SHELLS baked (5" dia)	1	59	3	1	49	8	1	1

ITEM DESCRIPTION	Serving Size	Calories	Total Fat (g)	Saturated Fat (g)	Sodium (mg)	Carbohydrates (g)	Fiber (g)	Protein (g)
TAMARIND								
Nectar, canned	1 cup	143	0	0	18	37	1	0
Fresh	1 fruit	5	0	0	1	1	0	0
TANGERINE JUICE								
Canned, sweetened	1 cup	124	1	0	2	30	1	1
Fresh	1 cup	106	0	0	2	25	1	1
Frozen concentrate, sweetened	1 cup	111	0	0	2	27	0	1
TANGERINES								
Canned in juice	1 cup	92	0	0	12	24	2	2
Canned in juice, drained	1 cup	72	0	0	9	18	2	1
Canned in light syrup	1 cup	154	0	0	15	41	2	1
Fresh (2-1/4" dia)	1 fruit	40	0	0	2	10	1	1
TAPIOCA (pearl, dry)	1 cup	544	0	0	2	135	1	0
TARO								
Cooked, slices	1 cup	187	0	0	20	46	7	1
Fresh, slices	1 cup	116	0	0	11	28	4	2
Leaves, fresh	1 cup	12	0	0	1	2	1	1
Leaves, steamed	1 cup	35	1	0	3	6	3	4
Shoots, cooked, slices	1 cup	20	0	0	3	4	0	1
Shoots, fresh, slices	1 cup	9	0	0	1	2	0	1
Tahitian, cooked, slices	1 cup	60	1	0	74	9	0	6
Tahitian, fresh, slices	1 cup	55	1	0	62	9	0	3
Tomatoes, green, fresh	1 cup	41	0	0	23	9	2	2
TARO CHIPS	1 oz	141	7	2	97	19	2	1
TEA								
Brewed w/ distilled water	6 fl oz	2	0	0	0	1	0	0
Brewed w/ tap water	8 fl oz	2	0	0	7	1	0	0
Chamomile	6 fl oz	2	0	0	2	0	0	0
Herbal, other than chamomile	6 fl oz	2	0	0	2	0	0	0
Instant, sweetened w/ saccharine, lemon	8 fl oz	5	0	0	14	1	0	0
Instant, sweetened w/ sugar, lemon	8 fl oz	91	0	0	5	22	0	0
Instant, unsweetened	8 fl oz	2	0	0	10	0	0	0
TEA SEED OIL	1 tbsp	120	14	3	0	0	0	0

ITEM DESCRIPTION	Serving Size	Calories	Total Fat (g)	Saturated Fat (g)	Sodium (mg)	Carbohydrates (g)	Fiber (g)	Protein (g)
TEMPEH	1 cup	320	18	4	15	16	0	31
TEQUILA SUNRISE (canned)	1 fl oz	34	0	0	18	4	0	0
TERIYAKI SAUCE	1 tbsp	16	0	0	690	3	0	1
THYME (fresh)	1 tsp	1	0	0	0	0	0	0
TILAPIA (Beacon Light)	3 oz	85	1	0	35	1	0	15
TILEFISH (cooked in dry heat)	3 oz	125	4	1	50	0	0	21
TOASTER PASTRIES								
Brown sugar cinnamon	1 pastry	206	7	2	212	34	1	3
Fruit	1 pastry	211	6	1	180	37	1	3
Fruit, frosted	1 pastry	215	6	1	172	39	0	2
Kellogg's Low Fat Pop Tarts, frosted brown sugar cinnamon	1 pastry	188	3	1	210	39	1	2
Kellogg's Low Fat Pop Tarts, frosted chocolate fudge	1 pastry	190	3	1	249	40	1	3
Kellogg's Low Fat Pop Tarts, frosted strawberry	1 pastry	191	3	1	201	40	1	2
Kellogg's Low Fat Pop Tarts, strawberry	1 pastry	192	3	1	220	40	1	2
Kellogg's Pop Tarts, apple cinnamon	1 pastry	205	5	1	174	37	1	2
Kellogg's Pop Tarts, blueberry	1 pastry	212	7	1	207	36	1	2
Kellogg's Pop Tarts, brown sugar cinnamon	1 pastry	219	9	1	214	32	1	3
Kellogg's Pop Tarts, cherry	1 pastry	204	5	1	220	37	1	2
Kellogg's Pop Tarts, frosted blueberry	1 pastry	203	5	1	207	37	1	2
Kellogg's Pop Tarts, frosted brown sugar cinnamon	1 pastry	211	7	1	184	34	1	3
Kellogg's Pop Tarts, frosted cherry	1 pastry	204	5	1	220	37	1	2
Kellogg's Pop Tarts, frosted chocolate fudge	1 pastry	201	5	1	203	37	1	3
Kellogg's Pop Tarts, frosted chocolate vanilla cream	1 pastry	203	5	1	229	37	1	3
Kellogg's Pop Tarts, frosted grape	1 pastry	203	5	1	198	38	1	2
Kellogg's Pop Tarts, frosted raspberry	1 pastry	205	6	1	211	37	1	2

ITEM DESCRIPTION	Serving Size	Calories	Total Fat (g)	Saturated Fat (g)	Sodium (mg)	Carbohydrates (g)	Fiber (g)	Protein (g)
Kellogg's Pop Tarts, frosted strawberry	1 pastry	203	5	1	169	38	1	2
Kellogg's Pop Tarts, frosted wild berry	1 pastry	210	5	1	168	39	1	2
Kellogg's Pop Tarts, s'mores	1 pastry	204	5	1	199	36	1	3
Kellogg's Pop Tarts, strawberry	1 pastry	205	5	2	185	37	1	2
Pillsbury Toaster Strudel, Apple	1	190	9	3.5	200	25	1	2
Pillsbury Toaster Strudel, Blueberry	1	190	9	3.5	190	26	0	3
Pillsbury Toaster Strudel, Cream Cheese	1	200	11	4.5	220	23	0	0
Pillsbury Toaster Strudel, Strawberry	1	190	9	3.5	190	25	1	3
TOFU								
Dried, frozen (koyadofu)	1 pc	82	5	1	1	2	1	8
Ex firm, prepared w/ nigari	1/5 block	83	5	0	7	2	0	9
Firm, prepared w/ nigari	1/5 block	64	4	1	11	2	1	7
Fried	1 pc	35	3	0	2	1	1	2
Hard, prepared w/ nigari	1/4 block	178	12	2	2	5	1	15
Okara	1 cup	94	2	0	11	15	0	4
Salted & fermented (fuyu)	1 block	13	1	0	316	1	0	1
Soft, prepared w/ nigari	1/5 block	55	3	0	7	2	0	6
Mori-Nu, silken, ex firm	1 slice	46	2	0	53	2	0	6
Mori-Nu, silken, firm	1 slice	52	2	0	30	2	0	6
Mori-Nu, silken, lite, ex firm	1 slice	32	1	0	82	1	0	6
Mori-Nu, silken, lite, firm	1 slice	31	1	0	71	1	0	5
Mori-Nu, silken, soft	1 slice	46	2	0	4	2	0	4
Nasoya Lite, firm	1/4 pkg	43	1	0	27	1	1	7
Nasoya Organic, ex firm	1/5 pkg	77	4	1	3	2	1	8
Nasoya Organic, firm	1/5 pkg	66	3	0	3	2	1	7
Nasoya Organic, super firm, cubed	1/5 pkg	96	5	1	5	3	2	10
TOFU YOGURT	1 cup	246	5	1	92	42	1	9
TOMATILLOS (fresh)	1 med	11	0	0	0	2	1	0
TOMATO CHILI SAUCE								
Bottled, w/o salt	1 tbsp	18	0	0	3	5	0	0
Bottled, w/ salt	1 tbsp	18	0	0	228	3	1	0

ITEM DESCRIPTION	Serving Size	Calories	Total Fat (g)	Saturated Fat (g)	Sodium (mg)	Carbohydrates (g)	Fiber (g)	Protein (g)
TOMATO JUICE								
Campbell's	8 oz	49	0	0	680	10	2	2
Campbell's Healthy Request	8 oz	51	0	0	481	10	2	2
Campbell's, low sodium	8 oz	49	0	0	141	10	2	2
Campbell's Organic	8 oz	49	0	0	680	10	2	2
Canned, w/o salt	1 cup	41	0	0	24	10	1	2
Canned, w/ salt	1 cup	41	0	0	654	10	1	2
Tomato & vegetable, low sodium	1 cup	53	0	0	169	11	2	1
TOMATO PASTE								
Canned, w/o added salt	1/2 cup	107	1	0	128	25	5	6
Canned, w/ salt	1/2 cup	107	1	0	1035	25	5	6
TOMATO PUREE								
Canned, w/o salt	1 cup	95	1	0	70	22	5	4
Canned, w/ salt	1 cup	95	1	0	998	22	5	4
TOMATOES								
Cherry	1 cup	27	0	0	7	6	2	1
Orange, fresh	1 tomato	18	0	0	47	4	1	1
Red, canned, packed in tomato juice	1 cup	41	0	0	343	10	2	2
Red, canned, packed in tomato juice, no salt added	1 cup	41	0	0	24	10	2	2
Red, canned, stewed	1 cup	66	0	0	564	16	3	2
Red, canned, w/ green chilies	1 cup	36	0	0	966	9	0	2
Red, cooked	1 cup	43	0	0	26	10	2	2
Red, stewed	1 cup	80	3	1	460	13	2	2
Red, w/ salt	1 cup	43	0	0	593	10	2	2
Sun-dried	1 cup	139	2	0	1131	30	7	8
Sun-dried, packed in oil, drained	1 cup	234	15	2	293	26	6	6
Yellow, fresh, chopped	1 cup	21	0	0	32	4	1	1
TOMATO SAUCE								
Canned	1 cup	59	0	0	1284	13	4	3
Canned, Spanish style	1 cup	81	1	0	1152	18	3	4
Canned, w/ herbs & cheese	1 cup	144	5	2	1325	25	5	5
Canned, w/ mushrooms	1 cup	86	0	0	1107	21	4	4
Canned, w/ onions	1 cup	103	0	0	1350	24	4	4

ITEM DESCRIPTION	Serving Size	Calories	Total Fat (g)	Saturated Fat (g)	Sodium (mg)	Carbohydrates (g)	Fiber (g)	Protein (g)
Canned, w/ onions, green peppers & celery	1 cup	102	2	0	1365	22	4	2
Canned, w/ tomato tidbits	1 cup	78	1	0	37	17	3	3
No salt	1 cup	102	0	0	27	21	4	3
TOMATO SEED OIL	1 tbsp	120	14	3	0	0	0	0
TONIC WATER	1 fl oz	10	0	0	4	3	0	0
TORTILLA CHIPS								
Low fat, baked w/o fat	1 oz	118	2	0	119	23	2	3
Low fat, made w/ Olestra, nacho cheese	1 oz	90	1	0	171	18	2	2
Low fat, unsalted	1 oz	118	2	0	4	23	2	3
Nacho cheese	1 oz	146	7	1	174	18	1	2
Nacho, made w/ masa flour	1 oz	141	7	1	201	18	2	2
Nacho, reduced fat	1 oz	126	4	1	284	20	1	2
Plain	1 oz	139	7	1	119	19	2	2
Plain, yellow corn	1 oz	139	6	1	80	19	1	2
Ranch flavor	1 oz	142	7	1	147	18	1	2
Taco flavor	1 oz	136	7	1	223	18	2	2
Unsalted, white corn	1 cup	131	6	1	4	17	1	2
TORTILLAS								
Corn (6" dia)	1 tortilla	58	1	0	3	12	1	1
Flour (6" dia)	1 tortilla	94	2	1	191	15	1	2
Mission Foods Flour Tortillas, soft taco (8")	1 serv	146	3	0	249	25	0	4
TOWEL GOURD								
Boiled (1" pcs)	1 cup	100	1	0	37	26	0	1
Fresh (1" pcs)	1 cup	19	0	0	3	4	0	1
TRAIL MIX								
Regular	1 cup	693	44	8	344	67	0	21
Reg, unsalted	1 cup	693	44	8	15	67	0	21
Reg, w/ chocolate chips, salted nuts & seeds	1 cup	707	47	9	177	66	0	21
Reg, w/ chocolate chips, unsalted nuts & seeds	1 cup	707	47	9	39	66	0	21
Tropical	1 cup	570	24	12	14	92	0	9

ITEM DESCRIPTION	Serving Size	Calories	Total Fat (g)	Saturated Fat (g)	Sodium (mg)	Carbohydrates (g)	Fiber (g)	Protein (g)
TREE FERN (cooked, chopped)	1/2 cup	28	0	0	4	8	3	0
TROUT								
Cooked in dry heat	3 oz	162	7	1	57	0	0	23
Rainbow, farmed, cooked in dry heat	3 oz	144	6	2	36	0	0	21
Rainbow, wild, cooked in dry heat	3 oz	128	5	1	48	0	0	19
TUNA								
Bluefin, fresh, cooked in dry heat	3 oz	156	5	1	42	0	0	25
Canned in oil, drained	3 oz	158	7	1	337	0	0	23
Canned in oil, w/o salt, drained	3 oz	168	7	1	42	0	0	25
Canned in water, drained	3 oz	99	1	0	287	0	0	22
Canned in water, w/o salt, drained	3 oz	99	1	0	42	0	0	22
Skipjack, fresh, cooked in dry heat	3 oz	112	1	0	40	0	0	24
White, canned in oil, drained	3 oz	158	7	1	337	0	0	23
White, canned in oil, w/o salt, drained	3 oz	158	7	1	42	0	0	23
White, canned in water, drained	3 oz	109	3	1	320	0	0	20
White, canned in water, w/o salt, drained	3 oz	109	3	1	42	0	0	20
Yellowfin, fresh	3 oz	92	1	0	31	0	0	20
Yellowfin, fresh, cooked in dry heat	3 oz	118	1	0	40	0	0	25
TUNA SALAD	3 oz	159	8	1	342	8	0	14
TURBOT (European, cooked in dry heat)	3 oz	104	3	0	163	0	0	17
TURKEY								
Back, w/ skin, roasted, chopped	1 cup	340	20	6	102	0	0	37
Breast meat (3-1/2" sq)	1 slice	22	0	0	213	1	0	4
Breast, pre-basted, w/ skin, roasted	4 oz	143	4	1	450	0	0	25
Breast, smoked, lemon pepper flavor, 97% fat free	1 slice	27	0	0	325	0	0	6
Breast, w/ skin, roasted	4 oz	214	8	2	71	0	0	33
Canned, meat only, broth drained	1 cup	220	9	3	630	0	0	32
Cooked	1 cup, pcs	313	23	7	1874	3	0	24
Dark meat, roasted, chopped	1 cup	262	10	3	111	0	0	40
Dark meat, w/ skin, roasted, chopped	1 cup	309	16	5	106	0	0	38

ITEM DESCRIPTION	Serving Size	Calories	Total Fat (g)	Saturated Fat (g)	Sodium (mg)	Carbohydrates (g)	Fiber (g)	Protein (g)
fryer-roasters, breast, meat only, roasted	4 oz	153	1	0	59	0	0	34
fryer-roasters, breast, w/ skin, roasted	4 oz	174	4	1	60	0	0	33
fryer-roasters, dark meat, meat only, roasted, chopped	1 cup	227	6	2	111	0	0	40
fryer-roasters, leg, meat only, roasted	1 leg	356	8	3	181	0	0	65
fryer-roasters, leg, w/ skin, roasted	1 leg	416	13	4	196	0	0	70
fryer-roasters, light meat, meat only, roasted, chopped	1 cup	196	2	1	78	0	0	42
fryer-roasters, meat only, roasted, chopped	1 cup	210	4	1	94	0	0	41
fryer-roasters, wing, meat only, roasted	1 wing	98	2	1	47	0	0	19
fryer-roasters, wing, w/ skin, roasted	1 wing	186	9	2	66	0	0	25
Giblets, simmered, some giblet fat, chopped	1 cup	289	17	6	93	1	0	30
Gizzards, simmered	1 gizzard	108	3	1	56	0	0	18
Ground, cooked (4 oz)	1 patty	193	11	3	88	0	0	22
Heart, simmered	1 heart	29	1	0	19	0	0	5
Light & dark meat, seasoned, diced	3 oz	117	5	1	723	1	0	16
Light meat, roasted, chopped	1 cup	220	5	1	90	0	0	42
Light meat, w/ skin, roasted, chopped	1 cup	276	12	3	88	0	0	40
Liver, simmered	1 liver	227	17	6	46	1	0	17
Louis Rich	1 serv	35	3	1	170	0	0	2
Meat & skin, roasted, chopped	1 cup	291	14	4	95	0	0	39
Meat only, roasted, chopped	1 cup	238	7	2	98	0	0	41
Neck, meat only, simmered	1 neck	274	11	4	85	0	0	41
Patties, breaded, battered, fried (2-1/4 oz)	1 patty	181	12	3	512	10	0	9
Roast, boneless, frozen, seasoned, light & dark meat, roasted, chopped	1 cup	209	8	3	918	4	0	29
Sticks, breaded, battered, fried (2-1/4 oz)	1 stick	179	11	3	536	11	0	9

ITEM DESCRIPTION	Serving Size	Calories	Total Fat (g)	Saturated Fat (g)	Sodium (mg)	Carbohydrates (g)	Fiber (g)	Protein (g)
Thigh, pre-basted, w/ skin, roasted	1 thigh	493	27	8	1372	0	0	59
Wing, w/ skin, roasted	1 wing	426	23	6	113	0	0	51
TURKEY BOLOGNA (Louis Rich)	1 serv	52	4	1	302	1	0	3
TURKEY BREAST								
Carl Buddig, light & dark meat, smoked	2 oz	91	5	2	625	1	0	10
Louis Rich, Carving Board, smoked	1 serv	42	0	0	540	1	0	9
Louis Rich, fat free, oven roasted	1 serv	24	0	0	334	1	0	4
Louis Rich, honey roasted, fat free	1 serv	57	0	0	661	3	0	11
Louis Rich, oven roasted	1 serv	28	1	0	270	1	0	5
Louis Rich, portion fat free, oven roasted	1 serv	50	0	0	659	1	0	11
Louis Rich, portion fat free, smoked	1 serv	52	0	0	721	1	0	11
Louis Rich, smoked	1 serv	28	1	0	257	1	0	5
Oscar Mayer, fat free, smoked	1 slice	10	0	0	142	0	0	2
TURKEY FAT	1 tbsp	115	13	4	0	0	0	0
TURKEY HAM								
Cured, thigh meat	1 oz	35	1	0	312	1	0	5
Dark meat, smoked, frozen	1 oz	33	1	0	258	1	0	5
Ex lean, prepackaged or deli slices	1 cup, pcs	171	5	2	1432	4	0	27
Louis Rich Turkey Ham	1 serv	32	1	0	316	0	0	5
TURKEY NUGGETS (Louis Rich, breaded)	1 pc	77	5	1	190	4	0	4
TURKEY PASTRAMI	2 slices	76	4	1	559	1	0	9
TURKEY PEPPERONI (Hormel, slices)	1 serv	73	3	1	557	1	0	9
TURKEY POT PIE (frozen)	1 serv	699	35	11	1390	70	4	26
TURKEY ROLL								
Light & dark meat	2 slices	85	4	1	334	1	0	10
Light meat	1 slice, oval	25	0	0	271	1	0	4
TURKEY SALAMI								
Cooked	1 serv	47	3	1	281	0	0	5
Louis Rich Turkey Salami	1 serv	41	3	1	281	0	0	4
Louis Rich Turkey Salami Cotto	1 serv	42	3	1	285	0	0	4

ITEM DESCRIPTION	Serving Size	Calories	Total Fat (g)	Saturated Fat (g)	Sodium (mg)	Carbohydrates (g)	Fiber (g)	Protein (g)
TURKEY SAUSAGE								
Breakfast links, mild	1 oz link	65	5	1	164	0	0	4
Hot, smoked	1 oz link	44	2	1	260	1	0	4
Italian, smoked	1 oz link	44	2	0	260	1	0	4
Louis Rich Turkey Smoked Sausage	2 oz	90	6	1	530	2	0	8
Reduced fat, brown & serve	1 oz link	32	2	0	99	2	0	3
TURKEY TACO MEAT (frozen, cooked)	1 cup	271	14	3	1157	6	0	31
TURMERIC (ground)	1 tbsp	24	1	0	3	4	1	1
TURNIP GREENS								
Boiled, chopped	1 cup	29	0	0	42	6	5	2
Canned, no salt added	1 cup	27	0	0	42	4	2	2
Fresh, chopped	1 cup	18	0	0	22	4	2	1
Frozen, boiled	1 cup	48	1	0	25	8	6	5
TURNIPS								
Boiled, mashed	1 cup	51	0	0	37	12	5	2
Fresh	1 large	51	0	0	123	12	3	2
Frozen, boiled	1 cup	36	0	0	56	7	3	2
UCUHUBA BUTTER	1 tbsp	120	14	12	0	0	0	0
VANILLA EXTRACT								
Imitation, no alcohol	1 tbsp	7	0	0	0	2	0	0
Imitation, w/ alcohol	1 tbsp	31	0	0	1	0	0	0
Real	1 tbsp	37	0	0	1	2	0	0
VEAL								
Breast, fat, cooked	3 oz	443	45	18	42	0	0	8
Breast, plate half, boneless, braised	3 oz	240	16	6	54	0	0	22
Breast, point half, boneless, braised	3 oz	211	12	5	56	0	0	24
Breast, whole, boneless, braised	3 oz	226	14	6	55	0	0	23
Breast, whole, boneless, lean, braised	3 oz	185	8	3	58	0	0	26
Composite of retail cuts, fat, cooked	3 oz	546	57	28	48	0	0	8
Composite of retail cuts, lean & fat, cooked	3 oz	196	10	4	74	0	0	26
Composite of retail cuts, lean, cooked	3 oz	167	6	2	76	0	0	27
Cubed for stew, leg & shoulder, braised	3 oz	160	4	1	79	0	0	30

ITEM DESCRIPTION	Serving Size	Calories	Total Fat (g)	Saturated Fat (g)	Sodium (mg)	Carbohydrates (g)	Fiber (g)	Protein (g)
Ground, broiled	3 oz	146	6	3	71	0	0	21
Leg, top round, braised	3 oz	179	5	2	57	0	0	31
Leg, top round, pan fried, breaded	3 oz	202	8	3	386	8	0	23
Leg, top round, pan fried, not breaded	3 oz	179	7	3	65	0	0	27
Leg, top round, roasted	3 oz	136	4	2	58	0	0	24
Loin, braised	3 oz	241	15	6	68	0	0	26
Loin, lean, braised	3 oz	192	8	2	71	0	0	29
Loin, lean, roasted	3 oz	149	6	2	82	0	0	22
Loin, roasted	3 oz	184	10	4	79	0	0	21
Rib, braised	3 oz	213	11	4	81	0	0	28
Rib, roasted	3 oz	194	12	5	78	0	0	20
Shank, fore & hind, braised	3 oz	162	5	2	79	0	0	27
Shoulder, arm, braised	3 oz	201	9	3	74	0	0	29
Shoulder, arm, roasted	3 oz	156	7	3	76	0	0	22
Shoulder, blade, braised	3 oz	191	9	3	83	0	0	27
Shoulder, blade, roasted	3 oz	158	7	3	85	0	0	21
Sirloin, braised	3 oz	214	11	4	67	0	0	27
Sirloin, lean, braised	3 oz	173	6	2	69	0	0	29
Sirloin, lean, roasted	3 oz	143	5	2	72	0	0	22
Sirloin, roasted	3 oz	172	9	4	71	0	0	21
VEGETABLE BROTH								
Swanson	1 cup	12	0	0	940	3	0	0
Swanson Certified Organic	1 cup	12	0	0	550	3	0	0
VEGETABLE JUICE COCKTAIL								
(canned)	1 cup	46	0	0	653	11	2	2
VEGETABLE OIL (Enova)	1 tbsp	124	14	1	0	0	0	0
VEGETARIAN MEAT LOAF	1 slice	110	5	1	308	4	3	12
VEGETARIAN STEW	1 cup	304	7	1	988	17	3	42
VEGGIE BURGER								
Boca Meatless Burgers Original Vegan	1	70	.5	0	260	6	4	13
Fillets, vegetarian	1 fillet	246	15	2	416	8	5	20
Green Giant Harvest Burger, original, frozen	1 patty	138	4	1	411	7	6	18

ITEM DESCRIPTION	Serving Size	Calories	Total Fat (g)	Saturated Fat (g)	Sodium (mg)	Carbohydrates (g)	Fiber (g)	Protein (g)
Loma Linda Vege-Burger, canned	1/4 cup	63	1	0	122	2	1	12
Morningstar Farms Cheddar Burger, frozen	1 patty	142	7	2	458	10	3	13
Morningstar Farms Grillers, original, frozen	1 patty	136	6	1	270	5	3	15
Morningstar Farms Grillers, prime, frozen	1 patty	169	9	1	356	4	2	17
Morningstar Farms Grillers, recipe crumbles, frozen	2/3 cup	72	2	0	235	4	3	10
Morningstar Farms Grillers, vegan, frozen	1 patty	94	2	0	280	6	4	12
Morningstar Farms Mushroom Lover's Burger, frozen	1 patty	108	6	1	221	8	1	7
Morningstar Farms Spicy Black Bean Burger, frozen	1 patty	115	4	1	348	13	5	11
Morningstar Farms Tomato & Basil Pizza Burger, frozen	1 patty	121	6	1	261	7	3	10
Worthington Vegetarian Burger, canned	1/4 cup	69	2	0	248	3	2	10
Veggie or soy burgers	1 patty	124	4	1	398	10	3	11
VEGGIE PATTIES								
Morningstar Farms Asian Veggie Patties, frozen	1 patty	104	4	1	486	10	2	7
Morningstar Farms Breakfast Patties, frozen	1 patty	78	3	0	240	4	2	8
Morningstar Farms Garden Veggie Patties, frozen	1 patty	118	4	1	352	9	3	12
Morningstar Farms Veggie Medley, frozen	1 patty	119	4	0	264	11	2	11
Worthington Fripats, frozen	1 patty	134	6	1	331	5	2	15
VENISON								
Ground, pan fried	1 patty	174	8	4	73	0	0	25
Loin, steak, lean, broiled	1 serv	81	1	0	31	0	0	16
VINEGAR								
Balsamic	1 tbsp	14	0	0	4	3	0	0
Cider	1 tbsp	3	0	0	1	0	0	0

ITEM DESCRIPTION	Serving Size	Calories	Total Fat (g)	Saturated Fat (g)	Sodium (mg)	Carbohydrates (g)	Fiber (g)	Protein (g)
Distilled	1 tbsp	3	0	0	0	0	0	0
Red wine	1 tbsp	3	0	0	1	0	0	0
VODKA								
80 proof	1 fl oz	64	0	0	0	0	0	0
86 proof	1 fl oz	70	0	0	0	0	0	0
90 proof	1 fl oz	73	0	0	0	0	0	0
94 proof	1 fl oz	76	0	0	0	0	0	0
WAFFLES								
Buttermilk, frozen, microwaved (4" dia)	1	101	3	1	232	15	1	2
Buttermilk, frozen, toasted (4" dia)	1	102	3	1	234	16	1	2
Kashi Heart to Heart Waffles Original	2	160	3	0	370	31	3	6
Kellogg's Eggo Banana Bread Waffles	1	90	6	1	270	32	2	5
Kellogg's Eggo Golden Oat Waffles (4" dia)	1	69	1	0	135	13	1	2
Kellogg's Eggo Low Fat Blueberry Nutri-Grain Waffles (4" dia)	1	73	1	0	207	15	1	2
Kellogg's Eggo Low Fat Homestyle Waffles (4" dia)	1	83	1	0	155	15	0	2
Kellogg's Eggo Low Fat Nutri-Grain Waffles (4" dia)	1	71	1	0	215	14	1	2
Plain, frozen, microwaved (4" dia)	1	95	3	1	218	15	1	2
Plain, frozen, toasted (4" dia)	1	103	3	1	241	16	1	2
Plain, homemade (7" dia)	1	218	11	2	383	25	0	6
WALLEYE POLLOCK (cooked in dry heat)	3 oz	96	1	0	99	0	0	20
WALNUT OIL	1 tbsp	120	14	1	0	0	0	0
WALNUTS								
Black, dried, chopped	1 cup	772	74	4	2	12	9	30
English, chopped	1 cup	765	76	7	2	16	8	18
WASABI ROOT (fresh, slices)	1 cup	142	1	0	22	31	10	6
WATER								
Aquafina	1 fl oz	0	0	0	0	0	0	0
Calistoga	1 fl oz	0	0	0	0	0	0	0

ITEM DESCRIPTION	Serving Size	Calories	Total Fat (g)	Saturated Fat (g)	Sodium (mg)	Carbohydrates (g)	Fiber (g)	Protein (g)
Crystal Geyser	1 fl oz	0	0	0	0	0	0	0
Dannon	1 fl oz	0	0	0	0	0	0	0
Dannon Fluoride to Go	1 fl oz	0	0	0	0	0	0	0
Dasani	1 fl oz	0	0	0	0	0	0	0
Evian	1 fl oz	0	0	0	0	0	0	0
Fruit flavored, sweetened, w/ added vits & minerals	1 fl oz	0	0	0	0	2	0	0
Fruit flavored, sweetened, w/ low calorie sweetener	1 fl oz	0	0	0	1	0	0	0
Generic, bottled	1 fl oz	0	0	0	1	0	0	0
Naya	1 fl oz	0	0	0	0	0	0	0
Perrier	1 fl oz	0	0	0	0	0	0	0
Poland Spring	1 fl oz	0	0	0	0	0	0	0
Tap, municipal	1 fl oz	0	0	0	1	0	0	0
Tap, well	1 fl oz	0	0	0	1	0	0	0
WATER CHESTNUTS								
Canned, slices	1/2 cup	35	0	0	6	9	2	1
Fresh, slices	1/2 cup	60	0	0	9	15	2	1
WATERCRESS (fresh, chopped)	1 cup	4	0	0	14	0	0	1
WATERMELON								
Fresh, diced	1 cup	46	0	0	2	12	1	1
Seeds, dried	1 cup	602	51	11	107	17	0	31
WAXGOURD								
Boiled, cubed	1 cup	24	0	0	187	5	2	1
Fresh, cubed	1 cup	17	0	0	147	4	4	1
WHEAT								
Durum	1 cup	651	5	1	4	137	0	26
Hard red spring	1 cup	632	4	1	4	131	23	30
Hard red winter	1 cup	628	3	1	4	137	23	24
Hard white	1 cup	657	3	1	4	146	23	22
Soft red winter	1 cup	556	3	0	3	125	21	17
Soft white	1 cup	571	3	1	3	127	21	18
Sprouted	1 cup	214	1	0	17	46	1	8
WHEAT BRAN (crude)	1 cup	125	2	0	1	37	25	9

ITEM DESCRIPTION	Serving Size	Calories	Total Fat (g)	Saturated Fat (g)	Sodium (mg)	Carbohydrates (g)	Fiber (g)	Protein (g)
WHEAT FLOUR								
White, all purpose, enriched, bleached	1 cup	455	1	0	2	95	3	13
White, all purpose, enriched, self rising	1 cup	442	1	0	1588	93	3	12
White, all purpose, enriched, unbleached	1 cup	455	1	0	2	95	3	13
White, all purpose, unenriched	1 cup	455	1	0	2	95	3	13
White, bread, enriched	1 cup	495	2	0	3	99	3	16
White, cake, enriched	1 cup	496	1	0	3	107	2	11
White, tortilla mix, enriched	1 cup	450	12	5	751	75	0	11
Whole grain	1 cup	407	2	0	6	87	15	16
WHEAT GERM	1 cup	414	11	2	14	60	15	27
WHEAT GERM OIL	1 tbsp	120	14	3	0	0	0	0
WHELK (cooked in moist heat)	3 oz	234	1	0	350	13	0	41
WHIPPED CREAM (topping, pressurized)	1 tbsp	8	1	0	4	0	0	0
WHIPPED TOPPING (frozen, low fat)	1 cup	168	10	8	54	18	0	2
WHISKEY								
80 proof	1 fl oz	64	0	0	0	0	0	0
86 proof	1 fl oz	70	0	0	0	0	0	0
90 proof	1 fl oz	73	0	0	0	0	0	0
94 proof	1 fl oz	76	0	0	0	0	0	0
WHISKEY SOUR								
Canned	1 fl oz	37	0	0	14	4	0	0
Prepared from bottled mix	1 fl oz	47	0	0	19	4	0	0
Prepared from bottled mix, w/ sodium	1 fl oz	45	0	0	6	4	0	0
WHITE BEANS								
Boiled	1 cup	249	1	0	11	45	11	17
Canned	1 cup	299	1	0	13	56	13	19
Fresh	1 cup	673	1	0	32	122	31	47
Small, boiled	1 cup	254	1	0	4	46	19	16
Small, fresh	1 cup	722	3	1	26	134	54	45

ITEM DESCRIPTION	Serving Size	Calories	Total Fat (g)	Saturated Fat (g)	Sodium (mg)	Carbohydrates (g)	Fiber (g)	Protein (g)
WHITEFISH								
Cooked in dry heat	3 oz	146	6	1	55	0	0	21
Smoked	1 oz	30	0	0	285	0	0	7
WHITE SAUCE								
Homemade, med thick	1 cup	368	27	7	885	23	1	10
Homemade, thick	1 cup	465	35	9	932	29	1	10
Homemade, thin	1 cup	262	17	5	820	19	0	9
WHITING (cooked in dry heat)	3 oz	146	1	0	112	0	0	20
WINE								
All	1 fl oz	24	0	0	1	1	0	0
Cooking	1 fl oz	14	0	0	182	2	0	0
Dessert, dry	1 fl oz	45	0	0	3	3	0	0
Dessert, sweet	1 fl oz	47	0	0	3	4	0	0
Light	1 fl oz	14	0	0	2	0	0	0
Non-alcoholic	1 fl oz	2	0	0	2	0	0	0
Red	1 fl oz	25	0	0	1	1	0	0
Red, Barbera	1 fl oz	25	0	0	0	1	0	0
Red, Burgundy	1 fl oz	25	0	0	0	1	0	0
Red, Cabernet Franc	1 fl oz	24	0	0	0	1	0	0
Red, Cabernet Sauvignon	1 fl oz	24	0	0	0	1	0	0
Red, Carignane	1 fl oz	22	0	0	0	1	0	0
Red, Claret	1 fl oz	24	0	0	0	1	0	0
Red, Gamay	1 fl oz	23	0	0	0	1	0	0
Red, Lemberger	1 fl oz	24	0	0	0	1	0	0
Red, Merlot	1 fl oz	24	0	0	1	1	0	0
Red, Mouvedre	1 fl oz	26	0	0	0	1	0	0
Red, Petite Sirah	1 fl oz	25	0	0	0	1	0	0
Red, Pinot Noir	1 fl oz	24	0	0	0	1	0	0
Red, Sangiovese	1 fl oz	25	0	0	0	1	0	0
Red, Syrah	1 fl oz	24	0	0	0	1	0	0
Red, Zinfandel	1 fl oz	26	0	0	0	1	0	0
White	1 fl oz	24	0	0	1	1	0	0
White, Chenin Blanc	1 fl oz	24	0	0	0	1	0	0
White, Fume Blanc	1 fl oz	24	0	0	0	1	0	0

ITEM DESCRIPTION	Serving Size	Calories	Total Fat (g)	Saturated Fat (g)	Sodium (mg)	Carbohydrates (g)	Fiber (g)	Protein (g)
White, Gewarztraminer	1 fl oz	24	0	0	0	1	0	0
White, late harvest	1 fl oz	34	0	0	0	4	0	0
White, Muller Thurgau	1 fl oz	22	0	0	0	1	0	0
White, Muscat	1 fl oz	25	0	0	0	2	0	0
White, Pinot Blanc	1 fl oz	24	0	0	0	1	0	0
White, Pinot Gris (Grigio)	1 fl oz	24	0	0	0	1	0	0
White, Riesling	1 fl oz	24	0	0	0	1	0	0
White, Sauvignon Blanc	1 fl oz	24	0	0	0	1	0	0
White, Semillon	1 fl oz	24	0	0	0	1	0	0
WINGED BEANS								
Boiled	1 cup	253	10	1	22	26	0	18
Immature seeds, boiled	1 cup	24	0	0	2	2	0	3
Immature seeds, fresh, slices	1 cup	22	0	0	2	2	0	3
WINTER SQUASH								
All varieties, baked, cubed	1 cup	76	1	0	2	18	6	2
All varieties, fresh, cubed	1 cup	39	0	0	5	10	2	1
WOLFFISH								
(Atlantic, cooked in dry heat)	3 oz	105	3	0	93	0	0	19
WONTON WRAPPERS	1 wrapper	93	0	0	183	19	1	3
WORCESTERSHIRE SAUCE	1 tbsp	13	0	0	167	3	0	0
YAMS								
Boiled or baked, cubed	1 cup	158	0	0	11	37	5	2
Fresh, cubed	1 cup	177	0	0	14	42	6	2
Mountain, fresh, cubed	1 cup	91	0	0	18	22	0	2
Mountain, steamed, cubed	1 cup	119	0	0	17	29	0	3
YARD LONG BEANS								
Boiled, slices	1 cup	49	0	0	4	10	0	3
Fresh, slices	1 cup	43	0	0	4	8	0	3
Mature seeds, boiled	1 cup	202	1	0	9	36	6	14
Mature seeds, fresh	1 cup	579	2	1	28	103	18	41
YEAST								
Baker's, active dry	1 tsp	12	0	0	2	2	1	2
Baker's, compressed	0.6 oz cake	18	0	0	5	3	1	1
YEAST EXTRACT SPREAD	1 tsp	9	0	0	216	1	0	2

ITEM DESCRIPTION	Serving Size	Calories	Total Fat (g)	Saturated Fat (g)	Sodium (mg)	Carbohydrates (g)	Fiber (g)	Protein (g)
YELLOW BEANS								
Boiled	1 cup	255	2	0	9	45	18	16
Fresh	1 cup	676	5	1	24	119	49	43
YELLOWTAIL								
Cooked in dry heat	3 oz	159	6	0	43	0	0	25
Raw	3 oz	124	4	1	33	0	0	20
YOGURT								
Breyers Light n' Lively, strawberry	4.4 oz	135	1	1	56	27	0	4
Breyers Light, nonfat strawberry, w/ aspartame & fructose	8 oz	125	0	0	102	22	0	8
Breyers, low fat strawberry	8 oz	218	2	1	118	41	0	9
Breyers Smooth & Creamy, low fat strawberry	8 oz	232	2	1	125	45	1	9
Dannon Fruit on the Bottom, Blueberry	6 oz	140	1.5	1	130	26	1	6
Dannon Light & Fit, Blueberry	1 serv	80	0	0	75	16	0	5
Fruit, low fat, 10 grams protein	8 fl oz	250	3	2	142	47	0	10
Fruit, low fat, 11 grams protein	8 fl oz	250	3	2	159	46	0	11
Fruit, low fat, 9 grams protein	8 fl oz	243	3	2	130	46	0	9
Fruit, low fat, w/ low calorie sweetener	8 fl oz	257	3	2	142	46	0	12
Fruit varieties, nonfat	8 fl oz	233	0	0	142	47	0	11
La Yogurt, Banana	1	160	2	1	110	30	0	7
La Yogurt, Light Vanilla	1	90	0	0	90	15	0	6
Plain, low fat	8 fl oz	154	4	2	172	17	0	13
Plain, skim milk	8 fl oz	137	0	0	189	19	0	14
Plain, whole milk	8 fl oz	149	8	5	113	11	0	9
Stonyfield Organic Fat Free Yogurt, Lemon	1	130	0	0	115	26	0	7
Stonyfield Organic Fat Free Yogurt, Plain	1	80	0	0	120	11	0	8
Stonyfield Organic Fat Free Yogurt, Strawberry	1	130	0	0	115	26	0	7
Vanilla, low fat	8 fl oz	208	3	2	162	34	0	12
Yoplait Light, Harvest Peach	6 oz	100	0	0	85	19	0	5
Yoplait Original, Strawberry	6 oz	170	0	1	80	33	0	5

ITEM DESCRIPTION	Serving Size	Calories	Total Fat (g)	Saturated Fat (g)	Sodium (mg)	Carbohydrates (g)	Fiber (g)	Protein (g)
ZUCCHINI								
Baby, fresh	1 med	2	0	0	0	0	0	0
Boiled, w/ skin, slices	1 cup	29	0	0	5	7	3	1
Fresh, w/ skin	1 cup	18	0	0	11	4	1	1
Frozen, boiled, w/ skin	1 cup	38	0	0	4	8	3	3
Italian style, canned	1 cup	66	0	0	849	16	0	2

popular restaurants

ARBY'S

ITEM DESCRIPTION	Serving Size	Calories	Total Fat (g)	Saturated Fat (g)	Sodium (mg)	Carbohydrates (g)	Fiber (g)	Protein (g)
BEVERAGES								
Capri Sun Fruit Juice	1	80	0	0	25	21	0	0
Coffee	sm	0	0	0	0	0	0	0
Diet Pepsi®	sm	0	0	0	5	0	0	0
Dr Pepper®	sm	180	0	0	45	48	0	0
Milk, 1% Low Fat Chocolate	1	160	2	1.5	200	28	0	8
Milk, 2% Reduced Fat White	1	120	4.5	3	130	12	0	9
Mountain Dew®	sm	200	0	0	25	54	0	0
Pepsi®	sm	180	0	0	5	49	0	0
Sierra Mist®	sm	190	0	0	0	50	0	0
Tea, Sweet	sm	100	0	0	0	26	0	0
DESSERTS								
Apple Turnover w/o Icing	1	310	16	7	190	38	1	5
Cherry Turnover w/o Icing	1	310	16	7	240	37	2	5
Cookies, Chocolate Chunk	2	420	21	10	320	54	2	4
Icing (topping)	1 serv	130	1.5	1	5	30	0	0
Shake, Chocolate	sm	450	12	8	350	75	1	12
Shake, Jamocha	sm	440	12	8	350	75	1	11
Shake, Vanilla	sm	380	12	8	310	60	0	11
DRESSINGS AND SPREADS								
Arby's Sauce®	1 serv	15	0	0	180	3	0	0
Cheese Sauce, Cheddar	1 serv	50	3.5	.5	360	4	0	1
Dipping Sauce, Bronco Berry®	1 pkg	90	0	0	30	22	0	0
Dipping Sauce, Buffalo	1 pkg	10	1	0	720	1	0	0
Dipping Sauce, Honey Dijon Mustard	1 pkg	140	13	2	130	5	0	0
Dipping Sauce, Ranch	1 pkg	160	16	3.5	280	2	0	1
Dressing, Balsamic Vinaigrette	1 pkg	130	12	2	470	5	0	0
Dressing, Buttermilk Ranch	1 pkg	210	23	3.5	380	2	0	1
Dressing, Dijon Honey Mustard	1 pkg	180	16	2.5	260	8	0	0
Horsey Sauce®	1 serv	50	5	.5	160	3	0	0
Icing	1 serv	130	1.5	1	5	30	0	0
Sauce, Marinara	1 pkg	35	1.5	0	160	5	1	1

ITEM DESCRIPTION	Serving Size	Calories	Total Fat (g)	Saturated Fat (g)	Sodium (mg)	Carbohydrates (g)	Fiber (g)	Protein (g)
Tangy Barbeque Sauce®	1 serv	45	0	0	350	11	0	0
KIDS MENU								
Applesauce	1	80	0	0	10	21	2	0
Chicken Tenders	2 pcs	240	11	1.5	770	21	1	14
Curly Fries	1	270	14	2	700	33	2	3
Homestyle Fries	1	240	10	1.5	680	35	3	3
Potato Cakes	2 pcs	260	15	2	400	28	2	2
Roast Beef Sandwich, Jr.	1	200	6	2	530	24	1	12
SALADS								
Chopped Farmhouse Chicken Salad, Crispy	1	430	24	8	1150	30	4	27
Chopped Farmhouse Chicken Salad, Roast	1	250	13	7	680	11	3	23
Chopped Farmhouse Salad, Turkey and Ham	1	250	14	7	910	10	3	23
Chopped Side Salad	1	70	5	3	100	4	1	4
SANDWICHES								
Arby's Melt	1	390	16	6	1130	39	2	22
Beef 'n Cheddar	reg	450	21	7	1240	43	2	22
Chicken	jr	340	17	3	690	33	2	13
Chicken, Bacon & Swiss, Crispy	1	600	27	7	1750	55	4	33
Chicken, Bacon & Swiss, Roast	1	470	19	5	1310	43	2	32
Chicken, Cordon Bleu Sandwich, Crispy	1	620	30	6	2040	53	3	36
Chicken, Cordon Bleu Sandwich, Roast	1	490	21	5	1600	40	2	35
Chicken, Crispy	1	530	25	4	1310	52	4	25
Chicken, Roast	1	400	16	3	870	40	3	24
Chicken Salad w/ Pecans	1	750	34	4.5	1350	85	4	29
Corned Beef Reuben	1	700	32	9	1870	64	4	38
Deluxe	jr	270	14	4	560	25	2	12
Ham & Cheddar	jr	210	6	1.5	930	26	1	13
Ham & Swiss Melt	1	300	8	3.5	1070	37	2	18
Roast Beef	jr	210	8	3	520	24	1	12
Roast Beef	reg	360	14	6	950	37	2	22
Roast Beef Super	1	440	20	6	1060	44	3	22

ITEM DESCRIPTION	Serving Size	Calories	Total Fat (g)	Saturated Fat (g)	Sodium (mg)	Carbohydrates (g)	Fiber (g)	Protein (g)
Roast Beef & Swiss	1	800	39	12	1660	78	5	37
Roast Chicken Club	1	500	23	7	1320	41	2	31
Roast Ham & Swiss	1	710	30	8	2010	78	5	36
Roast Turkey & Swiss	1	710	28	7	1780	78	5	39
Roast Turkey, Ranch & Bacon	1	810	36	10	2270	78	5	46
Roastburger, All American	1	410	18	6	1710	43	2	19
Roastburger, Bacon Cheddar	1	430	19	9	1830	42	2	25
Toasted Sub, Angus Three Cheese & Bacon	1	660	33	13	1810	46	2	47
Toasted Sub, Classic Italian	1	520	28	8	1770	47	3	22
Toasted Sub, French Dip & Swiss	1	450	17	8	2110	51	2	26
Toasted Sub, Philly Beef	1	510	26	9	1380	46	3	25
Toasted Sub, Turkey Bacon Club	1	480	21	6	1620	47	2	30
Ultimate BLT	1	820	44	9	1690	78	5	32
SIDES AND SNACKS								
Bacon	4 pcs	90	6	2	340	1	0	7
Chicken Tenders	reg	360	17	2.5	1160	31	2	21
Curly Fries	med	600	31	4	1550	74	5	6
Double Meat for Roastburger	1 serv	130	9	4	510	1	0	12
Homestyle Fries	med	480	21	3	1360	69	5	5
Jalapeño Bites®	5 pcs	300	17	6	740	31	2	5
Loaded Potato Bites®	5 pcs	350	21	6	810	32	3	9
Mozzarella Sticks	4 pcs	440	23	9	1190	39	2	21
Onion Rings	5 pcs	460	24	3	1400	56	3	6
Potato Cakes	3 pcs	390	23	3.5	600	42	3	3

(+) The sodium value will vary based on the level of sodium in the local water supply. Recommended portion sizes.
Curly Fries and Homestyle Fries (where available) are individually portioned at every restaurant. Variations will exist from restaurant to restaurant.

AU BON PAIN

BAKED ITEMS

	Serving Size	Calories	Total Fat (g)	Saturated Fat (g)	Sodium (mg)	Carbohydrates (g)	Fiber (g)	Protein (g)
Bagel, Asiago Cheese	1	370	8	5	700	57	2	17
Bagel, Cinnamon Crisp	1	410	7	4	400	77	4	11
Bagel, Cinnamon Raisin	1	320	1	0	450	68	3	11
Bagel, Everything	1	320	4	1	530	60	3	12
Bagel, Honey 9 Grain	1	350	4	0	490	69	6	12
Bagel, Jalapeño Double Cheddar	1	340	10	6	640	53	2	17

ITEM DESCRIPTION	Serving Size	Calories	Total Fat (g)	Saturated Fat (g)	Sodium (mg)	Carbohydrates (g)	Fiber (g)	Protein (g)
Bagel, Onion Dill	1	280	1	0	430	57	3	11
Bagel, Plain	1	280	1	0	430	56	2	11
Bagel, Plain Skinny	1	90	1	0	230	22	4	4
Bagel, Poppy	1	320	4	1	430	58	4	12
Bagel, Sesame Seed	1	330	5	1	440	59	3	12
Bagel, Whole Wheat Skinny	1	90	1	0	230	21	6	5
Baguette, Artisan	sm	230	2	1	570	46	2	8
Baguette, Artisan	lg	310	3	1	760	61	2	10
Baguette, Artisan Honey Multigrain	sm	250	3	0	500	49	4	8
Baguette, Artisan Honey Multigrain	lg	340	5	0	670	66	6	11
Blondie	1	530	32	10	630	57	3	6
Bread Bowl	1	620	3	1	1720	123	6	26
Bread, Artisan Sundried Tomato	1	270	1	0	750	57	2	10
Bread, Country White	1	270	1	0	670	56	2	9
Bread, Whole Wheat Multigrain	1	260	3	0	630	53	9	11
Breadstick, Asiago	1	190	4	3	350	28	1	9
Breadstick, Cheddar Jalapeño	1	130	2	1	260	26	1	6
Breadstick, Cinnamon Raisin	1	190	1	0	230	41	2	6
Breadstick, Everything	1	180	3	0	310	31	2	7
Breadstick, Rosemary Garlic	1	190	5	1	720	31	2	6
Breadstick, Sesame	1	180	4	1	220	30	2	7
Brownie, Chocolate Cheesecake	1	420	21	7	250	57	1	5
Brownie, Chocolate Chip	1	440	21	6	240	62	2	4
Brownie, Hazelnut Mocha	1	450	23	7	220	62	2	5
Brownie, Rocky Road	1	440	22	6	240	61	2	5
Ciabatta	sm	180	1	0	480	38	2	6
Ciabatta	lg	310	1	0	820	64	3	11
Cinnamon Roll w/ Icing	1	410	15	8	270	60	2	8
Cookie, Chocolate Chip	1	280	13	7	210	40	2	3
Cookie, Confetti w/ M&M'S®	1	280	13	6	210	39	0	3
Cookie, English Toffee	1	250	14	6	170	27	1	2
Cookie, Mini Chocolate Chip	1	70	3	2	55	10	0	1
Cookie, Mini Oatmeal Raisin	1	60	3	1	50	10	1	1
Cookie, Oatmeal Raisin	1	250	9	5	200	40	2	4

ITEM DESCRIPTION	Serving Size	Calories	Total Fat (g)	Saturated Fat (g)	Sodium (mg)	Carbohydrates (g)	Fiber (g)	Protein (g)
Cookie, Shortbread	1	340	20	10	300	37	1	4
Cookie, White Chocolate Chunk Macadamia Nut	1	300	16	8	240	36	1	3
Crème de Fleur	1	500	25	14	440	56	2	11
Croissant, Almond	1	600	38	14	300	55	4	13
Croissant, Apple	1	280	11	7	160	44	3	5
Croissant, Chocolate	1	440	22	13	210	58	3	7
Croissant, Ham & Cheese	1	390	21	11	580	35	1	15
Croissant, Plain	1	310	17	9	220	31	1	7
Croissant, Raspberry Cheese	1	370	17	9	280	46	2	8
Croissant, Spinach & Cheese	1	290	17	10	330	28	2	10
Croissant, Sweet Cheese	1	400	19	11	320	49	1	9
Croissant, Turkey Cheddar	1	380	21	12	460	35	1	15
Crumb Cake	1	720	40	17	980	85	1	8
Cupcake, Carrot Cake	1	330	15	6	230	45	1	3
Cupcake, Double Chocolate	1	320	13	6	250	49	2	4
Cupcake, French Vanilla	1	350	17	7	220	43	0	3
Cupcake, Red Velvet	1	400	22	7	290	46	1	3
Danish, Cherry	1	420	20	10	340	54	1	7
Danish, Lemon	1	440	20	10	360	57	1	7
Danish, Sweet Cheese	1	470	24	12	410	54	2	9
Farm House Roll	1	360	7	1	670	63	3	12
Flatbread, Caraway Rye	1	280	5	2	680	49	7	12
Focaccia	1	360	7	1	700	62	3	12
Lavash	1	300	9	4	230	44	6	12
Macaroon, Chocolate Dipped Cranberry Almond	1	300	15	11	190	36	4	4
Muffin, Blueberry	1	490	17	2	510	74	2	9
Muffin, Carrot Walnut	1	560	27	6	820	72	4	9
Muffin, Chocolate Chip	1	580	23	6	480	83	3	9
Muffin, Corn	1	490	17	3	600	75	3	10
Muffin, Cranberry Walnut	1	540	25	3	500	66	4	10
Muffin, Double Chocolate Chunk	1	620	25	8	540	86	4	11
Muffin, Low-fat Triple Berry	1	300	3	0	720	65	2	4

ITEM DESCRIPTION	Serving Size	Calories	Total Fat (g)	Saturated Fat (g)	Sodium (mg)	Carbohydrates (g)	Fiber (g)	Protein (g)
Muffin, Pumpkin	1	530	19	4	570	80	4	10
Muffin, Raisin Bran	1	480	11	2	600	85	10	12
Muffin, Southwest Jalapeño	1	560	30	5	720	64	2	8
Palmier	1	440	23	15	330	53	1	1
Pecan Roll	1	810	41	14	430	99	3	12
Pound Cake, Lemon	1 pc	490	25	5	480	63	1	5
Pound Cake, Marble	1 pc	420	23	5	450	50	1	5
Scone, Cinnamon	1	530	28	17	400	60	2	9
Scone, Orange	1	480	23	14	420	57	1	10
Shortbread, Chocolate Dipped	1	380	22	12	310	42	1	4
Strudel, Apple	1	440	24	14	270	50	1	5
Strudel, Cherry	1	460	26	16	270	50	1	5
Torsade, Chocolate and Crème	1	250	12	7	220	30	1	4
Torsade, Golden Raisin and Créme	1	240	11	7	210	32	1	4
BEVERAGES								
Caffe Americano	med (16 oz)	10	0	0	25	2	0	0
Caffe Latte	med (16 oz)	250	14	9	180	21	0	14
Cappuccino	med (16 oz)	150	8	5	110	13	0	8
Caramel Macchiato	med (16 oz)	430	12	8	190	69	0	12
Chai Latte	med (16 oz)	380	14	8	170	52	0	14
Chocolate Milk	sm (12 oz)	320	9	5	100	54	3	10
Diet Pepsi	med (22 oz)	0	0	0	70	0	0	0
Diet Sierra Mist	med (22 oz)	0	0	0	70	0	0	0
Hot Chocolate	med (16 oz)	460	15	9	170	74	4	16
Iced Caffe Latte	med (16 oz)	150	8	5	115	13	0	8
Iced Caramel Macchiato	med (16 oz)	390	10	6	160	66	0	10
Iced Chai Latte	med (16 oz)	250	7	4	90	42	0	7
Iced Coffee, Decaf French Roast	med (22 oz)	10	0	0	20	2	0	0
Iced Coffee, French Roast	med (22 oz)	10	0	0	20	2	0	0
Iced Coffee, French Vanilla	med (22 oz)	10	0	0	20	2	0	1
Iced Latte, Mocha	med (16 oz)	300	14	8	115	40	2	10
Iced Latte, Vanilla	med (16 oz)	330	7	5	100	59	0	7
Iced Latte, White Chocolate	med (16 oz)	330	13	8	190	51	0	6
Iced Tea, Peach	med (22 oz)	240	0	0	0	61	0	0

ITEM DESCRIPTION	Serving Size	Calories	Total Fat (g)	Saturated Fat (g)	Sodium (mg)	Carbohydrates (g)	Fiber (g)	Protein (g)
Latte, Mocha	med (16 oz)	390	19	11	170	27	2	15
Latte, Vanilla	med (16 oz)	410	12	7	150	66	0	12
Latte, White Chocolate	med (16 oz)	410	16	10	260	57	0	12
Lemonade	med (22 oz)	310	0	0	0	82	0	0
Mountain Dew	med (22 oz)	300	0	0	110	85	0	0
Orange Juice	sm (8 oz)	110	0	0	0	26	0	2
Orange Soda	med (22 oz)	360	0	0	70	96	0	0
Pepsi	med (22 oz)	280	0	0	55	77	0	0
Pepsi, Caffeine Free	med (22 oz)	280	0	0	55	77	0	0
Root Beer	med (22 oz)	280	0	0	110	80	0	0
Sierra Mist	med (22 oz)	280	0	0	70	72	0	0
Smoothie, Caramel Blast	med (16 oz)	540	17	12	105	104	0	6
Smoothie, Coffee Blast	med (16 oz)	440	21	15	115	71	0	8
Smoothie, Mocha Blast	med (16 oz)	440	17	12	95	80	2	7
Smoothie, Peach	med (16 oz)	310	1	0	115	69	4	4
Smoothie, Strawberry	med (16 oz)	310	1	0	110	66	3	4
Smoothie, Vanilla Blast	med (16 oz)	540	17	12	100	104	0	6
BREAKFAST ITEMS								
Apple Croissants Tart	1	80	4	2	55	12	1	1
Bagel w/ Bacon	1	370	7	3	770	57	2	18
Bagel w/ Bacon & Egg	1	510	18	6	900	58	2	29
Bagel w/ Bacon, Egg & Cheese	1	600	25	10	1040	59	2	34
Bagel w/ Egg	1	430	12	4	580	58	2	22
Bagel w/ Egg & Cheese	1	510	18	8	710	59	2	27
Bagel w/ Ham & Egg	1	470	13	5	1080	59	2	30
Bagel, Asiago w/ Sausage, Egg & Cheddar	1	810	46	20	1340	57	2	41
Bagel, Onion Dill w/ Smoked Salmon & Wasabi	1	430	12	5	1090	62	3	23
Ciabatta Melt w/ Bacon & Egg	1	490	24	11	1100	39	2	29
Egg Sandwich w/ Broccoli & Swiss	1	430	19	8	740	42	2	25
Egg Sandwich w/ Pastrami & Swiss on Light Rye	1	480	22	10	990	36	4	35
Egg White Sandwich w/ Cheddar	1	250	11	6	550	23	6	20

ITEM DESCRIPTION	Serving Size	Calories	Total Fat (g)	Saturated Fat (g)	Sodium (mg)	Carbohydrates (g)	Fiber (g)	Protein (g)
Eggs, Scrambled	1 serv	35	3	1	90	1	0	3
French Pecan Toast	1	70	4	2	45	8	0	2
Oatmeal	med (12 oz)	260	5	1	10	47	6	10
Oatmeal, Apple Cinnamon	med (12 oz)	280	4	1	10	56	7	8
Pineapple Blueberry Cobbler	1	45	2	0	35	8	1	1
Potatoes, Roasted	1 serv	35	1	0	110	6	1	1
Quinoa, Cinnamon Walnut	1 serv	45	3	0	0	4	1	2
Sausage w/ Peppers & Onions	1 serv	50	5	2	90	1	0	2
Southwest Corn Casserole	1 serv	60	4	2	85	4	0	3
DRESSINGS AND SPREADS								
Artichoke Aioli	1 serv	70	6	1	220	2	0	1
Basil Pesto	1 serv	120	12	2	220	1	0	2
Chili Dijon	1 serv	130	13	2	250	4	0	1
Cream Cheese, Honey Pecan	1 serv	200	16	10	135	10	0	2
Cream Cheese, Lite	1 serv	120	9	6	280	5	0	4
Cream Cheese, Sundried Tomato	1 serv	140	11	7	170	5	1	4
Cream Cheese, Vegetable	1 serv	170	16	10	270	3	0	3
Dijon Mustard Sauce	1 serv	20	2	0	400	1	0	1
Dressing, Balsamic Vinaigrette	1 serv	120	9	2	360	8	0	0
Dressing, Blue Cheese	1 serv	310	33	6	460	2	0	2
Dressing, Caesar	1 serv	270	28	5	370	4	0	1
Dressing, Fat Free Raspberry Vinaigrette	1 serv	50	0	0	190	12	0	0
Dressing, Fat Free Sun Dried Tomato Vinaigrette	1 serv	110	0	0	430	28	0	0
Dressing, Feta Vinaigrette	1 serv	160	16	3	500	3	0	1
Dressing, Hazelnut Vinaigrette	1 serv	270	25	4	300	11	0	1
Dressing, Light Ranch	1 serv	120	11	2	410	3	0	2
Dressing, Lite Honey Mustard	1 serv	170	9	2	380	20	0	1
Dressing, Lite Olive Oil Vinaigrette	1 serv	110	10	2	420	6	0	0
Dressing, Pomegranate Vinaigrette	1 serv	250	22	4	160	12	0	0
Dressing, Sesame Ginger	1 serv	230	20	3	680	12	0	1
Dressing, Thai Peanut	1 serv	160	8	1	740	20	0	2
Honey Mustard Sauce	1 serv	200	3	0	240	41	1	2

ITEM DESCRIPTION	Serving Size	Calories	Total Fat (g)	Saturated Fat (g)	Sodium (mg)	Carbohydrates (g)	Fiber (g)	Protein (g)
Mayonnaise	1 serv	70	7	1	200	2	0	0
Mayonnaise, Herb	1 serv	110	11	2	160	1	0	0
Mayonnaise, Jalapeño	1 serv	50	5	1	290	1	0	2
Spread, Herb Bagel	1 serv	140	12	8	340	4	0	5
Spread, Sun-Dried Tomato	1 serv	45	4	0	70	1	0	0
KIDS MENU								
Cheese Sandwich	1	360	22	12	550	32	1	11
Chicken Sandwich, Grilled	1 serv	240	6	1	570	28	5	20
Macaroni & Cheese	sm	360	21	13	1000	26	1	15
Turkey Sandwich, Roasted	1	270	7	2	780	33	1	17
MAIN MENU								
Apple Cranberry Orzo, Roasted	1 oz	45	1	0	25	9	1	1
Carrots, Roasted	1 oz	15	0	0	60	3	1	0
Chicken, Cajun w/ Penne	1 oz	45	2	1	100	4	0	3
Chicken w/ Penne Broccoli Alfredo (salad bar)	1 oz	60	4	2	85	3	0	2
Chicken w/ Penne Broccoli Alfredo	12 oz	690	43	18	1040	38	2	29
Chicken Penne Pesto	1 oz	60	3	1	75	4	0	4
Chicken Provencal	1 oz	25	1	0	35	3	0	2
Eggplant Parmesan	1 oz	50	3	1	150	4	1	2
Fire Roasted Exotic Grains & Vegetables	1 oz	40	1	0	85	7	1	1
Green Beans w/ Almonds, Roasted	1 oz	20	1	0	25	1	1	0
Italian Sausage, Peppers & Onions	1 oz	25	1	0	80	1	0	2
Jambalaya	1 oz	25	1	0	85	2	0	1
Lasagna, Meat (salad bar)	1 oz	45	2	1	100	4	0	2
Lasagna, Meat	10.7 oz	470	24	11	1080	41	5	22
Lasagna, Vegetarian	1 oz	45	3	2	80	3	0	3
Macaroni & Cheese (salad bar)	1 oz	40	3	2	115	3	0	2
Macaroni & Cheese	12 oz	540	31	20	1500	39	2	22
Mayan Chicken Bowl w/ Brown Rice	1 serv	510	13	3	870	72	4	27
Mayan Chicken Bowl w/ White Rice	1 serv	550	11	3	910	87	3	27
Meatballs w/ Marinara	1 oz	50	4	2	125	2	1	2
Meatloaf w/ Wine Sauce	1 oz	50	3	1	75	2	0	2
Penne w/ Burgundy Beef	1 oz	30	1	0	95	4	0	2

ITEM DESCRIPTION	Serving Size	Calories	Total Fat (g)	Saturated Fat (g)	Sodium (mg)	Carbohydrates (g)	Fiber (g)	Protein (g)
Penne Marinara	1 oz	30	1	0	55	5	0	1
Peppers, Stuffed w/ Lentils	1 oz	20	0	0	35	3	1	1
Polenta Marinara	1 oz	25	1	0	90	3	0	1
Potato, Baked	1	25	0	0	20	5	1	1
Quesadilla, Ancho Chicken	12 oz	700	28	10	1610	62	6	49
Quinoa	1 oz	25	0	0	50	4	1	1
Rice, Brown	1 oz	30	0	0	20	6	0	1
Rice, White	1 oz	35	0	0	20	8	0	1
Spinach, Creamed	1 oz	30	2	2	125	2	1	1
Steak Teriyaki Bowl w/ Brown Rice	1 serv	620	19	5	1390	86	5	25
Steak Teriyaki Bowl w/ White Rice	1 serv	660	18	5	1430	101	3	25
Tsaziki	1 oz	15	0	0	40	2	0	1
Zucchini, Roasted w/ Summer Squash	1 oz	5	0	0	15	1	0	0
SALADS								
Barbecue Beef	1 oz	30	1	0	100	4	0	2
Brown Rice Waldorf Nut	1 oz	45	3	0	40	5	0	0
Caesar Asiago	side	130	6	3	270	12	2	6
Caesar Asiago	1	220	12	6	480	18	3	11
Chef's Salad	1	260	15	7	1080	8	3	24
Chicken Caesar Asiago, Grilled	1	300	13	6	660	18	3	29
Chicken, Mediterranean	1	290	16	6	1150	12	3	25
Chicken, Thai Peanut	1	200	5	1	300	18	4	22
Egg & Cucumber	1 oz	40	3	1	85	1	0	2
Garden	1	80	2	0	105	15	4	3
Garden	side	50	2	0	70	9	2	2
Greek Salad	1	230	15	5	1170	16	4	8
Oriental Noodle	1 oz	90	2	0	150	19	0	0
Orzo Toscano	1 oz	35	1	0	90	6	1	1
Panzanella, Southwest	1 oz	50	3	0	55	7	0	1
Pasta, Aegean	1 oz	90	4	1	115	10	1	2
Pasta, Southwest Fusilli	1 oz	45	3	0	65	4	0	1
Potato Bacon	1 oz	40	2	0	125	5	1	1
Potato, Red Bliss	1 oz	30	2	0	70	5	0	1
Sesame Brown Rice & Orange	1 oz	45	2	0	65	6	0	1

ITEM DESCRIPTION	Serving Size	Calories	Total Fat (g)	Saturated Fat (g)	Sodium (mg)	Carbohydrates (g)	Fiber (g)	Protein (g)
Sesame Chicken, Mandarin	1	310	11	2	440	31	4	20
Tomato Cucumber	1 oz	10	0	0	40	2	0	0
Tomato, Green Bean & Almond	1 oz	20	2	0	50	2	0	0
Tuna	1 oz	45	3	0	105	1	0	4
Tuna Garden	1	270	13	2	530	19	5	21
Turkey Cobb	1	330	18	8	970	16	4	27
Watermelon & Feta	1 oz	15	1	0	25	3	0	0
SANDWICHES								
Black Bean Burger	1	560	18	5	930	76	14	29
Black Bean Burger, Toasted Southwestern on Country White	1	670	32	11	1500	66	8	33
Caprese	1	680	32	15	1200	65	4	30
Chicken & Mozzarella	1	690	24	8	1320	66	4	50
Chicken Pesto	1	670	24	5	1430	66	4	45
Chicken Salad	1	490	11	2	1050	67	4	30
Chicken, Arizona	1	720	29	12	1580	62	3	50
Chicken, Baked BBQ	1	690	19	7	1480	80	3	46
Chicken, Grilled on Ciabatta	1	470	4	1	1660	67	4	39
Chicken, Toasted Arizona on Sun-Dried Tomato	1	630	28	11	480	46	2	45
Eggplant & Mozzarella	1	640	27	10	1280	74	6	25
Ham & Swiss on Baguette	1	650	19	10	2040	82	4	41
Ham & Swiss on Country White	1	530	16	9	1850	61	2	39
Ham & Swiss, Tomatoes & Romaine on Farmhouse Roll	half	320	12	5	910	34	2	20
Hummus & Olives on Sun-Dried Tomato Bread	1	300	7	1	890	49	4	10
Pastrami	1	590	23	11	2080	52	7	47
Pastrami & Swiss, Toasted on Light Rye	1	500	21	11	1770	38	4	42
Regio	1	810	41	15	2220	69	3	35
Roast Beef & Brie on Country White	1	560	18	10	1390	60	3	39
Roast Beef & Brie on Farmhouse Roll	half	330	13	6	680	34	2	20
Roast Beef on Baguette	1	500	12	3	1370	65	3	33
Roast Beef Caesar	1	650	25	8	1670	68	3	39

ITEM DESCRIPTION	Serving Size	Calories	Total Fat (g)	Saturated Fat (g)	Sodium (mg)	Carbohydrates (g)	Fiber (g)	Protein (g)
Roast Beef Montana on Toasted Cheese Baguette	1	550	21	10	1830	66	4	42
Steakhouse Ciabatta	1	590	18	8	1850	72	3	36
Tuna & Cheddar on Country White	1	630	25	10	1370	63	3	38
Tuna & Cheddar on Farmhouse Roll	half	370	17	5	680	35	2	20
Tuna, Spicy	1	490	16	3	1210	60	11	30
Turkey Club	1	730	33	13	2080	60	3	47
Turkey Cranberry Brie on Multigrain	1	590	20	10	1680	66	9	42
Turkey & Swiss on Country White	1	530	14	8	1410	60	2	42
Turkey & Swiss on Farmhouse Roll	half	320	11	5	700	34	2	22
Turkey, Baked	1	750	28	9	1990	79	3	44
Turkey, Roasted on Baguette	1	490	5	2	1510	80	4	32
Wrap, Chicken Caesar Asiago	1	640	32	11	940	49	7	39
Wrap, Hot Angus Steak Teriyaki	1	630	16	4	1450	100	5	24
Wrap, Hot Mayan Chicken	1	580	13	3	1190	93	5	25
Wrap, Mediterranean	1	630	34	9	1350	61	10	21
Wrap, Southwest Tuna	1	800	46	16	1190	54	8	42
Wrap, Thai Peanut Chicken	1	560	17	5	880	68	8	34
SIDES AND SNACKS								
Almonds, Chocolate Covered	1 serv	230	15	5	10	20	2	4
Apples, Blue Cheese & Cranberries	1 serv	200	10	4	270	27	3	4
Brie, Fruit & Crackers	1 serv	200	11	6	280	18	0	6
Cheddar, Fruit & Crackers	1 serv	200	12	6	280	18	0	8
Cheese, Herb w/ Fruit & Crackers	1 serv	190	11	6	450	20	1	4
Cinnamon Buttons, Sugar Free	1 serv	70	0	0	0	17	0	0
Fruit Cup	sm	70	0	0	15	18	1	1
Granola topping	1 serv	230	8	1	75	37	3	5
Grapes	1 serv	160	0	0	0	41	2	2
Hummus & Cucumber	1 serv	130	8	0	460	10	3	3
Jell-O®, Lemon	1 serv	130	0	0	140	30	0	2
Jell-O®, Lime	1 serv	130	0	0	140	30	0	2
Jell-O®, Orange	1 serv	130	0	0	140	30	0	2
Licorice, Red	1 serv	150	1	0	20	33	0	1
Mozzarella & Tomato	1 serv	180	14	7	240	5	1	10

ITEM DESCRIPTION	Serving Size	Calories	Total Fat (g)	Saturated Fat (g)	Sodium (mg)	Carbohydrates (g)	Fiber (g)	Protein (g)
Muesli	1 serv	390	8	2	50	76	7	11
Nonpareils	1 serv	200	8	5	20	31	0	2
Nuts, Mixed	1 serv	180	16	3	60	7	1	5
Pineapple	1 serv	110	0	0	0	30	3	1
Pretzels, Chocolate Covered	2	160	5	4	210	24	1	3
Raisins, Dark Chocolate Covered	1 serv	180	8	5	0	26	2	2
Snack Mix, The 19th Hole	1 serv	160	10	2	200	15	2	4
Strawberry, Chocolate Covered	1	35	2	2	5	5	1	0
Turkey, Asparagus, Cranberry Chutney & Gorgonzola	1 serv	140	5	3	550	10	1	15
Turkish Apricots	1 serv	100	0	0	0	23	2	1
Watermelon	1 serv	70	0	0	0	17	1	1
Yogurt, Blueberry w/ Blueberries	sm	250	3	2	135	50	0	8
Yogurt, Strawberry w/ Blueberries	sm	250	2	2	135	50	0	7
Yogurt, Vanilla w/ Blueberries	sm	220	3	2	180	41	0	9
SOUPS								
12 Veggie	med	180	6	1	1290	25	4	5
Baked Stuffed Potato	med	380	22	11	1090	32	2	10
Bisque, Corn & Green Chili	med	290	17	9	1370	29	3	6
Bisque, Lobster	med	390	28	17	1340	23	0	8
Bisque, Wild Mushroom	med	200	10	2	1080	24	2	5
Black Bean	med	280	2	0	1100	51	28	17
Black-Eyed Pea, Southern	med	190	2	0	1050	31	9	12
Broccoli Cheddar	med	320	22	10	1060	21	2	12
Butternut Squash and Apple	med	240	8	3	860	40	4	4
Carrot Ginger	med	140	5	0	1030	24	4	2
Chicken & Dumpling	med	230	8	3	1150	30	2	11
Chicken Florentine	med	270	14	6	1140	27	1	9
Chicken Gumbo	med	190	9	1	930	22	2	6
Chicken Noodle	med	140	3	1	1120	20	2	9
Chicken Pot Pie	med	370	22	10	1020	26	3	15
Chili, Beef	med	300	13	4	1110	28	7	18
Clam Chowder	med	340	19	8	1090	29	2	10
Corn Chowder	med	380	19	9	1230	44	4	9

ITEM DESCRIPTION	Serving Size	Calories	Total Fat (g)	Saturated Fat (g)	Sodium (mg)	Carbohydrates (g)	Fiber (g)	Protein (g)
Cream of Chicken & Wild Rice	med	250	15	5	1040	24	1	6
Curried Rice & Lentil	med	190	2	0	1390	33	9	9
French Moroccan Tomato Lentil	med	210	3	0	1180	35	11	11
French Onion	med	130	5	3	1380	20	2	4
Garden Vegetable	med	80	2	0	1120	14	3	3
Harvest Pumpkin	med	270	15	8	1440	31	4	5
Hearty Cabbage	med	120	5	2	1110	15	3	5
Italian Wedding	med	190	10	4	1010	16	2	8
Mediterranean Pepper	med	190	5	1	640	28	8	8
Pasta E Fagioli	med	280	9	2	1110	39	10	13
Portuguese Kale	med	130	5	1	1290	16	4	6
Potato Cheese	med	280	15	9	1380	27	2	7
Potato Leek	med	320	20	11	1060	29	2	5
Red Beans, Italian Sausage & Rice	med	300	7	2	1210	45	19	15
Split Pea w/ Ham	med	280	2	0	1340	46	16	20
Stew, BBQ Chicken and Beef	med	300	10	4	1150	35	3	19
Stew, Beef & Vegetable	med	330	17	3	1160	27	3	20
Stew, Chicken & Vegetable	med	310	18	5	1000	27	3	12
Thai Coconut Curry	med	170	8	2	1120	22	2	5
Tomato	med	210	8	3	1240	30	4	6
Tomato Basil Bisque	med	220	9	6	540	29	4	7
Tomato Cheddar	med	260	17	6	1140	19	2	9
Tomato Florentine	med	140	3	1	1090	20	3	7
Tomato Rice	med	120	1	0	290	25	2	4
Tortilla, Southwest	med	210	11	4	1290	26	4	4
Vegetable, Beef Barley	med	150	3	2	1070	22	4	9
Vegetable, Southwest	med	190	5	1	430	30	6	7
Vegetable, Tuscan	med	180	5	2	1260	24	3	7
Vegetarian Chili	med	240	3	0	1070	43	22	13
Vegetarian Lentil	med	190	2	0	1320	33	12	10
Vegetarian Minestrone	med	120	2	0	1220	22	5	5
White Bean, Tuscan	med	180	4	1	1240	28	6	8
TOPPINGS AND EXTRAS								
Bacon	1 serv	90	6	2	330	0	0	7

ITEM DESCRIPTION	Serving Size	Calories	Total Fat (g)	Saturated Fat (g)	Sodium (mg)	Carbohydrates (g)	Fiber (g)	Protein (g)
Cheese, Brie	1 serv	170	15	9	320	1	1	7
Cheese, Cheddar	2 pcs	160	13	7	270	1	0	10
Cheese, Feta	1 serv	80	6	4	320	1	0	5
Cheese, Goat	1 serv	45	4	2	110	1	0	3
Cheese, Gorgonzola	1 serv	200	16	12	770	2	0	12
Cheese, Mozzarella	1 serv	120	9	6	105	0	0	9
Cheese, Swiss	1 serv	150	12	8	90	2	0	12
Chicken Breast	1 serv	130	2	0	300	0	0	28
Croutons	1 pkg	190	6	1	310	29	1	5
Granola	1 serv	230	8	1	75	37	3	5
Guacamole	1 serv	50	5	1	115	2	2	0
Ham	1 serv	100	3	1	1090	1	0	17
Hummus, Roasted Red Pepper	1 serv	80	5	0	250	6	2	2
Pastrami	1 serv	140	5	2	910	1	0	21
Peppers, Roasted Red	1 serv	10	0	0	105	2	0	0
Roast Beef	1 serv	110	3	1	400	0	0	22
Sausage Patty	1 serv	210	20	7	360	0	0	8
Tuna Salad Mix	1 serv	180	11	2	430	3	1	18
Turkey Breast	1 serv	90	1	0	650	1	0	20
Whipped Cream	1 serv	20	2	1	0	0	0	0

BLIMPIE

BREAKFAST ITEMS

Bagel	1	290	1	0	700	58	3	11
Bagel w/ Cream Cheese	1	390	11	6	780	59	3	13
Biscuit w/ Bacon, Egg & Cheese	1	520	30	18	1940	38	1	22
Biscuit w/ Egg & Cheese	1	380	20	15	1380	37	1	13
Biscuit w/ Ham, Egg & Cheese	1	420	21	15	1660	39	1	19
Biscuit w/ Sausage, Egg & Cheese	1	530	34	20	1690	37	1	19
Biscuit w/ Sausage Gravy	1	460	27	14	1320	43	2	12
Bluffin w/ Bacon, Egg & Cheese	1	270	12	5	890	27	2	14
Bluffin w/ Egg & Cheese	1	240	10	5	770	27	2	12
Bluffin w/ Ham, Egg & Cheese	1	280	10	5	1050	29	2	17
Bluffin w/ Sausage, Egg & Cheese	1	390	24	10	1080	27	2	18

ITEM DESCRIPTION	Serving Size	Calories	Total Fat (g)	Saturated Fat (g)	Sodium (mg)	Carbohydrates (g)	Fiber (g)	Protein (g)
Muffin, Plain	1	130	1	0	240	25	2	5
Burrito w/ Bacon, Egg & Cheese	1	580	28	12	2320	57	5	26
Burrito w/ Egg & Cheese	1	500	23	10	2010	57	5	21
Burrito w/ Ham, Egg & Cheese	1	580	24	10	2560	60	5	32
Burrito w/ Sausage, Egg & Cheese	1	800	50	20	2620	57	5	33
Burrito w/ Turkey, Egg & Cheese	1	560	23	10	2530	59	5	29
Cinnamon Roll	1	450	20	9	730	60	2	9
Grilled Breakfast Sandwich, Bacon	1	480	23	10	1620	44	1	25
Grilled Breakfast Sandwich, Ham	1	480	19	9	1860	47	1	30
Grilled Breakfast Sandwich, Sausage	1	710	45	18	1920	44	1	32
Grilled Breakfast Sandwich, Turkey	1	460	18	8	1830	46	1	28
Roll w/ Egg & Cheese	1	200	9	4	650	22	1	10
DESSERTS								
Brownie	1	230	10	4	115	28	1	3
Cookie, Chocolate Chunk	1	200	10	5	150	25	0	2
Cookie, Oatmeal Raisin	1	180	7	3	150	27	0	3
Cookie, Peanut Butter	1	210	13	5	170	21	0	3
Cookie, Sugar	1	320	16	6	240	42	0	3
Cookie, White Chocolate Macadamia Nut	1	200	11	5	110	25	0	2
DRESSINGS AND SPREADS								
Dressing, Blue Cheese	1 serv	230	24	5	440	2	n/a	2
Dressing, Buttermilk Ranch	1 serv	150	16	3	250	1	n/a	1
Dressing, Creamy Caesar	1 serv	210	21	4	520	2	n/a	1
Dressing, Creamy Italian	1 serv	180	18	3	420	4	0	0
Dressing, Dijon Honey Mustard	1 serv	180	17	3	240	8	n/a	1
Dressing, Fat-Free Italian	1 serv	25	0	n/a	390	5	0	0
Dressing, Light Buttermilk Ranch	1 serv	70	4	1	310	8	n/a	1
Dressing, Light Italian	1 serv	20	1	0	770	2	n/a	0
Dressing, Peppercorn	1 serv	120	12	2	210	1	0	0
Dressing, Special	1 serv	40	5	0	0	0	n/a	0
Dressing, Thousand Island	1 serv	210	20	3	350	6	0	0
Honey Mustard	1 serv	20	1	0	85	4	1	1
Mayonnaise	1 serv	100	11	2	100	0	0	0

ITEM DESCRIPTION	Serving Size	Calories	Total Fat (g)	Saturated Fat (g)	Sodium (mg)	Carbohydrates (g)	Fiber (g)	Protein (g)
Mustard, Deli Style	1 serv	15	0	0	170	0	0	0
Mustard, Spicy Brown	1 serv	15	0	0	170	0	n/a	0
Oil Blend	1 serv	60	6	1	0	0	0	0
Red Wine Vinegar	1 serv	5	0	0	0	1	0	0
Sauce, Red Hot Original	1 serv	10	0	0	760	2	0	0
KIDS MENU								
Ham & American Cheese	3 in	260	8	5	900	32	2	14
Tuna	3 in	280	11	2	460	30	2	14
Turkey	3 in	190	3	0	600	31	2	10
SALADS								
Antipasto	1	250	14	6	1630	12	4	20
Buffalo Chicken	1	220	9	5	840	10	4	25
Chicken Caesar	1	190	8	4	460	6	3	25
Coleslaw	side	160	9	2	240	20	2	1
Garden	1	30	0	0	15	6	3	2
Macaroni	side	330	22	5	790	28	2	5
Northwest Potato	side	260	17	4	390	22	3	3
Potato	side	230	12	3	490	28	3	3
Tuna	reg	270	19	3	370	6	3	18
Ultimate Club	1	260	14	7	1070	10	3	23
SANDWICHES								
Blimpie Best	6 in	450	17	6	1330	49	3	24
Blimpie Best, Super Stacked	6 in	550	22	8	2090	52	3	36
Blimpie Trio, Super Stacked	6 in	510	15	5	1760	51	3	40
BLT	6 in	430	22	5	960	43	2	15
BLT, Super Stacked	6 in	640	41	9	1440	43	2	22
Burger	1	460	24	10	1280	42	1	21
Chicken Teriyaki	6 in	450	12	5	1280	52	2	33
Chicken Teriyaki on Wheat	6 in	450	14	6	1260	50	5	35
Chicken w/ Cheddar, Bacon & Ranch	6 in	600	29	10	1570	48	3	36
Ciabatta, Buffalo Chicken	1	540	23	7	1970	49	3	31
Ciabatta, French Dip	1	430	11	5	1820	49	2	31
Ciabatta, Grilled Chicken Caesar	1	580	20	5	1480	62	3	34
Ciabatta, Mediterranean	1	450	8	3	1720	65	3	26

ITEM DESCRIPTION	Serving Size	Calories	Total Fat (g)	Saturated Fat (g)	Sodium (mg)	Carbohydrates (g)	Fiber (g)	Protein (g)
Ciabatta, Roast Beef, Turkey & Cheddar	1	520	24	8	1780	51	3	25
Ciabatta, Sicilian	1	590	22	6	2170	66	3	29
Ciabatta, Spicy Chicken & Pepperoni	1	710	34	11	2070	65	3	33
Ciabatta, Tuscan	1	570	20	6	2030	65	3	28
Ciabatta, Ultimate Club	1	520	24	7	1600	47	2	27
Club	6 in	410	13	4	1050	49	3	23
Cuban	6 in	410	11	5	1630	43	1	29
French Dip	6 in	410	11	5	1650	46	1	30
Ham & Swiss	6 in	420	14	5	1020	49	3	23
Ham & Swiss on Wheat	6 in	420	15	5	1000	47	6	26
Ham, Salami & Provolone	6 in	470	20	7	1270	49	3	24
Hot Dog	1	510	29	12	1420	45	1	17
Meatball	6 in	580	31	13	1960	50	4	27
Pastrami, Hot	6 in	430	16	7	1350	42	1	30
Pastrami, Hot, Super Stacked	6 in	570	23	10	2110	43	1	46
Philly Steak & Onion	6 in	600	35	11	1410	46	1	25
Pretzel, Ham & Swiss	1	520	15	5	940	75	4	24
Pretzel, Turkey Bacon	1	560	18	8	1800	70	3	28
Reuben	6 in	530	20	6	1740	52	3	34
Roast Beef & Provolone	6 in	430	14	5	980	46	3	28
Roast Beef & Provolone on Wheat	6 in	430	16	5	1000	44	6	32
Tuna	6 in	470	21	3	770	43	2	24
Turkey & Avocado	6 in	360	7	1	1340	51	4	21
Turkey & Bacon, Super Stacked	6 in	640	29	10	2830	49	2	43
Turkey & Cranberry	6 in	350	4	1	1220	58	3	20
Turkey & Provolone	6 in	410	13	4	1310	49	3	24
Turkey & Provolone on Wheat	6 in	420	14	5	1350	47	6	27
Vegetarian Special	6 in	590	30	9	1170	66	4	16
Veggie & Cheese	6 in	460	21	9	1420	50	3	19
Veggie Supreme	6 in	550	27	13	1500	50	3	26
VegiMax	6 in	520	20	6	1270	56	5	28
VegiMax on Wheat	6 in	520	21	6	1250	54	9	31
Wrap, Chicken Caesar	reg	560	24	8	1480	56	4	30
Wrap, Southwestern	reg	530	22	6	1770	61	4	23

ITEM DESCRIPTION	Serving Size	Calories	Total Fat (g)	Saturated Fat (g)	Sodium (mg)	Carbohydrates (g)	Fiber (g)	Protein (g)
SIDES AND SNACKS								
Cheetos, Crunchy	1 pkg	160	10	3	290	15	1	2
Chips, Baked Potato	1 pkg	120	2	0	170	26	2	2
Chips, Cheddar Sour Cream	1 pkg	240	15	5	280	21	2	3
Chips, KC Master Barbecue	1 pkg	240	15	5	300	22	1	3
Chips, KC Master Barbecue, Baked	1 pkg	130	4	0	240	25	2	2
Chips, Multigrain Harvest Cheddar	1 pkg	210	9	2	280	28	3	3
Chips, Multigrain Original	1 pkg	210	9	1	140	29	4	3
Chips, Potato	1 pkg	220	15	5	270	22	1	3
Doritos, Cooler Ranch	1 pkg	240	12	3	300	31	2	3
Doritos, Nacho Cheese	1 pkg	240	12	3	330	30	2	3
Fritos	1 pkg	320	20	2	210	30	2	4
Pretzels, Classic Thin Style	1 pkg	220	2	0	n/a	47	2	4
SOUPS								
Bean w/ Ham	1	140	1	0	1070	23	11	8
Beef Steak & Noodle	1	120	4	2	780	14	0	8
Beef Stew	1	170	4	4	890	18	2	17
Captain's Corn Chowder	1	210	7	3	890	29	4	6
Chicken & Dumpling	1	170	7	3	970	19	3	11
Chicken Gumbo	1	90	2	0	1280	13	2	6
Chicken Noodle	1	130	4	1	1040	18	2	7
Chicken w/ White & Wild Rice	1	250	10	3	1030	15	4	14
Cream of Broccoli w/ Cheese	1	250	19	11	1040	13	0	7
Cream of Potato	1	190	9	3	860	24	3	5
French Onion	1	80	4	1	1020	11	1	2
Garden Vegetable	1	80	1	0	620	14	3	5
Grande Chili w/ Bean & Beef	1	310	9	4	1440	31	9	20
Harvest Vegetable	1	100	1	0	920	19	3	4
Italian Style Wedding	1	130	4	2	900	17	0	7
Minestrone	1	90	3	0	1150	14	4	4
New England Clam Chowder	1	170	3	2	1060	28	2	7
Pasta Fagioli w/ Sausage	1	150	5	2	910	22	4	7
Split Pea w/ Ham	1	130	2	0	1090	21	6	8
Tomato Basil w/ Raviolini	1	110	1	0	720	22	0	4

ITEM DESCRIPTION	Serving Size	Calories	Total Fat (g)	Saturated Fat (g)	Sodium (mg)	Carbohydrates (g)	Fiber (g)	Protein (g)
Vegetable Beef	1	80	2	1	1010	13	2	4
Yankee Pot Roast	1	80	2	1	750	12	1	5
TOPPINGS AND EXTRAS								
Bacon	1 serv	110	8	3	450	0	0	7
Bread, Cheddar Jalapeño	6 in	210	5	2	470	36	1	8
Bread, Ciabatta	1 serv	230	3	0	590	43	2	8
Bread, Honey Oat	6 in	260	8	2	400	41	5	10
Bread, Marble Rye	6 in	240	3	1	590	46	2	9
Bread, Pretzel	1 serv	320	4	1	350	65	2	8
Bread, Wheat	6 in	210	4	1	400	38	5	10
Bread, White	6 in	210	3	1	420	40	1	7
Bread, Zesty Parmesan	6 in	240	5	2	490	39	2	9
Cappacola	1 serv	20	1	0	160	0	n/a	3
Cheese, American	1 serv	100	9	5	510	1	n/a	5
Cheese, Cheddar Shredded	1 serv	110	9	6	180	0	0	7
Cheese, Cheddar, Smoked	1 serv	80	6	4	380	1	n/a	4
Cheese, Parmesan Shredded	1 serv	50	4	2	150	1	0	4
Cheese, Pepper Jack	1 serv	80	7	4	135	0	0	6
Cheese, Provolone	1 serv	80	6	4	190	0	n/a	5
Cheese, Swiss	1 serv	80	6	4	45	0	0	6
Chicken Strips, Grilled	1 serv	110	4	1	300	0	0	19
Corned Beef	1 serv	35	1	0	250	1	0	6
Guacamole	1 serv	45	4	1	135	2	1	0
Ham	1 serv	35	1	0	280	2	n/a	5
Lettuce	1 serv	5	0	0	0	1	0	0
Meatballs	1 serv	220	16	6	1010	8	2	11
Olives	1 serv	15	2	0	125	1	0	0
Onion	3 pcs	10	0	0	0	3	0	0
Pastrami	1 serv	45	3	1	250	1	0	6
Pepperoni	1 serv	70	6	3	230	1	n/a	3
Peppers, Hot Ring	12 pcs	0	0	0	450	1	0	0
Peppers, Jalapeño	18 pcs	10	0	0	490	1	0	0
Peppers, Red Roasted	1 serv	10	0	0	100	2	0	0
Peppers, Sweet Strips	6 pcs	20	0	0	115	5	0	0

ITEM DESCRIPTION	Serving Size	Calories	Total Fat (g)	Saturated Fat (g)	Sodium (mg)	Carbohydrates (g)	Fiber (g)	Protein (g)
Philly Steak & Onion	1 serv	210	15	6	630	5	n/a	13
Prosciuttini	1 serv	15	0	0	180	1	0	2
Roast Beef	1 serv	30	1	0	150	0	0	8
Salami	1 serv	35	3	1	135	0	0	2
Seafood Salad	1 serv	90	4	1	410	10	1	4
Tomato	1 serv	5	0	0	0	2	0	0
Tuna	1 serv	240	18	3	350	0	0	16
Turkey	1 serv	30	0	0	316	1	n/a	5
Wrap, Spinach Herb	12 in	310	8	3	840	52	3	9
Wrap, Traditional	12 in	310	8	3	670	52	5	9

The Nutritional Information Blimpie has provided is based on standard product formulations. Product variations may occur based on regional differences, ingredient substitutions, seasonal conditions, differences in product production at the store, and suppliers. Some items listed may not be available in all stores. This list may not include test products, limited time offers, and regional menu variations.

BOSTON MARKET

DESSERTS

ITEM DESCRIPTION	Serving Size	Calories	Total Fat (g)	Saturated Fat (g)	Sodium (mg)	Carbohydrates (g)	Fiber (g)	Protein (g)
Brownie, Chocolate Chip Fudge	1	470	19	4	340	74	3	8
Cake, Chocolate	1 serv	580	34	11	360	67	3	5
Cookie, Chocolate Chip	1	370	19	10	340	50	1	3
Cornbread	1	200	6	2	300	34	1	3
Pie, Apple	1 serv	580	30	13	690	74	3	4

DRESSINGS AND SPREADS

ITEM DESCRIPTION	Serving Size	Calories	Total Fat (g)	Saturated Fat (g)	Sodium (mg)	Carbohydrates (g)	Fiber (g)	Protein (g)
Sauce, Beef Au Jus	1 serv	20	0	0	730	4	0	0
Sauce, Honey Habanero	1 serv	60	0	0	240	13	0	0
Sauce, Sweet Thai Chili Garlic	1 serv	60	1	0	210	13	1	0
Sauce, Zesty Barbecue	1 serv	60	0	0	240	13	0	0

MAIN MENU

ITEM DESCRIPTION	Serving Size	Calories	Total Fat (g)	Saturated Fat (g)	Sodium (mg)	Carbohydrates (g)	Fiber (g)	Protein (g)
Beef Brisket	reg	230	13	3.5	570	0	0	28
Chicken Pot Pie, Pastry Top	1	800	48	24	1120	60	4	32
Chicken, 1/2 Rotisserie	1	640	33	10	1380	2	0	84
Chicken, 1/4 White Rotisserie	1	320	13	4	710	1	0	51
Chicken, 1/4 White Rotisserie, Skinless	1	220	2.5	1	700	1	0	49
Chicken, Dark Rotisserie	3 pcs	390	22	6	1270	1	0	51
Chicken, Dark (2 Thighs & Drumstick)	3 pcs	540	36	11	1080	1	0	53

ITEM DESCRIPTION	Serving Size	Calories	Total Fat (g)	Saturated Fat (g)	Sodium (mg)	Carbohydrates (g)	Fiber (g)	Protein (g)
Chicken, Dark Skinless (2 Thighs & Drumstick)	3 pcs	340	17	5	720	1	0	47
Chicken, Dark Skinless (Thigh & 2 Drumsticks)	3 pcs	290	11	3.5	1010	0	0	45
Chicken, Thigh & Drumstick	2 pcs	310	20	6	670	1	0	33
Meatloaf	lg	720	45	20	1635	38	9	42
Meatloaf	reg	480	30	13	1090	25	6	28
Turkey Pot Pie, Pastry Top	1	790	46	23	1220	60	4	34
Turkey, Roasted	lg	260	5	2	870	0	0	54
Turkey, Roasted	reg	180	3	1	620	0	0	38
SALADS								
Caesar	entrée	500	39	9	1190	25	3	14
Caesar	side	310	20	5	745	13	2	20
Caesar w/ Chicken	entrée	620	40	10	1490	26	3	40
Caesar, no Dressing	side	50	2.5	1.5	85	3	1	4
Mediterranean	entrée	640	44	10	1190	27	3	36
Mediterranean	side	320	22	5	595	14	1	18
Southwest Santa Fe	entrée	660	40	9	1370	40	4	36
Southwest Santa Fe	side	330	20	4.5	685	20	2	18
SANDWICHES								
Brisket Dip Carver	1	840	45	12	1660	62	3	46
Chicken Carver, Rotisserie	1	820	36	9	1890	66	3	56
Chicken, Pulled BBQ	1	690	17	6	1880	93	5	41
Chicken Salad, Rotisserie	1	1050	64	10	1700	87	11	39
Meatloaf Carver	1	940	40	18	2430	96	10	46
Slider, BBQ Chicken	1 serv	210	5	1	520	35	0	10
Slider, Meatloaf	1 serv	270	11	3.5	630	34	2	11
Slider, Turkey	1 serv	260	14	2.5	500	24	0	12
Turkey BLT	1	1030	57	11	2190	89	11	48
Turkey Carver, Roasted	1	790	35	9	1810	66	3	50
SIDES AND SNACKS								
Apples w/ Cinnamon	1	210	3	0	15	47	3	0
Corn, Sweet	1	170	4	1	95	37	2	6
Creamed Spinach	1	280	23	15	580	12	4	9

ITEM DESCRIPTION	Serving Size	Calories	Total Fat (g)	Saturated Fat (g)	Sodium (mg)	Carbohydrates (g)	Fiber (g)	Protein (g)
Gravy, Beef	3 oz	35	1.5	0.5	500	4	0	1
Gravy, Poultry	4 oz	50	1	0	350	8	0	2
Green Beans	1	60	3.5	1.5	180	7	3	2
Green Beans, Mediterranean	1	120	9	2.5	220	10	4	3
Macaroni & Cheese	1	300	11	7	1100	35	2	11
Potatoes, Garlic Dill New	1	140	3	1	120	24	3	3
Potatoes, Loaded Mashed	1	300	15	8	800	30	3	9
Potatoes, Mashed	1	270	11	5	820	36	4	51
Soup, Broccoli Cheese	1	480	33	21	1490	25	4	22
Soup, Chicken Noodle	1	240	8	2.5	1360	23	2	21
Soup, Chicken Tortilla w/ Toppings	1	410	25	7	2040	30	2	17
Soup, Chicken Tortilla w/o Toppings	1	160	8	1.5	1640	13	2	10
Spinach, Garlicky Lemon	1	140	10	6	440	9	5	6
Squash Casserole	1	270	17	7	1120	20	3	9
Sweet Potato Casserole	1	460	16	4.5	270	77	3	4
Vegetable Stuffing	1	190	8	1	580	25	2	3
Vegetables, Steamed	1	60	2	0	40	8	3	2

Nutrition information and ingredients are current as of the date this resource was printed. Nutrition calculations and ingredients are based on standard product formulations and recipes. Variations can be expected due to slight differences in product assembly by employees, local vendors, and other factors. This information is provided as a reference only. The allergen information provided refers to the big 8 required allergens for labeling.

BURGER KING

BEVERAGES

Apple Juice, Minute Maid	1	100	0	0	15	23	0	0
Cherry Coke®‡	sm (16 oz)	150	0	0	5	42	0	0
Chocolate Milk, 1% Low Fat	8 oz	160	2.5	1.5	150	26	0	8
Coca-Cola Classic‡	sm (16 oz)	140	0	0	0	39	0	0
Coffee, Iced	21 oz	130	4	3	105	21	0	3
Coffee, Iced Mocha	21 oz	290	4.5	3	240	61	2	3
Coffee, Iced Vanilla	21 oz	230	3.5	2.5	90	50	0	3
Coffee‡ , Decaf	sm (16 oz)	0	0	0	0	0	0	0
Coffee‡ , Regular	sm (16 oz)	0	0	0	0	0	0	0
Diet Coke‡	sm (16 oz)	0	0	0	15	0	0	0
Dr Pepper‡	sm (16 oz)	140	0	0	35	39	0	0
Fanta Cherry	16 oz	110	0	0	5	31	0	0

ITEM DESCRIPTION	Serving Size	Calories	Total Fat (g)	Saturated Fat (g)	Sodium (mg)	Carbohydrates (g)	Fiber (g)	Protein (g)
Fanta Orange	16 oz	160	0	0	0	42	0	0
Flavor Shot, Chocolate Syrup	1	90	.5	0	75	22	1	0
Flavor Shot, Vanilla Syrup	1	70	0	0	0	17	0	0
Fruit Punch‡ Hi-C®	sm (16 oz)	150	0	0	15	42	0	0
Iced Tea, Southern Style	sm (16 oz)	180	0	0	20	50	0	0
Iced Tea, Sweetened	sm (16 oz)	90	0	0	20	24	0	0
Iced Tea, Unsweetened	sm (16 oz)	0	0	0	20	0	0	0
Icee Coca-Cola/Frozen Coke	16 oz	90	0	0	10	25	0	0
Lemonade	sm (16 oz)	140	0	0	60	39	0	0
Lemonade, Light	sm (16 oz)	5	0	0	0	1	0	0
Milk Shake, Chocolate	med (16 oz)	590	15	12	470	99	1	12
Milk Shake, Strawberry	med (16 oz)	560	15	11	400	98	0	11
Milk Shake, Vanilla	med (16 oz)	480	15	11	390	78	0	11
Milk, Fat Free	8 oz	90	0	0	125	13	0	9
Orange Juice, Minute Maid	10 oz	140	0	0	20	33	0	2
Root Beer, Barq's®‡	sm (16 oz)	160	0	0	20	46	0	0
Sprite‡	sm (16 oz)	140	0	0	30	39	0	0
Tea, Sweet	sm (16 oz)	120	0	0	0	31	0	0
Tea, Sweet Green	sm (16 oz)	120	0	0	0	31	0	0
Tea, Unsweetened	sm (16 oz)	0	0	0	0	0	0	0
Vault‡	sm (16 oz)	160	0	0	15	42	0	0
Whipped Topping (for coffee)	1 serv	100	7	7	30	10	0	1
BREAKFAST ITEMS								
Biscuit w/ Bacon, Egg & Cheese	1	420	25	16	1360	34	1	16
Biscuit w/ Breakfast Steak	1	650	38	21	1780	50	2	21
Biscuit w/ Chicken Fritter	1	400	20	12	1320	39	1	15
Biscuit w/ Country Ham, Egg & Cheese	1	470	26	16	2010	33	1	18
Biscuit w/ Ham, Egg, & Cheese	1	420	22	15	1410	33	1	16
Biscuit w/ Sausage	1	420	27	15	1090	32	1	13
Biscuit w/ Sausage, Egg, & Cheese	1	570	37	19	1510	34	1	20
Biscuits & Sausage Gravy Platter	1 serv	680	35	28	2350	76	2	16
BK™ Breakfast Bowl	1	540	42	13	1020	17	2	24
BK™ Breakfast Ciabatta Club Sandwich	1	480	23	7	1270	41	2	24
BK® Breakfast Muffin Sandwich	1	410	26	9	860	24	1	17

ITEM DESCRIPTION	Serving Size	Calories	Total Fat (g)	Saturated Fat (g)	Sodium (mg)	Carbohydrates (g)	Fiber (g)	Protein (g)
BK™ Breakfast Platter	1	810	54	22	1790	57	4	25
BK® Kids Breakfast Muffin Sandwich	1	240	11	4	550	23	1	9
BK™ Ultimate Breakfast Platter	1	1310	72	26	2490	134	5	32
BK Wrapper™ w/ Cheesy Bacon	1	380	24	7	1020	28	2	13
Breakfast Burrito w/ Bacon, Egg, Cheese & Salsa	1	300	16	6	910	24	1	15
Breakfast Burrito w/ Potato, Egg, Cheese & Salsa	1	320	17	6	900	29	2	13
Breakfast Burrito w/ Sausage, Egg, Cheese & Salsa	1	440	29	10	1120	25	1	20
Cini-Minis	4 pcs	400	18	7	380	52	2	7
Croissan'wich® w/ Bacon, Egg & Cheese	1	360	19	8	830	26	0	14
Croissan'wich® w/ Egg & Cheese	1	320	16	7	680	26	0	11
Croissan'wich® w/ Ham, Egg & Cheese	1	350	17	7	1110	27	0	18
Croissan'wich® w/ Sausage & Cheese	1	380	24	10	780	26	0	14
Croissan'wich® w/ Sausage, Egg & Cheese	1	490	31	11	990	27	0	18
Double Croissan'wich™ w/ Bacon, Egg, & Cheese	1	440	25	11	1190	27	0	20
Double Croissan'wich™ w/ Ham, Bacon, Egg, & Cheese	1	440	24	10	1470	28	0	23
Double Croissan'wich™ w/ Ham, Egg, & Cheese	1	440	22	10	1740	28	0	26
Double Croissan'wich™ w/ Ham, Sausage, Egg, & Cheese	1	570	35	14	1630	28	0	28
Double Croissan'wich™ w/ Sausage, Bacon, Egg, & Cheese	1	570	37	15	1350	28	0	24
Double Croissan'wich™ w/ Sausage, Egg, & Cheese	1	700	49	18	1510	29	0	29
Eggs	side	160	12	3	320	3	0	10
Enormous Omelet Sandwich	1	760	44	15	1840	44	2	35
French Toast Sticks	3 pcs	230	11	2	260	29	1	3
French Toast Sticks	5 pcs	380	18	3	430	49	2	5
French Toast Sticks Platter w/ Bacon & Syrup	1	550	22	4.5	650	79	2	10

ITEM DESCRIPTION	Serving Size	Calories	Total Fat (g)	Saturated Fat (g)	Sodium (mg)	Carbohydrates (g)	Fiber (g)	Protein (g)
French Toast Sticks Platter w/ Sausage & Syrup	1	670	33	8	760	80	2	13
Hash Browns	sm	250	16	3.5	410	24	3	2
Mini Blueberry Biscuits w/ icing	4 pcs	390	15	15	830	57	1	5
Pancakes w/ 1 oz syrup	3	500	19	4.5	700	77	1	7
Pancake Platter w/ Sausage & 1 oz Syrup	1 serv	670	34	9	1010	78	1	14
Scrambled Egg Platter w/ Bacon	1	700	42	19	1650	56	4	23
Scrambled Egg Platter w/ Sausage	1	810	53	22	1760	57	4	26
Southwest Potatoes	side	90	3.5	1	220	12	2	2
Vanilla Icing	1 pkg	90	0	0	25	22	0	0
DESSERTS								
Cheesecake, Strawberry Swirl	1 serv	300	16	8	250	35	0	3
Cone, Soft Serve	1	180	7	4	110	29	0	4
Cookies, Chocolate Chip	2 pcs	330	15	8	250	47	1	3
Cookies, Oatmeal Raisin	2 pcs	310	13	8	260	46	3	4
Funnel Cake Sticks w/ Icing	9 pcs	300	11	3	210	49	1	2
Pie, Dutch Apple	1 serv	320	14	6	300	46	1	2
Pie, HERSHEY®'s Sundae	1 serv	300	18	12	210	31	1	3
Sundae, Caramel	1	300	7	5	260	55	0	5
Sundae, Chocolate Fudge	1	290	8	7	230	53	1	6
Sundae, OREO® BK® Fusion	1	530	17	10	460	90	2	9
DRESSINGS AND SPREADS								
Caramel Sauce	1 pkg	45	0.5	0	35	10	0	0
Dipping Sauce, Barbecue	1 pkg	40	0	0	310	11	0	0
Dipping Sauce, Buffalo	1 pkg	80	8	1.5	360	2	0	0
Dipping Sauce, Honey Mustard	1 pkg	90	6	1	180	8	0	0
Dipping Sauce, Ranch	1 pkg	140	15	2.5	230	1	0	1
Dipping Sauce, Sweet & Sour	1 pkg	45	0	0	55	11	0	0
Dipping Sauce, Zesty Onion Ring	1 pkg	150	15	2.5	210	3	1	0
Dressing, Ken's® Creamy Caesar	1 pkg	210	21	4	610	4	0	3
Dressing, Ken's® Fat Free Ranch	1 pkg	60	0	0	740	15	2	0
Dressing, Ken's® Honey Mustard	1 pkg	270	23	3	510	15	0	1
Dressing, Ken's® Light Italian	1 pkg	120	11	1.5	440	5	0	0
Dressing, Ken's® Ranch	1 pkg	190	20	3	550	2	0	1

ITEM DESCRIPTION	Serving Size	Calories	Total Fat (g)	Saturated Fat (g)	Sodium (mg)	Carbohydrates (g)	Fiber (g)	Protein (g)
French Fry Sauce	1 serv	90	7	1	250	5	0	0
Jam, Strawberry or Grape	1 pkg	30	0	0	0	7	0	0
Ketchup	1 pkg	10	0	0	125	3	0	0
Marinara Sauce	1 serv	15	0	0	170	4	1	1
Mayonnaise	1 pkg	80	9	0.5	75	1	0	0
Picante Taco Sauce	1 serv	10	0	0	115	2	0	0
Syrup	1 pkg	120	0	0	15	30	0	0
MAIN MENU								
Big Fish® Sandwich	1	640	31	5	1560	67	3	23
Big Fish® Sandwich, no Tartar Sauce	1	460	13	2.5	1320	64	3	23
BK Stuffed Steakhouse™	1	590	34	12	1240	48	2	26
BK Wrapper™, Spicy Chicken	1	360	19	5	1010	32	2	14
Buck Double	1	410	22	10	740	28	1	24
Cheeseburger	1	300	14	6	710	28	1	16
Cheeseburger w/ Bacon	1	330	16	7	810	28	1	18
Cheeseburger, Rodeo	1	350	11	7	600	37	2	16
Chicken Fries	6 pcs	250	15	2.5	820	16	1	14
Chicken Fries	9 pcs	380	22	4	1220	24	2	21
Chicken Sandwich, American Original	1	730	47	12	1830	49	3	29
Chicken Sandwich, Italian Original	1	520	22	7	1670	50	3	32
Chicken Sandwich, Original	1	630	39	7	1390	46	3	24
Chicken Sandwich, Original Club	1	690	43	9	1590	48	3	29
Chicken Sandwich, Original, no Mayo	1	420	16	3.5	1210	46	3	24
Chicken Sandwich, Tendercrisp®	1	800	46	8	1640	68	3	32
Chicken Sandwich, Tendercrisp®, no Mayo	1	590	22	4	1450	68	3	31
Chicken Sandwich, Tendergrill®	1	470	18	3.5	1100	40	2	37
Chicken Sandwich, Tendergrill®, no Mayo	1	360	7	1.5	1010	40	2	37
Chicken Tenders®	4 pcs	180	11	2	310	13	0	9
Chicken Tenders®	6 pcs	270	16	3	460	19	0	14
Chicken Tenders Sandwich	1	440	28	4.5	610	35	1	12
Chick'n Crisp® Sandwich, Spicy	1	460	30	5	810	34	2	13
Chick'n Crisp® Sandwich, Spicy, no Mayo	1	300	12	2.5	670	35	2	12
Country Pork Sandwich	1	810	42	13	1910	78	4	29
Double Cheeseburger	1	450	26	12	960	29	1	26

ITEM DESCRIPTION	Serving Size	Calories	Total Fat (g)	Saturated Fat (g)	Sodium (mg)	Carbohydrates (g)	Fiber (g)	Protein (g)
Double Cheeseburger w/ Bacon	1	510	30	14	1150	29	1	31
Double Hamburger	1	360	18	8	520	28	1	22
Double Stacker	1	500	31	12	780	28	1	27
Double Whopper® Sandwich	1	900	57	19	1050	51	3	47
Double Whopper® Sandwich w/ Cheese	1	990	65	24	1480	53	3	52
Double Whopper® Sandwich w/ Cheese, no Mayo	1	830	47	21	1340	53	3	52
Double Whopper® Sandwich, no Mayo	1	740	39	16	910	51	3	47
Hamburger	1	260	10	4	490	28	1	13
Macaroni & Cheese, Kraft®	1	160	5	1.5	340	22	1	7
Quad Stacker	1	800	55	24	1270	30	1	49
Single Stacker	1	380	22	8	700	28	1	17
Steakhouse XT™	1	770	46	17	1330	52	3	36
Steakhouse XT™, A1®	1	970	61	23	1920	54	4	42
Tacos	2	330	23	8	750	18	5	14
Texas Double Whopper® Sandwich	1	1040	69	26	1770	50	3	56
Texas Triple Whopper® Sandwich	1	1270	86	33	1840	50	3	76
Texas Whopper® Sandwich	1	800	51	18	1700	50	3	37
Triple Stacker	1	650	43	18	1020	29	1	38
Triple Whopper® Sandwich	1	1140	75	27	1110	51	3	67
Triple Whopper® Sandwich w/ Cheese	1	1230	82	32	1550	53	3	71
Triple Whopper® Sandwich w/ Cheese, no Mayo	1	1070	64	29	1410	53	3	71
Triple Whopper® Sandwich, no Mayo	1	980	57	24	970	51	3	66
Veggie® Burger**	1	410	16	2.5	1030	44	7.	22
Veggie® Burger** w/ Cheese	1	450	20	5	1250	44	7	24
Veggie® Burger**, no Mayo	1	320	7	1	960	43	7	22
Whopper Jr.® Sandwich	1	340	19	5	510	28	2	14
Whopper Jr.® Sandwich w/ Cheese	1	380	23	8	730	29	2	16
Whopper Jr.® Sandwich w/ Cheese, no Mayo	1	300	14	6	710	31	1	16
Whopper Jr.® Sandwich, no Mayo	1	260	10	4	440	28	2	13
Whopper® Sandwich	1	670	40	11	980	51	3	29
Whopper® Sandwich w/ Cheese	1	760	47	16	1410	53	3	33
Whopper® Sandwich w/ Cheese, no Mayo	1	600	30	14	1270	53	3	32

ITEM DESCRIPTION	Serving Size	Calories	Total Fat (g)	Saturated Fat (g)	Sodium (mg)	Carbohydrates (g)	Fiber (g)	Protein (g)
Whopper® Sandwich, no Mayo	1	510	23	9	840	51	3	28
Whopper® Sandwich w/ Mustard	1	530	23	9	1080	52	3	29
SALADS								
Chicken Garden, Tendercrisp®	1	410	22	5	1060	28	4	26
Chicken Garden, Tendergrill™	1	230	7	3	920	9	3	33
Garden	1	70	3.5	2	90	7	3	2
Side	1	40	2	1	45	2	1	3
SIDES AND SNACKS								
Apple Sauce, Motts® Harvest Plus	1 serv	50	0	0	0	13	1	0
BK™ Fresh Apple Fries	1 serv	25	0	0	0	6	1	0
French Fries, Salted•	med	440	22	4.5	670	56	5	5
Mozzarella Sticks	4 pcs	280	15	5	650	24	2	11
Onion Rings	med	400	21	3.5	630	47	4	6
TOPPINGS AND EXTRAS								
Bacon	1 pc	15	1	0	50	0	0	1
Butter	2 pats	70	8	2.5	65	0	0	0
Cheese, American	1 pc	45	4	2.5	220	1	0	2
Croutons, Garlic Parmesan	1 serv	60	2	0	120	9	0	1
Green Chilies	1 serv	5	0	0	0	1	0	0
Pickles	2	0	0	0	100	0	0	0

™ & © 2010 Burger King Brands, Inc. All Rights Reserved. © 2010 The Coca-Cola Company. "Coca-Cola," "Coca-Cola Classic," "Diet Coke," "Sprite," "ICEE" and "Minute Maid" are registered trademarks of the Coca-Cola Company. All Rights Reserved. DR PEPPER is a registered trademark of Dr Pepper/Seven Up, Inc. © 2010. "NESTLE PURE LIFE" is a registered trademark of Nestle Waters North America, Inc. The HERSHEY®'S trademark and trade dress are used under license. A.1.® Thick & Hearty Steak Sauce, KRAFT® Macaroni and Cheese, and OREO® are registered trademarks of Kraft Foods Holdings, Inc. Ken's Steak House and the associated marks are registered trademarks owned by Ken's Foods, Inc.

** Burger King Corporation makes no claim that the BK VEGGIE® Burger or any other of its products meets the requirements of a vegan or vegetarian diet. The patty is cooked in the microwave.

• The sodium content of French Fries may vary based on level added after cooking. To reduce sodium, HAVE IT YOUR WAY® and order your french fries without salt.

"†": These values represent Sodium derived from ingredients other than water. The actual amount of Sodium in the beverages will vary depending on the quantity contained in the water supply where the finished beverages are produced.

CARL'S JR.

BEVERAGES

Cherry Coca-Cola®	20 oz	170	0	0	10	47	0	0
Coca-Cola® Classic	20 oz	160	0	0	10	45	0	0
Coca-Cola Zero™	20 oz	0	0	0	10	0	0	0
Coffee, Decaf	16 oz	10	0	0	10	2	0	0
Coffee, Regular	16 oz	10	0	0	10	2	0	0
Diet Coke®	20 oz	0	0	0	20	0	0	0

ITEM DESCRIPTION	Serving Size	Calories	Total Fat (g)	Saturated Fat (g)	Sodium (mg)	Carbohydrates (g)	Fiber (g)	Protein (g)
Diet Dr Pepper®	20 oz	0	0	0	90	0	0	0
Dr Pepper®	20 oz	150	0	0	55	43	0	0
Fanta® Orange	20 oz	180	0	0	30	50	0	0
Fanta® Strawberry	20 oz	190	0	0	20	52	0	0
Hi-C® Flashin' Fruit Punch	20 oz	170	0	0	20	47	0	0
Hi-C® Poppin' Pink Lemonade	20 oz	160	0	0	75	42	0	0
Iced Tea, Fresh Brewed	20 oz	5	0	0	25	1	0	0
Iced Tea, Raspberry Nestea®	20 oz	100	0	0	20	27	0	0
Lemonade, Minute Maid Light™	20 oz	5	0	0	10	1	0	0
Powerade® Mountain Blast	20 oz	90	0	0	90	25	0	0
Root Beer, Barq's®	20 oz	180	0	0	45	50	0	0
Sprite®	20 oz	160	0	0	40	43	0	0
Squirt®	20 oz	170	0	0	65	43	0	0
BREAKFAST ITEMS								
Biscuit 'N' Gravy™	1	420	21	8	1380	50	1	8
Biscuit w/ Bacon, Egg & Cheese	1	430	25	11	1170	37	1	16
Biscuit w/ Ham, Egg & Cheese	1	430	22	10	1590	38	1	19
Biscuit w/ Sausage	1	420	26	11	1140	37	1	11
Biscuit w/ Sausage & Egg	1	500	32	12	1190	37	1	17
Biscuit w/ Sausage, Egg & Cheese	1	550	36	15	1420	38	1	19
Breakfast Burger™	1	780	41	15	1410	65	4	38
Burrito w/ Bacon & Egg	1	550	31	12	970	37	1	29
Burrito w/ Steak & Eggs	1	650	36	15	1730	42	2	41
Burrito, Loaded	1	780	48	17	1460	51	3	35
French Toast Dips®, no Syrup	5 pcs	460	21	4	570	60	3	9
Hash Brown Nuggets	1 serv	350	23	4	440	32	3	3
Made From Scratch Biscuit™	1	270	12	6	790	36	1	5
Monster Biscuit™	1	710	48	19	1790	38	1	31
Sourdough Breakfast Sandwich	1	450	21	8	1470	38	1	29
Strawberry Biscuit	1	360	12	6	810	60	1	5
Sunrise Croissant®	1	590	44	17	810	28	1	20
DESSERTS								
Cake, Chocolate	1 pc	300	12	3	350	48	1	3
Cheesecake, Strawberry Swirl	1 pc	290	16	9	230	32	0	6

ITEM DESCRIPTION	Serving Size	Calories	Total Fat (g)	Saturated Fat (g)	Sodium (mg)	Carbohydrates (g)	Fiber (g)	Protein (g)
Cookie, Chocolate Chip	1	370	19	10	350	48	2	3
Malt, Chocolate	1	770	35	24	390	98	1	15
Malt, Oreo® Cookie	1	780	39	25	450	93	1	17
Malt, Strawberry	1	760	35	24	330	98	0	15
Malt, Vanilla	1	770	35	24	330	100	0	15
Shake, Chocolate	1	700	34	23	310	84	1	14
Shake, Oreo® Cookie	1	720	38	25	370	79	1	15
Shake, Strawberry	1	690	34	23	260	84	0	14
Shake, Vanilla	1	700	34	23	250	85	0	14
DRESSINGS AND SPREADS								
Blue Cheese Dressing	1 serv	320	34	7	410	1	0	2
House Dressing	1 serv	220	22	3.5	440	3	0	1
Low Fat Balsamic Dressing	1 serv	35	1.5	0	480	5	0	0
Raspberry Vinaigrette	1 serv	160	12	2	150	12	0	0
Sesame Asian Dressing	1 serv	120	8	1.5	480	12	0	1
KIDS MENU								
Cheeseburger	1	290	15	7	790	25	1	12
Chicken Tenders	2 pcs	220	12	2.5	770	10	1	19
Hamburger	1	230	10	3.5	510	24	1	9
MAIN MENU								
Burger, Big Hamburger	1	470	17	8	1010	55	3	24
Burger, Famous Star™ w/ Cheese	1	660	39	13	1240	53	3	27
Burger, Guacamole Bacon Six Dollar Burger™	1	1040	72	24	2240	51	4	49
Burger, Jalapeño Burger™	1	720	47	14	1350	51	6	27
Burger, Jalapeño Six Dollar Burger™	1	930	63	21	2200	51	6	45
Burger, Low Carb Six Dollar Burger™	1	570	43	19	1460	9	1	38
Burger, Original Six Dollar Burger™	1	900	54	21	2000	59	3	45
Burger, Portobello Mushroom Six Dollar Burger™	1	870	53	19	1730	52	4	47
Burger, Super Star® w/ Cheese	1	920	58	24	1580	55	3	47
Burger, Teriyaki	1	610	29	11	1020	60	3	28
Burger, The Big Carl™	1	910	58	23	1350	52	2	47
Burger, Western Bacon Six Dollar Burger®	1	1000	53	22	2370	77	4	52

ITEM DESCRIPTION	Serving Size	Calories	Total Fat (g)	Saturated Fat (g)	Sodium (mg)	Carbohydrates (g)	Fiber (g)	Protein (g)
Cheeseburger, Double Western Bacon™	1	960	52	23	1770	71	4	52
Cheeseburger, Western Bacon Cheeseburger®	1	710	33	13	1430	70	4	32
Chicken Club™ Sandwich, Charbroiled	1	560	27	7	1330	46	3	36
Chicken Sandwich, Charbroiled BBQ	1	380	7	1.5	1070	51	3	30
Chicken Sandwich, Charbroiled Santa Fe™	1	630	35	8	1460	46	3	32
Chicken™ Sandwich, Crispy w/ Bacon & Swiss	1	750	40	9	1990	62	4	36
Chicken Sandwich, Spicy	1	420	26	5	1260	37	3	12
Chicken Tenders	5 pcs	560	31	6	1930	24	2	47
Chicken Tenders	3 pcs	340	19	3.5	1160	14	1	28
Fish Sandwich, Carl's Catch™	1	680	37	6	1260	70	4	20
SALADS								
Chicken, Grilled w/ Cranberry Apple Walnut	1	310	11	3.5	840	27	4	26
Chicken, Hawaiian Grilled	1	260	8	0	560	34	4	22
Chicken, Original Grilled	1	270	9	3	780	21	3	25
Side Salad	side	120	5	1.5	250	13	2	4
SIDES AND SNACKS								
Chicken Stars™	4 pcs	170	10	2	360	12	1	8
Chicken Stars™	6 pcs	260	16	3.5	540	18	2	12
Chicken Stars™	9 pcs	390	23	5	810	26	3	18
Chili Cheese Fries	1 serv	950	55	18	1950	83	8	27
CrissCut® Fries	1 serv	450	29	5	900	42	4	5
Fish & Chips	1 serv	710	38	6	1410	69	7	22
French Fries	med	430	21	4	870	56	5	5
Fried Zucchini	1 serv	330	18	3	610	36	2	6
Onion Rings	1 serv	530	28	4.5	590	61	3	8

CHILI'S

APPETIZERS

ITEM DESCRIPTION	Serving Size	Calories	Total Fat (g)	Saturated Fat (g)	Sodium (mg)	Carbohydrates (g)	Fiber (g)	Protein (g)
Corn Guacamole w/ Chips	1 serv	1400	84	15	2250	151	25	17
Fried Cheese w/ Marinara	1 serv	660	35	15	2040	54	1	32
Fries, Texas Cheese w/ Chili & Ranch	half	1350	94	42	3620	72	9	59
Fries, Texas Cheese w/ Chili & Ranch	1 serv	2120	144	69	5920	117	14	97
Fries, Texas Cheese w/ Ranch	1 serv	1960	136	65	5370	109	12	84
Fries, Texas Cheese w/ Ranch	half	1260	89	40	3300	67	7	51
Nachos, Beef	8	1170	74	38	2430	59	8	67
Nachos, Beef	12	1720	108	55	3560	86	12	99
Nachos, Chicken	8	1140	71	35	1940	57	8	71
Nachos, Chicken	12	1670	103	51	2830	83	12	106
Nachos, Classic	8	980	67	34	1780	55	42	8
Nachos, Classic	12	1440	97	50	2590	81	62	11
Onion String & Crispy Jalapeño Stack	1 serv	1050	81	18	2230	71	4	12
Skillet Queso w/ Chips	1 serv	1710	101	37	3490	147	13	45
Southwestern Eggrolls w/ Avocado Ranch	1 serv	780	41	10	1830	81	7	24
Spinach & Artichoke Dip w/ Chips	1 serv	1610	102	42	1610	139	14	33
Tostada Chips w/ Salsa	1 serv	1020	51	10	1210	125	11	12
Triple Dipper Big Mouth Bites w/ Ranch	1 serv	850	58	16	1870	51	1	30
Triple Dipper™ Boneless Buffalo Wings w/ Bleu Cheese	1 serv	810	54	10	2320	43	1	35
Triple Dipper™ Chicken Crispers®, No Dressing	1 serv	340	15	4	1130	21	1	30
Triple Dipper™ Fried Cheese w/ Marinara	1 serv	390	21	9	1250	33	1	19
Triple Dipper™ Hot Spinach & Artichoke Dip w/ Chips	1 serv	1290	77	26	870	128	12	21
Triple Dipper™ Southwestern Eggrolls w/ Avocado Ranch	1 serv	560	32	8	1320	54	5	16
Triple Dipper™ Wings Over Buffalo® w/ Bleu Cheese	1 serv	480	41	8	1790	5	1	24
Wings Over Buffalo® w/ Bleu Cheese	1 serv	690	53	11	2100	7	1	46

ITEM DESCRIPTION	Serving Size	Calories	Total Fat (g)	Saturated Fat (g)	Sodium (mg)	Carbohydrates (g)	Fiber (g)	Protein (g)
Wings, Boneless Buffalo w/ Bleu Cheese	1 serv	1490	88	16	4590	94	2	76
DESSERTS								
Brownie Sundae	1	1290	61	30	930	195	8	14
Cake, Molten Chocolate	1 pc	1020	46	27	710	144	5	11
Cheesecake	1 pc	710	42	26	460	68	0	12
Pie, Chocolate Chip Paradise	1 pc	1250	64	33	660	163	4	15
Shake, Frosty Chocolate	1	690	33	21	210	92	0	8
DRESSINGS AND SPREADS								
Barbecue Sauce	1 serv	50	0	0	500	12	1	1
Dressing, Ancho Chile Ranch	1 serv	190	19	4	420	3	0	1
Dressing, Avocado Ranch	1 serv	140	14	2	310	3	1	1
Dressing, Bleu Cheese	1 serv	240	26	5	310	1	0	1
Dressing, Citrus Balsamic Vinaigrette	1 serv	250	25	4	220	6	0	0
Dressing, Honey Lime	1 serv	200	17	3	250	13	0	0
Dressing, Honey Mustard	1 serv	200	22	3	400	1	0	1
Dressing, Honey Mustard, Fat Free	1 serv	70	0	0	510	11	0	0
Dressing, Low Fat Ranch	1 serv	80	5	1	360	9	0	1
Dressing, Ranch	1 serv	180	19	3	380	2	0	1
Guacamole	1 serv	45	4	0	140	3	2	1
Honey Chipotle Sauce	1 serv	140	0	0	530	34	0	0
Ranch, for Chips	1 serv	480	50	8	1010	6	0	3
Salsa, for Chips	1 serv	50	0	0	1090	8	0	2
KIDS MENU								
Apples w/ Cinnamon	side	280	11	2	130	48	9	0
Broccoli, Steamed	side	30	0	0	30	6	3	3
Celery Sticks w/ Ranch	side	80	5	1	380	10	0	1
Chicken Crispers, Crispy	1 serv	380	22	4	630	19	2	26
Chicken Platter, Grilled	1 serv	160	4	1	170	2	0	30
Chicken Sandwich, Grilled	1 serv	230	5	1	230	21	1	22
Corn	side	130	2	0	5	22	6	4
Corn Dog	1 serv	270	14	5	600	31	0	6
Corn on the Cob, no Butter	1 serv	150	2	0	5	32	3	5
French Fries	side	190	7	2	600	30	3	2
Grilled Cheese	1 serv	530	42	12	1020	30	1	11

ITEM DESCRIPTION	Serving Size	Calories	Total Fat (g)	Saturated Fat (g)	Sodium (mg)	Carbohydrates (g)	Fiber (g)	Protein (g)
Little Chicken Crispers	1 serv	340	15	4	1130	21	1	30
Little Mouth Burger	1 serv	330	18	7	630	23	1	19
Little Mouth Cheeseburger	1 serv	400	24	10	950	24	1	22
Macaroni & Cheese	1 serv	500	18	6	930	69	3	16
Mandarin Oranges	side	35	0	0	0	8	0	0
Mashed Potatoes w/o Gravy	side	120	7	2	430	14	1	2
Pineapple	side	35	0	0	0	9	1	0
Pizza, Cheese	1 serv	570	24	9	1120	67	3	23
Quesadilla, Cheese	1 serv	470	24	13	1010	42	2	21
Rice	side	190	7	2	580	30	1	3
Salad w/ Low Fat Ranch	side	130	8	2	460	14	1	4
Shake, Chocolate	1 serv	460	22	14	140	61	0	6
LUNCH MENU								
Big Mouth Burger Bites w/ Fries	1 serv	970	58	17	2100	80	4	31
Chili's Terlingua Chili w/ Toppings	1 bowl	360	20	10	1170	17	5	29
Pasta, Cajun w/ Grilled Chicken	1 serv	870	44	19	2310	71	4	48
Quesadilla, Bacon Ranch Chicken w/ Fries	1 serv	1070	67	21	2480	71	6	41
Salad, Cobb w/ Avocado Ranch	1	430	33	8	680	12	6	23
Salad, House, no Dressing	1	90	5	3	150	7	1	5
Sandwich, California Club w/ Fries	1	740	38	10	1970	73	7	23
Sandwich, Fajita Chicken w/ Fries	1	730	38	8	1140	70	6	28
Sandwich, Grilled Ham & Swiss w/ Fries	1	680	36	10	2010	68	5	22
Sandwich, Southwestern BLT w/ Fries	1	630	33	8	1370	68	5	11
Sandwich, Turkey w/ Fries	1	690	34	10	1610	69	5	22
Soup, Chicken Enchilada	1 bowl	400	25	10	1630	23	3	21
Soup, Chicken & Green Chile	1 bowl	200	7	3	1250	21	3	15
Soup, Sweet Corn	1 bowl	450	36	20	960	31	1	4
MAIN MENU								
Big Mouth® Bites w/ Ranch	1	2120	133	38	4810	163	7	66
Burger, Avocado on Wheat Bun	1	1570	90	29	3170	138	15	54
Burger, Bacon	1	1570	91	28	3690	125	9	61
Burger, Jalapeño Smokehouse w/ Ranch	1	2210	144	46	6600	136	11	92
Burger, Mushroom-Swiss	1	1540	88	28	3710	126	10	59

ITEM DESCRIPTION	Serving Size	Calories	Total Fat (g)	Saturated Fat (g)	Sodium (mg)	Carbohydrates (g)	Fiber (g)	Protein (g)
Burger, Oldtimer®	1	1310	65	20	3230	128	10	51
Burger, Shiner Bock® BBQ	1	1680	87	27	4050	166	10	58
Burger, Southern Smokehouse w/ Ancho Chile BBQ	1	2290	139	46	6500	163	11	93
Chicken Crispers® w/ Honey Mustard	1 serv	1350	68	13	3910	129	11	61
Chicken Crispers®, Crispy Honey-Chipotle w/ Ranch	1 serv	1660	76	13	4110	196	13	54
Chicken Crispers®, Crispy no Dressing	1 serv	1210	57	10	2670	125	52	13
Chicken, Margarita Grilled	1 serv	550	14	4	1870	62	3	46
Chicken, Margarita Grilled, Custom Combination	1 serv	260	7	2	720	15	2	38
Chicken, Monterey	1 serv	890	48	21	2920	51	8	66
Chicken, Monterey, Custom Combination	1 serv	530	25	14	1130	13	2	59
Fajita Condiments	1 serv	230	19	10	490	7	3	10
Fajita, Chicken, no Tortillas or Condiments	1 serv	360	10	3	1330	24	7	44
Fajitas, Beef, no Tortillas or Condiments	1 serv	390	14	5	1950	27	7	38
Fajitas, Buffalo Chicken, no Tortillas or Condiments	1 skillet	950	59	16	5120	51	11	52
Fajita, Trio	1 serv	530	20	7	2340	30	8	56
Guiltless Salmon w/ Garlic & Herbs	1 serv	480	17	4	1590	37	5	49
Guiltless Sandwich, Grilled Chicken w/ Steamed Broccoli	1	610	13	5	1320	78	8	43
Guiltless Sirloin, Classic	1 serv	370	9	4	3680	20	6	53
Guiltless Wrap, Santa Fe Chicken w/ Steamed Broccoli	1	680	25	8	2110	80	8	37
Pasta, Cajun w/ Grilled Chicken	1 serv	1500	76	36	4130	124	6	79
Pasta, Cajun w/ Grilled Shrimp	1 serv	1480	81	38	4480	125	6	64
Quesadilla, Bacon Ranch Chicken	1 serv	1650	107	39	3450	96	5	78
Quesadilla, Bacon Ranch Steak	1 serv	1680	111	41	3940	98	5	74
Ribeye, Flame-Grilled	1 serv	1570	116	50	3560	57	7	78
Ribs, Baby Back, Custom Combination	1/2 rack	760	49	20	2590	14	2	64
Ribs, Memphis Dry Rub	1/2 rack	1080	57	19	4080	82	8	62
Ribs, Original	1/2 rack	1140	63	23	3800	75	9	69
Ribs, Shiner Bock® BBQ	1/2 rack	1200	63	23	3710	91	8	69

ITEM DESCRIPTION	Serving Size	Calories	Total Fat (g)	Saturated Fat (g)	Sodium (mg)	Carbohydrates (g)	Fiber (g)	Protein (g)
Salmon, Grilled w/ Garlic & Herbs	1 serv	580	28	10	1660	38	5	49
Salmon, Grilled w/ Garlic & Herbs, Custom Combination	1 serv	310	15	5	590	1	1	42
Sandwich, BBQ Pulled Pork	1	1670	85	16	4240	172	13	54
Sandwich, Buffalo Chicken Ranch	1 serv	1410	68	12	3940	143	12	52
Sandwich, California Club	1	1490	76	20	3950	147	15	46
Sandwich, Grilled Chicken	1 serv	1280	63	15	2580	121	9	57
Sandwich, Grilled Ham & Swiss	1	1360	71	20	4010	137	9	45
Sandwich, Turkey	1	1340	64	17	3140	138	11	41
Sandwich, Steakhouse	1	1010	45	19	3450	115	11	38
Shrimp, Fried w/ Cocktail Sauce	1 serv	990	52	11	3650	108	9	26
Shrimp, Fried w/ Cocktail Sauce, Custom Combination	1 serv	270	12	3	1500	25	0	14
Shrimp, Spicy Garlic & Lime Grilled Custom Combination	1 serv	150	8	3	700	4	0	15
Sirloin, Chili's Classic	1 serv	1010	60	24	3370	59	7	62
Sirloin, Chili's Classic Custom Combination	1 serv	360	18	9	1420	7	0	42
Steak, Country Fried	1 serv	1270	71	14	3700	120	9	41
Tacos, Crispy Chicken	1 serv	1630	78	22	4320	171	13	63
Tacos, Chicken Club	1 serv	1260	60	18	4320	120	11	59
Tacos, Crispy Shrimp	1 serv	1500	68	20	4760	174	11	51
Tortillas, Flour	3 pcs	390	10	3	1040	63	3	10
Wrap, Santa Fe Chicken w/ Ancho-Chile Ranch	1	1320	73	20	3200	126	11	45
SALADS								
Boneless Buffalo Chicken	1	990	68	14	4310	48	8	46
Caribbean Salad w/ Grilled Chicken	1	610	25	4	800	65	6	33
Caribbean Salad w/ Grilled Shrimp	1	620	31	6	1060	66	6	19
Chicken Caesar	1	650	44	8	1130	26	5	40
Cobb Salad	1	710	52	15	1050	22	11	46
House, no Dressing	1	180	11	6	290	15	2	10
Quesadilla Explosion	1 serv	1400	89	28	2360	90	9	65
SOUPS								
Broccoli Cheese	1 cup	110	7	4	600	8	1	5

ITEM DESCRIPTION	Serving Size	Calories	Total Fat (g)	Saturated Fat (g)	Sodium (mg)	Carbohydrates (g)	Fiber (g)	Protein (g)
Chicken Enchilada	1 cup	200	13	5	820	11	1	11
Chicken & Green Chile	1 cup	100	4	1	620	11	1	8
Chili's Terlingua Chili w/ Toppings	1 cup	180	10	5	580	9	3	14
Potato, Loaded Baked	1 cup	210	15	9	590	11	1	8
Sweet Corn	1 cup	230	18	10	480	16	1	2
TOPPINGS AND EXTRAS								
Avocado Slices	1 serv	80	7	1	0	4	3	1
Bacon, Applewood Smoked	3 pcs	90	7	3	370	0	0	7
Black Beans	1 serv	100	1	0	620	18	5	6
Black Bean Patty	1	200	2	0	800	25	7	21
Broccoli, Steamed	1 serv	80	6	3	490	6	3	3
Bun, Plain Wheat	1	360	9	4	350	62	3	9
Cheese, American	1 pc	70	6	4	320	1	0	3
Cheese, Cheddar	1 pc	80	7	4	135	0	0	5
Cheese, Provolone	1 pc	80	6	4	190	0	0	5
Cheese, Swiss	1 pc	80	6	4	105	0	0	6
Cinnamon Apples	1 serv	280	11	2	130	48	9	0
Cole Slaw	1 serv	240	20	4	490	15	2	1
Corn on the Cob w/ Butter	1	200	7	1	420	32	3	5
French Fries	1 serv	380	13	3	1210	61	6	4
Gravy	1 serv	30	2	0	350	4	1	0
Mashed Potatoes w/ Black Pepper Gravy	1 serv	280	15	4	1300	31	3	4
Mashed Potatoes, Loaded	1 serv	390	25	10	1160	28	3	13
Rice	1 serv	190	7	2	580	30	1	3
Rice & Black Beans, added to Entrée	1 serv	290	7	2	1200	48	6	9
Shrimp, Fried, added to Entrée	3 pcs	110	6	2	450	7	0	6
Shrimp, Spicy Garlic & Lime, added to Entrée	3 pcs	80	4	2	350	2	0	8
Sour Cream	1 serv	60	6	4	55	1	0	1

The nutritional analysis is comprised of data from Analytical Food Laboratories (an independent testing facility commissioned by Chili's) combined with nutrient data from Chili's suppliers, the U.S. Agriculture and nutrient database analysis of Chili's recipes using Genesis SQL Nutritional Analysis Program from ESHA Research in Salem, Oregon. The rounding of figures is based on FDA guidelines. Chili's attempts to provide nutritional information regarding its products that is as complete as possible. Some menu items may not be at all restaurants; test products, test recipes, limited time offers, or regional items may not be included. While menu item ingredients information is based on standard product recipes, variations may occur due to ordinary differences inherent in the preparation of menu items, local suppliers, region of the country, and season of the year. Additionally, no products are certified as vegetarian. This listing is updated periodically in an attempt to reflect the current status of Chili's products. 04222010

ITEM DESCRIPTION	Serving Size	Calories	Total Fat (g)	Saturated Fat (g)	Sodium (mg)	Carbohydrates (g)	Fiber (g)	Protein (g)
CHIPOTLE								
Barbacoa	1 serv (4 oz)	170	7	2.5	510	2	0	24
Beans, Black	1 serv (4 oz)	120	1	0	250	23	11	7
Beans, Pinto	1 serv (4 oz)	120	1	0	330	22	10	7
Carnitas	1 serv (4 oz)	190	8	2.5	540	1	0	27
Cheese	1 serv (1 oz)	100	8.5	5	180	0	0	8
Chicken	1 serv (4 oz)	190	6.5	2	370	1	0	32
Chips	1 serv (4 oz)	570	27	3.5	420	73	8	8
Crispy Taco Shell	1	60	2	0.5	10	9	1	<1
Fajita Vegetables	1 serv (2.5 oz)	20	0.5	0	170	4	1	1
Guacamole	1 serv (3.5 oz)	150	13	2	190	8	6	2
Rice, Cilantro-Lime	1 serv (3 oz)	130	3	0.5	150	23	0	2
Romaine Lettuce (salad)	2.5 oz	10	0	0	5	2	1	1
Romaine Lettuce (tacos)	1 oz	5	0	0	0	1	1	0
Salsa, Corn	1 serv (3.5 oz)	80	1.5	0	410	15	3	3
Salsa, Green Tomatillo	1 serv (2 oz)	15	0	0	230	3	1	1
Salsa, Red Tomatillo	1 serv (2 oz)	40	1	0	510	8	4	2
Salsa, Tomato	1 serv (3.5 oz)	20	0	0	470	4	<1	1
Sour Cream	1 serv (2 oz)	120	10	7	30	2	0	2
Steak	1 serv (4 oz)	190	6.5	2	320	2	0	30
Tortilla (burrito)	1	290	9	3	670	44	2	7
Tortilla (taco)	1	90	2.5	1	200	13	<1	2
Vinaigrette	1 serv (2 oz)	260	24.5	4	700	12	1	0

We got these facts from analyzing our food. But nutritional content may vary because of changes in growing seasons, different suppliers, slight variations in our recipes, or the different places that we buy our ingredients. We may update this chart from time to time.

CHUCK E. CHEESE

DESSERTS

ITEM DESCRIPTION	Serving Size	Calories	Total Fat (g)	Saturated Fat (g)	Sodium (mg)	Carbohydrates (g)	Fiber (g)	Protein (g)
Cake, Chocolate	1 pc	290	13	4	220	41	2	3
Cake, Chocolate 1/4 Sheet	1 pc	310	14	5	200	41	2	3
Cake, Vanilla Buttercream	1 pc	310	18	6	230	35	0	2
Cinnamon Sticks w/ Cinnamon Topping & Sugar Icing	1 pc	70	2	1	87	11	0	1

ITEM DESCRIPTION	Serving Size	Calories	Total Fat (g)	Saturated Fat (g)	Sodium (mg)	Carbohydrates (g)	Fiber (g)	Protein (g)
Dessert Pizza w/ Cinnamon Apples, Shortbread & Sugar Icing	1 pc	192	5	2	164	33	1	2
MAIN MENU								
Ciabatta w/ Chicken	1	715	28	7	1940	80	3	44
Pizza, Individual Cheese	1	540	19	8	1255	69	3	21
Pizza, Large All Meat Combo	1 pc	240	11	4	566	24	1	10
Pizza, Large Barbecue Chicken	1 pc	205	7	3	447	27	1	7
Pizza, Large Cheese	1 pc	170	6	3	404	23	1	7
Pizza, Large Super Combo	1 pc	205	9	3	508	24	1	8
Pizza, Large Veggie Combo	1 pc	175	6	2	402	24	1	10
Pizza, Medium All Meat Combo	1 pc	215	11	4	608	22	1	9
Pizza, Medium Barbecue Chicken	1 pc	185	6	2	460	24	1	8
Pizza, Medium Cheese	1 pc	155	5	2	360	21	1	6
Pizza, Medium Super Combo	1 pc	185	8	3	453	22	1	7
Pizza, Medium Veggie Combo	1 pc	160	6	2	366	22	2	6
Pizza, Small All Meat Combo	1 pc	180	9	3	508	19	1	9
Pizza, Small Barbecue Chicken	1 pc	150	5	2	394	21	1	7
Pizza, Small Cheese	1 pc	130	4	2	308	19	1	5
Pizza, Small Super Combo	1 pc	160	7	3	393	19	1	6
Pizza, Small Veggie Combo	1 pc	135	5	2	319	20	1	5
Sandwich Platter (Chicken, Ham & Cheese, or Italian)	1 pc	183	8	2	543	20	1	9
Sandwich w/ Ham & Cheese	1	685	27	8	2206	79	3	33
Sub, Italian	1	790	39	12	2374	78	3	34
Wings Platter	4 pcs	300	20	8	1308	16	4	16
SIDES AND SNACKS								
Breadsticks w/ Marinara & Light Ranch Dressing	1 pc	175	9	2	412	18	1	6
Buffalo Wings	1 pc	75	5	1	327	4	1	4
Carrot Sticks w/ Ranch	side	183	15	2	451	12	2	2
Celery & Bleu Cheese	4 pcs	269	26	5	606	6	2	3
French Fries w/ Ketchup & Light Ranch	1 serv	420	20	2	929	55	6	6
Fruit Garnish	1 serv	65	0	0	2	9	1	0

ITEM DESCRIPTION	Serving Size	Calories	Total Fat (g)	Saturated Fat (g)	Sodium (mg)	Carbohydrates (g)	Fiber (g)	Protein (g)
Hot Dogs w/ Mustard & Relish	1	310	19	7	1084	35	2	11
Mandarin Oranges	1 serv	56	0	0	6	15	1	0
Mozzarella Sticks w/ Marinara Sauce	1 pc	93	6	2	211	6	0	4
Pasta Salad	side	150	4	0.5	280	24	1	4
Sampler Platter	1 serv/ 7	329	19	5	840	25	2	13
Veggie Platter	1 serv/ 8	129	11	2	264	7	2	2

** All sandwiches served with Lettuce, Tomatoes, Onion, Balsamic Vinaigrette, Mayonnaise **

Chuck E. Cheese's attempts to provide nutrition and ingredient information regarding its products that is as complete as possible. While the nutrition and ingredient information is based on standard product formulations, variations may occur depending on the local supplier, the region of the country, and the season of the year. Further, product formulations change periodically. Serving sizes may vary from the quantity on which the analysis was completed. If you need further information or have food sensitivities and/or dietary concerns regarding specific ingredients in specific menu items, please visit our website (www.chuckecheese.com) or call us at 972-258-4255. This listing is effective as of January 2009.

DAIRY QUEEN

BEVERAGES

Coca-Cola	sm	160	0	0	10	43	0	0
Coffee	12 oz	5	0	0	5	0	0	0
Diet Coca-Cola	sm	0	0	0	10	0	0	0
Diet Pepsi®	sm	0	0	0	30	0	0	0
Dr Pepper®	sm	160	0	0	55	43	0	0
Lemonade Chiller, Classic	sm	270	0	0	20	69	0	0
Lemonade Chiller, Strawberry	sm	320	0	0	40	82	0	0
Limeade	sm	200	0	0	0	41	1	0
Mountain Dew®	sm	190	0	0	80	51	0	0
Mug®	sm	160	0	0	65	47	0	0
Pepsi®	sm	160	0	0	40	44	0	0
Root Beer, Barq's®	sm	180	0	0	40	48	0	0
Sierra Mist®	sm	170	0	0	45	43	0	0
Sprite®	sm	150	0	0	40	42	0	0

DESSERTS

Arctic Rush, All Flavors	sm	230	0	0	25	58	0	0
Banana Split	1 serv	520	14	10	150	94	4	9
Blizzard, Banana Cream Pie	sm	570	21	14	330	85	1	11
Blizzard, Banana Split	sm	440	14	9	190	71	1	11
Blizzard, Butterfinger®	sm	470	16	10	220	71	0	11
Blizzard, Chocolate Xtreme	sm	650	29	16	380	88	2	12
Blizzard, Cookie Dough	sm	710	28	16	400	104	1	13

ITEM DESCRIPTION	Serving Size	Calories	Total Fat (g)	Saturated Fat (g)	Sodium (mg)	Carbohydrates (g)	Fiber (g)	Protein (g)
Blizzard, Double Fudge Cookie Dough	sm	750	32	16	420	107	2	13
Blizzard, French Silk Pie	sm	670	30	19	310	90	1	12
Blizzard, Georgia Mud Fudge™	sm	680	35	13	430	82	3	13
Blizzard, Hawaiian	sm	440	15	10	180	67	1	10
Blizzard, Heath®	sm	600	26	16	310	83	1	11
Blizzard, M&M's® Chocolate Candy	sm	660	23	14	230	101	1	13
Blizzard, Midnight Truffle	sm	750	37	21	280	99	3	15
Blizzard, Mint Oreo®	sm	560	18	10	360	87	1	11
Blizzard, Oreo® Cookies	sm	550	20	10	410	81	1	12
Blizzard, Reese's® Peanut Butter Cups®	sm	530	21	11	260	74	1	13
Blizzard, Snickers®	sm	670	26	13	310	99	1	15
Blizzard, Strawberry CheeseQuake®	sm	510	21	13	280	69	0	12
Blizzard, Turtle Pecan Cluster	sm	700	33	18	310	89	2	13
Buster Bar® Treat	1	480	31	15	220	45	2	11
Cake, 10"	1 pc /12	410	15	11	200	60	1	8
Cake, 10" Chocolate Xtreme Blizzard	1 pc /12	630	29	21	320	84	2	10
Cake, 10" Oreo Blizzard	1 pc /12	540	23	15	320	76	1	9
Cake, 10" Reese's® Peanut Butter Cups Blizzard	1 pc /12	590	27	19	270	77	2	11
Cake, 8"	1 pc /8	410	15	11	210	59	1	9
Cake, 8" Chocolate Xtreme Blizzard	1 pc /8	620	29	20	310	83	2	10
Cake, 8" Oreo Blizzard	1 pc /8	550	24	17	310	75	1	9
Cake, 8" Reese's® Peanut Butter Cups Blizzard	1 pc /8	580	27	19	260	75	2	10
Cake, Heart	1 pc /10	290	11	8	150	42	1	6
Cake, Log	1 pc /8	310	12	8	170	44	1	6
Cake, Sheet	1 pc /24	320	13	9	170	47	1	6
Cone, Chocolate	sm	240	7	5	115	37	0	6
Cone, Chocolate Coated Waffle w/ Soft Serve	1	540	21	13	170	77	1	10
Cone, Plain Waffle w/ Soft Serve	1	420	13	7	135	67	0	10
Cone, Vanilla	sm	230	7	4.5	100	36	0	6
Dilly® Bar, Butterscotch	1	210	11	9	105	24	0	3

ITEM DESCRIPTION	Serving Size	Calories	Total Fat (g)	Saturated Fat (g)	Sodium (mg)	Carbohydrates (g)	Fiber (g)	Protein (g)
Dilly® Bar, Cherry	1	210	12	8	80	24	0	3
Dilly® Bar, Chocolate	1	240	15	9	70	24	1	4
Dilly® Bar, Chocolate Mint	1	240	15	9	70	24	1	4
Dilly® Bar, Heath	1	220	13	10	95	25	0	3
Dilly® Bar, no Sugar Added	1	190	13	10	60	24	5	3
Dipped Cone, Chocolate	sm	330	15	12	110	42	0	6
DQ Fudge Bar	1	50	0	0	70	13	6	4
DQ Home-Pak™	1	1150	38	25	510	171	0	31
DQ Sandwich	1	190	5	3	135	31	1	4
DQ Vanilla Orange Bar	1	60	0	0	40	18	6	2
Float, Arctic Rush	sm	330	6	4	95	65	0	5
Freeze, Arctic Rush	sm	380	10	6	140	65	0	8
Malt, Banana	sm	540	20	15	230	80	1	13
Malt, Caramel	sm	620	21	15	290	95	0	14
Malt, Cherry	sm	570	20	15	250	84	0	13
Malt, Chocolate	sm	600	20	15	250	92	1	13
Malt, Hot Fudge	sm	620	24	18	280	90	1	14
Malt, Peanut Butter	sm	710	35	17	400	83	2	16
Malt, Strawberry	sm	570	20	15	240	83	1	13
Malt, Vanilla	sm	590	20	15	240	89	0	13
MooLatté, Cappuccino	16 oz	460	16	12	160	72	0	8
MooLatté, Caramel	16 oz	530	16	13	210	89	0	8
MooLatté, French Vanilla	16 oz	510	15	12	160	87	0	8
MooLatté, Mocha	16 oz	510	18	13	180	81	1	8
Oreo Brownie Earthquake®	1 serv	740	27	15	350	149	2	11
Parfait, Peanut Buster®	1 serv	710	31	18	350	96	3	17
Peanut Butter Bash	1	580	27	15	300	73	2	11
Pecan Mudslide	1	640	30	12	310	83	2	11
Shake, Banana	sm	500	20	14	190	70	1	12
Shake, Caramel	sm	570	21	15	260	85	0	13
Shake, Cherry	sm	520	20	15	220	74	0	12
Shake, Chocolate	sm	550	20	15	220	82	1	13
Shake, Hot Fudge	sm	580	23	18	240	80	1	13
Shake, Peanut Butter	sm	660	35	17	370	73	2	15

ITEM DESCRIPTION	Serving Size	Calories	Total Fat (g)	Saturated Fat (g)	Sodium (mg)	Carbohydrates (g)	Fiber (g)	Protein (g)
Shake, Strawberry	sm	520	20	15	210	73	1	12
Shake, Vanilla	sm	550	20	15	200	80	0	12
StarKiss® Bar, Cherry	1	80	0	0	10	21	0	0
StarKiss® Bar, Stars & Stripes™	1	80	0	0	10	21	0	0
Strawberry Shortcake	1	480	17	13	370	75	1	8
Sundae, Banana	sm	230	7	4.5	90	37	1	6
Sundae, Caramel	sm	300	8	5	140	50	0	6
Sundae, Cherry	sm	240	7	4.5	100	39	0	6
Sundae, Chocolate	sm	280	8	4.5	115	48	1	6
Sundae, Hot Fudge	sm	300	10	8	135	46	0	6
Sundae, Marshmallow	sm	290	7	4.5	100	50	0	5
Sundae, Peanut Butter	sm	390	22	7	260	39	1	9
Sundae, Pineapple	sm	230	7	4.5	100	38	0	6
Sundae, Strawberry	sm	260	7	4.5	105	44	0	6
Waffle Bowl Sundae, Chocolate Covered Strawberry	1	760	38	30	170	96	2	10
Waffle Bowl Sundae, Fudge Brownie Temptation	1	940	48	23	440	122	6	13
Waffle Bowl Sundae, Turtle	1	810	35	18	300	115	2	11
DRESSINGS AND SPREADS								
Dipping Sauce, BBQ	1 serv	80	0	0	430	1	1	1
Dipping Sauce, Bleu Cheese	1 serv	210	21	4	690	5	0	2
Dipping Sauce, Honey Mustard	1 serv	250	21	3	380	16	0	1
Dipping Sauce, Ranch	1 serv	310	32	5	360	3	0	1
Dipping Sauce, Sweet & Sour	1 serv	90	0	0	240	24	0	0
Dipping Sauce, Wild Buffalo	1 serv	110	12	2	900	1	0	0
Dressing, Fat-Free Italian	1 serv	15	0	0	360	4	0	0
Dressing, Fat-Free Ranch	1 serv	35	0	0	430	5	0	1
Dressing, Fat-Free Red French	1 serv	40	0	0	320	10	0	0
Dressing, Fat-Free Thousand Island	1 serv	60	0	0	390	16	0	0
Gravy	1 serv	90	6	2	480	8	0	1
KIDS MENU								
Cheeseburger Meal w/ Applesauce	1	490	18	9	930	56	2	20
Cheeseburger Meal w/ Banana	1	510	19	9	900	63	4	21

ITEM DESCRIPTION	Serving Size	Calories	Total Fat (g)	Saturated Fat (g)	Sodium (mg)	Carbohydrates (g)	Fiber (g)	Protein (g)
Cheeseburger Meal w/ Fries	1	580	26	10	1310	60	3	21
Chicken Strip Meal w/ Applesauce	1	360	11	1	810	40	3	16
Chicken Strip Meal w/ Banana	1	380	10	1	750	45	5	16
Chicken Strip Meal w/ Fries	1	470	18	2.5	1170	44	4	18
Grilled Cheese Meal w/ Applesauce	1	400	13	8	1050	53	3	13
Grilled Cheese Meal w/ Banana	1	430	13	8	1020	59	5	14
Grilled Cheese Meal w/ Fries	1	510	21	9	1410	57	3	15
Hot Dog Meal w/ Applesauce	1	380	18	7	930	45	2	11
Hot Dog Meal w/ Banana	1	400	18	7	900	51	4	12
Hot Dog Meal w/ Fries	1	470	25	8	1270	48	3	12
MAIN MENU								
Breaded Mushrooms	1 serv	250	9	1	500	36	2	7
Burger, Bacon Cheese GrillBurger	1/4 lb	630	35	13	1280	44	2	36
Burger, Cheeseburger	1	400	18	9	920	34	1	19
Burger, Cheeseburger Deluxe	1	400	18	9	930	35	1	20
Burger, Deluxe Hamburger	1	350	14	7	680	34	1	17
Burger, Double Cheeseburger	1	640	34	18	1230	34	1	34
Burger, Double Cheeseburger Deluxe	1	640	34	18	1240	35	1	34
Burger, Double Hamburger	1	540	26	13	750	34	1	29
Burger, DQ Ultimate	1	780	48	22	1390	33	1	41
Burger, FlameThrower GrillBurger	1/2 lb	1010	71	25	1540	42	2	56
Burger, GrillBurger w/ Cheese	1/2 lb	820	49	20	1190	44	3	52
Burger, GrillBurger w/ Cheese	1/4 lb	530	26	12	910	42	2	31
Burger, Mushroom Swiss GrillBurger	1/4 lb	590	35	12	700	39	2	30
Chicken Strip Basket	4 pcs	1160	47	7	2960	120	9	40
Chicken Strip Basket	6 pcs	1370	57	8	3650	123	10	52
Chili	cup	470	16	7	2600	54	2	29
Chili Cheese Fries	1 serv	1020	51	15	2360	117	9	25
Corn Dog	1	460	19	5	970	56	1	17
French Fries	reg	310	13	2	640	43	3	4
Hot Dog	1	290	17	7	900	22	1	11
Hot Dog, Chili	1	330	20	8	1050	24	1	13
Hot Dog, Chili Cheese	1	380	24	11	980	23	1	16
Hot Dog, Foot-Long	1	560	35	14	1600	39	2	20

ITEM DESCRIPTION	Serving Size	Calories	Total Fat (g)	Saturated Fat (g)	Sodium (mg)	Carbohydrates (g)	Fiber (g)	Protein (g)
Hot Dog, Foot-Long Chili Cheese	1	670	43	19	1720	41	2	28
Onion Rings	1 serv	360	16	2	840	47	2	6
Popcorn Shrimp Basket	1 serv	1000	49	22	3650	116	8	19
Quesadilla Basket, Chicken	1 serv	1200	60	27	2740	115	9	47
Quesadilla Basket, Veggie	1 serv	1030	50	21	2270	114	9	28
Salad	side	25	0	0	20	17	2	11
Salad, Crispy Chicken	1	460	19	6	1230	31	6	29
Salad, Grilled Chicken	1	280	11	5	890	14	4	31
Sandwich, Barbecue Beef	1	270	6	1.5	970	41	1	16
Sandwich, Barbecue Pork	1	310	9	2.5	830	41	2	17
Sandwich, Classic Club	1	580	29	9	1750	42	2	32
Sandwich, Crispy Chicken	1	560	27	3.5	1010	47	3	20
Sandwich, Crispy Fish	1	430	18	2.5	1160	51	2	16
Sandwich, FlameThrower Chicken	1	860	55	11	1850	51	3	30
Sandwich, Grilled Cheese	1	290	13	8	1020	30	1	13
Sandwich, Grilled Chicken	1	370	16	2.5	810	32	1	24
Sandwich, Supreme BLT	1	590	34	9	1380	40	2	28
Sandwich, Turkey	1	520	25	7	1550	42	2	29
White Cheese Curds	1 serv	550	45	25	900	0	0	35
Wrap, Crispy Chicken	1	290	17	3.5	620	17	2	11
Wrap, FlameThrower Chicken	1	300	18	4	620	17	2	11
Wrap, Grilled Chicken	1	200	13	3.5	450	9	1	12
TOPPINGS AND EXTRAS								
Banana Slices	1 serv	25	0	0	0	6	1	0
Brownie Pieces	1 serv	130	6	3	150	17	1	1
Butterfinger Pieces	1 serv	110	4.5	2	55	18	0	1
Caramel Topping	1 serv	90	1	0.5	50	20	0	1
Cheesecake Pieces	1 serv	100	6	3.5	80	10	0	2
Choco Chunks	1 serv	150	10	8	0	17	1	1
Chocolate Topping	1 serv	70	1.5	0	25	17	1	0
Cocoa Fudge	1 serv	140	10	2	70	16	0	1
Coconut Flakes	1 serv	80	7	6	35	7	2	1
Cookie Dough Pieces	1 serv	130	6	3	95	18	0	1
Heath Pieces	1 serv	150	9	5	95	17	0	1

ITEM DESCRIPTION	Serving Size	Calories	Total Fat (g)	Saturated Fat (g)	Sodium (mg)	Carbohydrates (g)	Fiber (g)	Protein (g)
Hot Fudge Topping	1 serv	90	3.5	3.5	45	15	0	1
M&M's Chocolate Candies	1 serv	140	6	3.5	20	20	1	1
Oreo Cookie Pieces	1 serv	140	6	1.5	190	20	1	1
Peanut Butter Topping	1 serv	180	15	2	170	8	1	3
Peanuts	1 serv	80	7	1	55	3	1	4
Pecan Pieces	1 serv	100	11	1	55	2	1	1
Reese's® Peanut Butter Cups Pieces	1 serv	150	9	3	85	16	1	3
Snickers Pieces	1 serv	130	7	2.5	70	17	1	2
Strawberry Topping	1 serv	25	0	0	5	6	0	0
Whipped Topping	1 serv	90	7	7	0	7	0	0

DOMINO'S PIZZA

DOMINO'S BREAD BOWL PASTA™

ITEM DESCRIPTION	Serving Size	Calories	Total Fat (g)	Saturated Fat (g)	Sodium (mg)	Carbohydrates (g)	Fiber (g)	Protein (g)
Chicken Alfredo in Bread Bowl	half	700	26	11	1040	93	3	25
Chicken Carbonara in Bread Bowl	half	740	28	12	1110	94	3	28
Italian Sausage Marinara in Bread Bowl	half	730	27	10	1380	97	4	26
Pasta Primavera in Bread Bowl	half	670	24	11	880	94	4	20
Three Cheese Mac-N-Cheese in Bread Bowl	half	730	28	14	1390	95	3	27

DOMINO'S PASTA IN A DISH™

ITEM DESCRIPTION	Serving Size	Calories	Total Fat (g)	Saturated Fat (g)	Sodium (mg)	Carbohydrates (g)	Fiber (g)	Protein (g)
Chicken Alfredo	1 bowl	600	29	16	1080	58	2	27
Chicken Carbonara	1 bowl	670	35	18	1220	59	2	32
Italian Sausage Marinara	1 bowl	670	32	15	1760	66	5	28
Mac-N-Cheese	1 bowl	670	34	21	1770	61	2	30
Pasta Primavera	1 bowl	540	27	16	770	59	3	16

DRESSINGS AND SPREADS

ITEM DESCRIPTION	Serving Size	Calories	Total Fat (g)	Saturated Fat (g)	Sodium (mg)	Carbohydrates (g)	Fiber (g)	Protein (g)
Dipping Sauce, Blue Cheese	1 pkg	240	25	4.5	310	2	0	1
Dipping Sauce, Garlic	1 pkg	250	28	5	160	0	0	0
Dipping Sauce, Hot	1 pkg	50	4.5	0.5	1480	3	0	0
Dipping Sauce, Italian	1 pkg	220	24	3.5	460	1	0	0
Dipping Sauce, Marinara	1 pkg	25	0	0	270	5	1	1
Dipping Sauce, Parmesan Peppercorn	1 pkg	310	33	5	510	3	0	2
Dipping Sauce, Ranch	1 pkg	200	21	3	340	2	0	0

ITEM DESCRIPTION	Serving Size	Calories	Total Fat (g)	Saturated Fat (g)	Sodium (mg)	Carbohydrates (g)	Fiber (g)	Protein (g)
Dipping Sauce, Sweet Icing	1 pkg	250	2.5	0.5	0	57	0	0
Dressing, Blue Cheese	1 pkg	230	24	4.5	440	2	0	2
Dressing, Buttermilk Ranch	1 pkg	230	24	3.5	390	2	0	1
Dressing, Creamy Caesar	1 pkg	210	21	3.5	520	2	0	1
Dressing, Golden Italian	1 pkg	210	22	3.5	360	2	0	0
Dressing, Light Italian	1 pkg	20	1	0	770	3	0	0
FEAST PIZZAS								
America's Favorite Feast: Pepperoni, Mushroom, Sausage	lg, 1 pc /8	120	10	4	470	4	1	6
Bacon Cheeseburger Feast: Beef, Bacon, Cheddar Cheese	lg, 1 pc /8	140	11	5	450	3	1	8
Deluxe Feast Pepperoni: Green Pepper, Onion, Mushroom, Sausage	lg, 1 pc /8	100	8	3.5	380	4	1	5
ExtravaganZZa (Toppings Only): Pepperoni, Ham, Green Pepper, Onion, Black Olive, Mushroom, Sausage, Beef, Extra Cheese	lg, 1 pc /8	150	12	5	590	5	1	9
MeatZZa Feast: Pepperoni, Ham, Sausage, Beef, Extra Cheese	lg, 1 pc /8	150	11	5	580	4	1	9
Ultimate Pepperoni Feast (Toppings Only): Extra Pepperoni & Extra Cheese	lg, 1 pc /8	130	11	5	530	4	1	7
PIZZAS								
Brooklyn w/ Cheese	lg, 1 pc /6	380	15	7	810	45	2	18
Brooklyn w/ Pepperoni	lg, 1 pc /6	460	22	9.5	107	45	2	21
Deep Dish w/ BBQ Sauce & Cheese	lg, 1 pc /8	400	18	7.5	910	48	4	14
Deep Dish w/ Beef	lg, 1 pc /8	380	18.5	7	860	40	5	15
Deep Dish w/ Cheese	lg, 1 pc /8	330	14	5	760	40	5	12
Deep Dish w/ Ham & Pineapple	lg, 1 pc /8	350	14.5	5	870	42	5	14
Deep Dish w/ Pepperoni	lg, 1 pc /8	380	18.5	6.5	950	40	5	14
Hand Tossed w/ Beef	lg, 1 pc /8	290	12.5	5	590	34	2	13
Hand Tossed w/ Cheese	lg, 1 pc /8	240	8	3	490	34	2	10
Hand Tossed w/ Green Pepper, Onion & Mushroom	lg, 1 pc /8	245	8	3	490	34	2	10

ITEM DESCRIPTION	Serving Size	Calories	Total Fat (g)	Saturated Fat (g)	Sodium (mg)	Carbohydrates (g)	Fiber (g)	Protein (g)
Hand Tossed w/ Ham & Pineapple	lg, 1 pc /8	260	8.5	3	600	36	2	12
Hand Tossed w/ Pepperoni	lg, 1 pc /8	300	13	5	670	36	3	12
Hand Tossed Wisconsin 6 Cheese	lg, 1 pc /8	340	16	8	690	34	2	15
Thin Crust w/ Beef	lg, 1 pc /8	230	14.5	5.5	440	19	1	10
Thin Crust w/ Cheese	lg, 1 pc /8	180	10	3.5	340	19	1	7
Thin Crust w/ Green Pepper, Onion & Mushroom	lg, 1 pc /8	185	10	3.5	340	19	1	7
Thin Crust w/ Ham & Pineapple	lg, 1 pc /8	200	10.5	3.5	450	21	1	9
Thin Crust w/ Pepperoni	lg, 1 pc /8	230	14.5	5	530	19	1	9
SANDWICHES								
Buffalo Chicken w/ Blue Cheese	1	840	42	17	2690	74	3	43
Chicken Bacon Ranch	1	880	46	17	2370	71	2	45
Chicken Parm	1	760	32	17	2200	72	3	48
Italian	1	880	48	23	2680	69	3	43
Italian Sausage & Peppers	1	900	49	23	2240	72	4	42
Mediterranean Veggie	1	680	29	17	2050	72	4	32
Philly Cheese Steak	1	690	28	15	2120	70	3	39
Sweet & Spicy Chicken Habanero	1	810	34	18	2160	82	3	47
SIDES AND SNACKS								
Breadsticks	1 pc	110	6	1.3	100	11	0	2
Buffalo Chicken Kickers	2 pcs	100	4.5	1	280	7	1	9
Buffalo Wings, Barbecue	2 pcs	230	14	3.5	410	6	0	17
Buffalo Wings, Hot	2 pcs	200	14	3.5	690	2	0	16
Buffalo Wings, Plain	2 pcs	200	14	3.5	320	1	0	16
Cakes, Chocolate Lava Crunch	1	350	17	10	170	47	1	4
Cheesy Bread	1 pc	120	6	2	140	11	0	4
Chicken Caesar Salad, Grilled	half	90	3.5	1.5	290	5	2	9
Cinna Stix	1 pc	120	6	1	85	14	1	2
Croutons	1 pkg	90	3.5	0	140	11	0	2
Salad, Garden Fresh	half	70	3.5	2.5	80	5	2	4
Salad, Grilled Chicken Caesar	half	90	3.5	1.5	290	5	2	9
TOPPINGS AND EXTRAS (PER SLICE OR SANDWICH)								
Anchovies*, Pizza Topping	1 serv	14	1	0	414	79	0	1.6
Bacon, Pizza Topping	1 serv	59	4.5	1.6	221.3	1.1	0	3.6

ITEM DESCRIPTION	Serving Size	Calories	Total Fat (g)	Saturated Fat (g)	Sodium (mg)	Carbohydrates (g)	Fiber (g)	Protein (g)
Banana Peppers, Pizza Topping	1 serv	3.1	0	0	51.3	0.6	0.4	0.1
Beef, Pizza Topping	1 serv	53.8	4.6	2	101.3	0	0.1	2.8
Cheese, American, Pizza Topping	1 serv	45	3.8	2.4	222.5	0.4	0	2.4
Cheese, Cheddar, Pizza Topping	1 serv	36.3	2.9	1.9	55	0.1	0	2.3
Cheese, Feta, Pizza Topping	1 serv	15	1	0.6	63.8	0.1	0	1.3
Cheese, Parmesan, Shredded, Pizza Topping	1 serv	27.5	2	1.4	76.3	0.3	0	2.1
Cheese, Provolone, Pizza Topping	1 serv	31.3	2.5	1.5	73.8	0.1	0	1.9
Chicken, Pizza Topping	1 serv	25	0.8	0.2	130	0.6	0	3.9
Chorizo*, Pizza Topping	1 serv	16.3	0.8	0.3	106.2	0.1	0	2.1
Garlic*, Pizza Topping	1 serv	6.3	0	0	0.6	1.5	0.1	0.3
Green Chile Peppers*, Pizza Topping	1 serv	1.9	0	0	1.9	0.5	0.4	0.1
Green Peppers, Pizza Topping	1 serv	1.9	0	0	0	0.5	0.1	0.1
Ham, Pizza Topping	1 serv	15	0.8	0.3	170	0	0	1.9
Jalapeños, Pizza Topping	1 serv	3.1	0	0	180	0.6	0.3	0.1
Mushrooms, Pizza Topping	1 serv	3.8	0	0	4.4	0.4	0.1	0.5
Olives, Black, Pizza Topping	1 serv	18.8	1.9	0.4	77.5	0.4	0.4	0.1
Olives, Green, Pizza Topping	1 serv	18.8	1.9	0.4	233.8	0.4	0.4	0.1
Onions, Pizza Topping	1 serv	3.1	0	0.1	1.2	0.6	0.1	0.1
Pepperoni, Pizza Topping	1 serv	40	3.5	1.3	171.3	0	0	1.9
Philly Steak, Pizza Topping	1 serv	15	0.6	0.3	86.3	0.4	0	2.1
Pineapple, Pizza Topping	1 serv	11.3	0	0	1.9	2.9	0.1	0.1
Red Pepper, Roasted, Pizza Topping	1 serv	1.9	0	0	17.5	0.4	0.1	0.1
Salami, Pizza Topping	1 serv	36.3	3	1.1	158.8	0.3	0	2.3
Sausage, Italian, Pizza Topping	1 serv	62.5	5.3	2	183.8	1.6	0	2.1
Sausage, Italian, Sliced, Pizza Topping	1 serv	48.8	4.3	1.5	117.5	0	0	2.5
Spinach, Pizza Topping	1 serv	1.9	0	0	5.6	0.3	0.1	0.3
Tomato, Pizza Topping	1 serv	3.8	0	0	56.3	0.9	0.4	0.1
Wing Sauce, Pizza Topping	1 serv	1.9	0	0	172.5	0.4	0.1	0

DUNKIN' DONUTS

BAKED ITEMS

ITEM DESCRIPTION	Serving Size	Calories	Total Fat (g)	Saturated Fat (g)	Sodium (mg)	Carbohydrates (g)	Fiber (g)	Protein (g)
Bagel, Blueberry	1	330	3	1	620	65	5	11
Bagel, Cinnamon Raisin	1	330	3.5	0.5	450	65	5	11
Bagel, Everything	1	350	4.5	0.5	660	66	5	13
Bagel, Garlic	1	340	2.5	0.5	660	68	6	12
Bagel, Multigrain	1	390	8	0.5	560	65	9	14
Bagel, Onion	1	310	2	0	380	63	3	11
Bagel, Plain	1	320	2.5	0.5	660	63	5	11
Bagel, Poppy Seed	1	350	6	0.5	660	64	5	13
Bagel, Salt	1	320	2.5	0.5	3420	63	5	11
Bagel, Sesame	1	360	6	0.5	660	63	5	13
Bagel, Sour Cream & Onion	1	330	2.5	0.5	930	66	3	12
Bagel, Wheat	1	320	3.5	0	550	61	5	12
Bagel Twist, Cheddar Cheese	1	400	9	4.5	800	63	5	17
Bagel Twist, Chocolate Chip	1	340	4	1.5	530	66	4	10
Bagel Twist, Cinnamon Raisin	1	350	3.5	0.5	460	72	5	11
Biscuit	1	280	14	8	620	32	1	5
Bow Tie	1	310	15	7	400	39	1	4
Brownie	1	440	23	5	250	58	1	3
Coffee Roll	1	400	18	7	400	53	3	7
Coffee Roll, Cocoa	1	310	14	6	360	44	3	5
Coffee Roll, Double Cocoa	1	320	15	6	370	44	3	5
Coffee Roll w/ Chocolate Frosting	1	410	19	8	420	53	3	7
Coffee Roll w/ Maple Frosting	1	410	19	8	410	54	3	7
Coffee Roll w/ Vanilla Frosting	1	410	19	8	410	54	3	7
Cookie, Oatmeal Raisin	1	320	9	4.5	210	54	3	5
Cookie, Reverse Chocolate Chunk	1	380	18	10	320	50	2	5
Cookie, Triple Chocolate Chunk	1	360	15	8	380	53	2	5
Croissant	1	310	16	7	350	35	1	7
Danish, Apple Cheese	1	330	16	7	270	41	1	4
Danish, Cheese	1	330	17	8	270	39	1	5
Danish, Strawberry Cheese	1	320	16	7	260	40	1	4

ITEM DESCRIPTION	Serving Size	Calories	Total Fat (g)	Saturated Fat (g)	Sodium (mg)	Carbohydrates (g)	Fiber (g)	Protein (g)
Donut, Apple Crumb	1	490	18	9	350	80	2	4
Donut, Apple N' Spice	1	270	14	6	350	32	1	3
Donut, Apple Pie	1	320	15	7	360	42	1	3
Donut, Bavarian Kreme	1	270	15	7	350	31	1	4
Donut, Blueberry Cake	1	340	17	8	570	44	1	4
Donut, Blueberry Crumb	1	500	18	9	350	84	2	4
Donut, Boston Kreme	1	310	16	7	370	39	1	3
Donut, Chocolate Coconut Cake	1	550	39	25	390	47	2	5
Donut, Chocolate Dipped Banana	1	290	12	5	260	41	2	5
Donut, Chocolate Frosted	1	270	15	7	340	31	1	3
Donut, Chocolate Frosted Cake	1	370	23	10	320	45	1	4
Donut, Chocolate Frosted Cocoa	1	250	11	4.5	260	32	2	4
Donut, Chocolate Glazed Cake	1	370	24	11	390	35	1	3
Donut, Chocolate Kreme Filled	1	370	21	10	370	42	1	4
Donut, Cinnamon Cake	1	340	22	10	300	38	1	4
Donut, Cocoa Boston Kreme	1	280	13	5	270	39	2	5
Donut, Cocoa Butternut	1	260	11	5	250	36	2	4
Donut, Cocoa Coconut	1	260	13	6	260	33	2	5
Donut, Cocoa Confetti	1	270	12	5	260	35	2	4
Donut, Cocoa Glazed	1	240	11	4.5	240	32	2	4
Donut, Cocoa Jelly	1	300	12	5	260	45	2	5
Donut, Cocoa Kreme Puff	1	300	16	7	260	34	2	4
Donut, Cupid's Choice	1	310	14	6	270	43	1	4
Donut, Cupid's Cocoa	1	320	14	6	290	47	2	4
Donut, Double Chocolate Cake	1	380	25	11	410	36	2	4
Donut, Double Cocoa Kreme	1	300	16	7	260	36	2	5
Donut, Double Cocoa Kreme Puff	1	290	16	6	260	34	2	5
Donut, Dulce de Chocolate	1	350	17	7	360	45	1	4
Donut, Dulce de Leche	1	290	16	7	340	31	1	4
Donut, Glazed	1	260	14	6	330	31	1	3
Donut, Glazed Cake	1	360	22	10	300	44	1	3
Donut, Glazed Cocoa Jelly	1	290	11	4.5	250	44	2	4
Donut, Guayaba Burst	1	300	15	7	330	38	1	4
Donut, Jelly Filled	1	290	14	7	340	36	1	3

ITEM DESCRIPTION	Serving Size	Calories	Total Fat (g)	Saturated Fat (g)	Sodium (mg)	Carbohydrates (g)	Fiber (g)	Protein (g)
Donut, Lemon Filled	1	270	15	7	350	31	1	4
Donut, Lemon Meringue Pie	1	320	16	7	360	42	1	3
Donut, Maple Frosted	1	270	15	7	340	32	1	3
Donut, Maple Frosted Cocoa	1	250	11	4.5	250	33	2	4
Donut, Marble Frosted	1	270	15	7	340	32	1	3
Donut, Marble Frosted Cocoa	1	260	11	4.5	250	36	2	4
Donut, Old Fashioned Cake	1	320	22	10	300	33	1	3
Donut, Pina Boom	1	270	15	7	350	32	1	4
Donut, Pina Colada	1	330	17	9	380	42	1	4
Donut, Powdered Cake	1	340	22	10	300	38	1	4
Donut, Powdered Cocoa	1	220	11	4.5	240	25	2	5
Donut, Reverse Boston Kreme	1	290	12	5	260	42	2	4
Donut, Strawberry Frosted	1	280	15	7	340	32	1	3
Donut, Strawberry Frosted Cocoa	1	250	11	4.5	250	33	2	4
Donut, Strawberry Shortcake	1	330	15	7	360	47	1	3
Donut, Sugar Raised	1	230	14	6	330	22	1	3
Donut, Sugared Cocoa	1	200	11	4.5	240	23	2	4
Donut, Triple Cocoa	1	260	12	5	260	35	2	5
Donut, Vanilla Cocoa Kreme	1	310	17	7	260	36	2	5
Donut, Vanilla Frosted Cocoa Donut	1	250	11	4.5	250	33	2	4
Donut, Vanilla Kreme Filled	1	380	23	10	370	42	1	4
Eclair	1	390	19	8	360	52	2	5
English Muffin	1	160	2	0	350	31	1	5
French Cruller	1	250	20	9	105	18	0	2
Fritter, Apple	1	410	17	7	380	60	2	6
Fritter, Double Cocoa	1	430	19	8	430	62	3	5
Fritter, Glazed	1	410	17	7	380	60	2	6
Fritter, Vanilla Cocoa	1	440	20	8	420	63	2	5
Muffin, Blueberry	1	500	16	3	500	83	2	7
Muffin, Chocolate Chip	1	610	23	7	520	92	3	8
Muffin, Coffee Cake	1	650	27	9	530	95	1	8
Muffin, Corn	1	510	18	3.5	840	80	1	7
Muffin, Honey Bran Raisin	1	490	15	3	450	82	5	7
Muffin, Reduced Fat Blueberry	1	450	11	2	700	81	2	7

ITEM DESCRIPTION	Serving Size	Calories	Total Fat (g)	Saturated Fat (g)	Sodium (mg)	Carbohydrates (g)	Fiber (g)	Protein (g)
Muffin, Triple Chocolate	1	640	32	9	460	81	3	7
Munchkin, Cinnamon Cake	1	60	3.5	1.5	65	6	0	1
Munchkin, Cocoa Glazed	1	35	1	0	40	6	0	1
Munchkin, Cocoa Kreme Puff	1	50	2.5	1	50	7	0	1
Munchkin, Double Cocoa Kreme Puff	1	50	2.5	1	45	7	0	1
Munchkin, Glazed	1	70	4	2	80	7	0	1
Munchkin, Glazed Cake	1	70	3.5	1.5	65	8	0	1
Munchkin, Glazed Chocolate Cake	1	70	3.5	1.5	85	8	0	1
Munchkin, Jelly Filled	1	80	4	2	85	9	0	1
Munchkin, Plain Cake	1	60	3.5	1.5	65	6	0	1
Munchkin, Powdered Cake	1	60	3.5	1.5	65	7	0	1
Munchkin, Sugar	1	60	3.5	1.5	65	6	0	1
Stick, Cinnamon Cake	1	350	18	8	420	44	2	4
Stick, Glazed Cake	1	370	18	8	420	48	1	4
Stick, Glazed Chocolate Cake	1	390	25	11	540	40	2	3
Stick, Jelly	1	420	18	8	440	60	1	4
Stick, Plain Cake	1	330	18	8	420	36	1	4
Stick, Powdered Cake	1	360	18	8	420	43	2	5
BEVERAGES								
Cappuccino	sm (10 oz)	80	4	2.5	70	7	0	4
Cappuccino w/ Sugar	sm (10 oz)	140	4	2.5	70	24	0	4
Chai, Vanilla	med (14 oz)	330	8	8	180	53	8	11
Coffee	sm (10 oz)	5	0	0	5	1	0	0
Coffee w/ Cream	sm (10 oz)	60	6	4	20	2	0	1
Coffee w/ Cream and Sugar	sm (10 oz)	120	6	4	20	19	0	1
Coffee w/ Milk	sm (10 oz)	25	1	1	20	2	0	1
Coffee w/ Milk and Sugar	sm (10 oz)	80	1	1	20	20	0	1
Coffee w/ Skim Milk	sm (10 oz)	15	0	0	25	3	0	2
Coffee w/ Skim Milk and Splenda	sm (10 oz)	25	0	0	25	5	0	2
Coffee w/ Skim Milk and Sugar	sm (10 oz)	70	0	0	25	20	0	2
Coffee w/ Splenda	sm (10 oz)	15	0	0	5	3	0	0
Coffee w/ Sugar	sm (10 oz)	60	0	0	5	18	0	0
Coffee, Blueberry	sm (10 oz)	15	0	0	5	2	0	0
Coffee, Caramel	sm (10 oz)	10	0	0	5	2	0	0

ITEM DESCRIPTION	Serving Size	Calories	Total Fat (g)	Saturated Fat (g)	Sodium (mg)	Carbohydrates (g)	Fiber (g)	Protein (g)
Coffee, Cinnamon	sm (10 oz)	15	0	0	5	2	0	0
Coffee, Coconut	sm (10 oz)	10	0	0	5	1	0	0
Coffee, French Vanilla	sm (10 oz)	10	0	0	5	1	0	0
Coffee, Hazelnut	sm (10 oz)	10	0	0	5	1	0	0
Coffee, Mocha	sm (10 oz)	110	0	0	20	26	1	1
Coffee, Mocha w/ Cream	sm (10 oz)	170	6	4	30	27	1	2
Coffee, Raspberry	sm (10 oz)	15	0	0	5	2	0	0
Coffee, Toasted Almond	sm (10 oz)	10	0	0	5	1	0	0
Coolatta®, Coffee w/ Cream	sm (16 oz)	400	23	14	75	49	0	3
Coolatta®, Coffee w/ Milk	sm (16 oz)	240	4	2.5	90	50	0	4
Coolatta®, Coffee w/ Skim Milk	sm (16 oz)	210	0	0	90	51	0	4
Coolatta®, Strawberry	sm (16 oz)	310	0	0	45	75	0	0
Coolatta®, Tropicana Orange	sm (16 oz)	230	0	0	40	57	0	1
Coolatta®, Vanilla Bean	sm (16 oz)	430	6	3.5	170	91	0	3
Dunkaccino®	sm (10 oz)	240	11	9	220	35	1	2
Espresso	1	5	0	0	5	1	0	0
Espresso w/ Sugar	1	30	0	0	5	7	0	0
Hot Chocolate	sm (10 oz)	220	7	7	270	39	2	2
Iced Caramel Swirl Latte	sm (16 oz)	220	6	3.5	150	35	0	8
Iced Caramel Swirl Latte w/ Skim Milk	sm (16 oz)	180	0	0	150	36	0	9
Iced Coffee	sm (16 oz)	10	0	0	5	2	0	1
Iced Coffee w/ Cream	sm (16 oz)	70	6	4	20	3	0	1
Iced Coffee w/ Cream & Sugar	sm (16 oz)	120	6	4	20	20	0	1
Iced Coffee w/ Milk	sm (16 oz)	30	1	1	20	3	0	2
Iced Coffee w/ Milk and Sugar	sm (16 oz)	90	1	1	20	21	0	2
Iced Coffee w/ Skim Milk	sm (16 oz)	20	0	0	25	3	0	2
Iced Coffee w/ Skim Milk & Splenda	sm (16 oz)	30	0	0	25	5	0	2
Iced Coffee w/ Skim Milk & Sugar	sm (16 oz)	80	0	0	25	21	0	2
Iced Coffee w/ Sugar	sm (16 oz)	70	0	0	5	19	0	1
Iced Coffee, Mocha w/ Cream	sm (16 oz)	180	6	4	35	28	1	2
Iced Dunkin' Dark® Roast Coffee w/ Cream & Sugar	sm (16 oz)	130	6	3.5	20	20	0	1
Iced Dunkin' Dark® Roast Coffee w/ Skim Milk & Splenda	sm (16 oz)	30	0	0	25	5	0	2

ITEM DESCRIPTION	Serving Size	Calories	Total Fat (g)	Saturated Fat (g)	Sodium (mg)	Carbohydrates (g)	Fiber (g)	Protein (g)
Iced Latte	sm (16 oz)	120	6	3.5	105	10	0	6
Iced Latte Lite	sm (16 oz)	80	0	0	110	13	0	7
Iced Latte Lite, Vanilla	sm (16 oz)	90	0	0	110	14	0	7
Iced Latte w/ Skim Milk	sm (16 oz)	70	0	0	110	11	0	7
Iced Latte w/ Skim Milk & Sugar	sm (16 oz)	130	0	0	110	28	0	7
Iced Latte w/ Sugar	sm (16 oz)	170	6	3.5	100	27	0	6
Iced Latte, Mocha Raspberry	sm (16 oz)	230	6	4	110	36	1	7
Iced Latte, Mocha Spice	sm (16 oz)	220	6	4	95	35	1	7
Iced Mocha Swirl Latte	sm (16 oz)	220	6	4	115	35	1	7
Iced Mocha Swirl Latte w/ Skim Milk	sm (16 oz)	180	0	0	125	36	1	8
Iced Tea, Freshly Brewed Sweetened	16 fl oz	80	0	0	0	20	0	0
Iced Tea, Freshly Brewed Unsweetened	16 fl oz	5	0	0	0	1	0	0
Iced Tea, Peach Flavored	16 fl oz	15	0	0	0	2	0	0
Iced Tea, Peach Flavored Sweetened	16 fl oz	90	0	0	0	21	0	0
Iced Tea, Raspberry Flavored	16 fl oz	15	0	0	0	2	0	0
Iced Tea, Raspberry Flavored Sweetened	16 fl oz	90	0	0	0	21	0	0
Latte	sm (10 oz)	120	6	3.5	105	10	0	6
Latte Lite	sm (10 oz)	80	0	0	110	13	0	7
Latte w/ Sugar	sm (10 oz)	170	6	3.5	100	27	0	6
Latte, Caramel Swirl	sm (10 oz)	220	6	3.5	150	35	0	8
Latte, Mocha Raspberry	sm (10 oz)	230	6	4	110	36	1	7
Latte, Mocha Spice	sm (10 oz)	220	6	4	95	35	1	7
Latte, Mocha Swirl	sm (10 oz)	220	6	4	115	35	1	7
Latte, Vanilla Lite	sm (10 oz)	90	0	0	110	14	0	7
Tea, Decaffeinated	10 oz	0	0	0	5	0	0	0
Tea, Decaffeinated w/ Milk	10 oz	20	1	0.5	20	1	0	1
Tea, Decaffeinated w/ Milk & Sugar	10 oz	80	1	0.5	20	19	0	1
Tea, Decaffeinated w/ Skim Milk	10 oz	10	0	0	20	2	0	1
Tea, Decaffeinated w/ Skim Milk & Sugar	10 oz	70	0	0	20	19	0	1
Tea, Decaffeinated w/ Sugar	10 oz	60	0	0	5	17	0	0
Tea, Earl Grey	10 oz	0	0	0	5	0	0	0
Tea, Earl Grey w/ Milk	10 oz	20	1	0.5	20	1	0	1

ITEM DESCRIPTION	Serving Size	Calories	Total Fat (g)	Saturated Fat (g)	Sodium (mg)	Carbohydrates (g)	Fiber (g)	Protein (g)
Tea, Earl Grey w/ Milk & Sugar	10 oz	80	1	0.5	20	19	0	1
Tea, Earl Grey w/ Skim Milk	10 oz	10	0	0	20	2	0	1
Tea, Earl Grey w/ Skim Milk & Sugar	10 oz	70	0	0	20	19	0	1
Tea, Earl Grey w/ Sugar	10 oz	60	0	0	5	17	0	0
Tea, English Breakfast	10 oz	0	0	0	5	0	0	0
Tea, English Breakfast w/ Milk	10 oz	20	1	0.5	20	1	0	1
Tea, English Breakfast w/ Milk & Sugar	10 oz	80	1	0.5	20	19	0	1
Tea, English Breakfast w/ Skim Milk	10 oz	10	0	0	20	2	0	1
Tea, English Breakfast w/ Skim Milk & Sugar	10 oz	70	0	0	20	19	0	1
Tea, English Breakfast w/ Sugar	10 oz	60	0	0	5	17	0	0
Tea, Freshly Brewed Unsweetened	10 oz	0	0	0	5	0	0	0
Tea, Freshly Brewed w/ Milk	10 oz	20	1	0.5	20	1	0	1
Tea, Freshly Brewed w/ Milk & Sugar	10 oz	80	1	0.5	20	19	0	1
Tea, Freshly Brewed w/ Skim Milk	10 oz	10	0	0	20	2	0	1
Tea, Freshly Brewed w/ Skim Milk & Sugar	10 oz	70	0	0	20	19	0	1
Tea, Freshly Brewed w/ Sugar	10 oz	60	0	0	5	17	0	0
Tea, Green	10 oz	0	0	0	5	0	0	0
Tea, Green w/ Milk	10 oz	20	1	0.5	20	1	0	1
Tea, Green w/ Milk & Sugar	10 oz	80	1	0.5	20	19	0	1
Tea, Green w/ Skim Milk	10 oz	10	0	0	20	2	0	1
Tea, Green w/ Skim Milk & Sugar	10 oz	70	0	0	20	19	0	1
Tea, Green w/ Sugar	10 oz	60	0	0	5	17	0	0
Tea, Sweet	16 oz	120	0	0	0	29	0	0
Turbo Shot™	1.75 oz	5	0	0	5	1	0	0
Turbo Shot™	2.5 oz	5	0	0	10	1	0	0
Turbo Shot™	3.5 oz	10	0	0	15	2	0	0
Turbo Shot™	4 oz	10	0	0	15	2	0	0
White Hot Chocolate	sm (10 oz)	230	8	8	310	38	1	2
BREAKFAST ITEMS								
Bagel w/ Bacon, Egg & Cheese	1	530	19	7	1340	66	5	24
Bagel w/ Egg & Cheese	1	480	15	5	1130	66	5	20
Bagel w/ Ham, Egg & Cheese	1	510	16	6	1390	66	5	26

ITEM DESCRIPTION	Serving Size	Calories	Total Fat (g)	Saturated Fat (g)	Sodium (mg)	Carbohydrates (g)	Fiber (g)	Protein (g)
Bagel w/ Sausage, Egg & Cheese	1	690	35	13	1650	66	5	29
Big n' Toasty	1	580	35	11	1370	41	1	26
Biscuit w/ Bacon, Egg & Cheese	1	490	30	14	1300	35	1	18
Biscuit, Chicken	1	500	25	10	1260	48	2	20
Biscuit w/ Egg & Cheese	1	440	27	13	1090	35	1	14
Biscuit w/ Ham, Egg & Cheese	1	480	28	14	1350	35	1	19
Biscuit, Sausage	1	490	33	16	1140	33	1	13
Biscuit w/ Sausage, Egg & Cheese	1	650	46	20	1610	36	1	22
Croissant w/ Bacon, Egg & Cheese	1	530	33	13	1030	38	2	20
Croissant w/ Egg & Cheese	1	480	29	12	820	38	2	16
Croissant w/ Ham, Egg & Cheese	1	510	31	12	1080	38	2	21
Croissant w/ Sausage, Egg & Cheese	1	690	48	19	1340	39	2	24
English Muffin w/ Bacon, Egg & Cheese	1	370	18	6	1030	34	1	18
English Muffin w/ Egg & Cheese	1	320	15	5	820	34	1	14
English Muffin w/ Ham, Egg & Cheese	1	360	165	6	1080	34	1	20
English Muffin w/ Sausage, Egg & Cheese	1	530	34	13	1340	34	1	23
Flatbread w/ Egg White Turkey Sausage	1	280	8	3	770	32	3	19
Flatbread w/ Egg White Veggie	1	280	10	4	690	32	3	16
Flatbread w/ Grilled Cheese	1	380	18	9	840	36	1	16
Flatbread w/ Ham & Cheese	1	310	11	4.5	880	35	1	19
Flatbread w/ Turkey, Cheddar & Bacon	1	410	20	7	1140	36	1	22
Hash Browns	9 pcs	200	11	1.5	730	22	3	2
Wrap w/ Bacon, Egg & Cheese	1	210	12	5	580	14	1	10
Wrap w/ Egg & Cheese	1	180	11	4	470	14	1	8
Wrap w/ Egg White & Turkey Sausage	1	150	5	2.5	400	14	1	11
Wrap w/ Egg White & Veggie	1	150	6	3	340	14	1	10
Wrap w/ Ham, Egg & Cheese	1	200	11	4.5	600	14	1	11
Wrap w/ Sausage, Egg & Cheese	1	290	20	8	730	14	1	12

Allergy sufferers should always read the product ingredient statement and allergen information available at www.DunkinDonuts.com/Nutrition. Please note that our restaurants prepare and serve products that contain allergens other than the products you select.

Dunkin' Donuts has made a reasonable effort to provide nutritional and ingredient information based upon standard product formulations and following the FDA guidelines using formulation and nutrition labeling software. Variations may occur due to: seasonal conditions; regional differences; ingredient substitutions; and differences in product assembly or size at the restaurant. Test products, limited time offers, and regional menu variations may not be included and not all items listed may be available in all restaurants. The information on these printed materials may vary from that which may be available in our restaurants. We will update www.DunkinDonuts.com/Nutrition frequently, so please revisit this site for the most current information. Any customers with specific dietary concerns are advised to www.DunkinDonuts.com/Nutrition or call our customer care line at 800-859-5339.

HARDEE'S

ITEM DESCRIPTION	Serving Size	Calories	Total Fat (g)	Saturated Fat (g)	Sodium (mg)	Carbohydrates (g)	Fiber (g)	Protein (g)
BREAKFAST ITEMS								
Big Country® Breakfast Platter w/ Bacon*	1	910	48	12	2210	91	4	27
Biscuit 'N' Gravy™	1	530	33	8	1510	48	1	9
Biscuit 'N' Gravy Breakfast Bowl™	1	770	54	14	1950	49	1	20
Biscuit w/ Bacon, Egg & Cheese	1	530	36	11	1390	36	0	15
Biscuit w/ Chicken Fillet	1	600	34	7	1680	50	1	24
Biscuit w/ Country Ham	1	440	26	6	1710	36	0	14
Biscuit w/ Country Steak	1	630	43	11	1330	45	0	16
Biscuit w/ Ham, Egg & Cheese	1	540	33	10	1830	36	0	23
Biscuit w/ Jelly	1	520	34	7	1020	44	0	5
Biscuit w/ Loaded Omelet	1	610	42	14	1540	36	0	20
Biscuit w/ Pork Chop	1	690	42	8	1330	48	1	29
Biscuit w/ Sausage	1	530	38	10	1240	36	0	11
Biscuit w/ Sausage & Egg	1	590	42	11	1300	36	0	16
Biscuit, Cinnamon 'N' Raisin™	1	300	15	3	680	40	1	3
Biscuit, Made from Scratch™	1	370	23	5	890	35	0	5
Biscuit, Monster Biscuit™	1	770	55	18	2310	37	0	29
Breakfast Burrito, Loaded	1	760	49	21	1700	39	1	39
Croissant, Sunrise Croissant™ w/ Ham	1	400	23	10	1070	27	1	21
Frisco Breakfast Sandwich®	1	400	18	7	1350	27	2	23
Grits	1 serv	110	5	1	490	16	1	2
Hash Rounds™	med	350	22	5	490	34	3	4
Low Carb Breakfast Bowl™	1	620	50	21	1380	6	2	36
Pancakes, no Syrup	3 pcs	300	5	1	830	55	2	8
DESSERTS								
Apple Turnover	1	290	15	5	350	36	1	2
Cookie, Chocolate Chip	1	290	11	5	280	44	0	4
Ice Cream Bowl†	1 scoop	235	13	8	85	27	0	5
Ice Cream Cone†	1 scoop	285	13	8	140	37	0	6
Malt †	1	780	35	24	330	98	0	17
Peach Cobbler	sm	285	7	1	230	56	1	1
Shake †	1	705	33	23	260	86	0	14

ITEM DESCRIPTION	Serving Size	Calories	Total Fat (g)	Saturated Fat (g)	Sodium (mg)	Carbohydrates (g)	Fiber (g)	Protein (g)
KIDS MENU								
Cheeseburger	kid	600	27	6	930	68	4	21
Chicken Strips, no Sauce	kid	500	25	5	1050	50	3	19
Hamburger	kid	560	24	6	710	67	4	18
SANDWICHES								
Big Hot Ham 'N' Cheese™	1	460	20	8	2040	40	2	36
Burger, Bacon Cheese Thickburger®**	1/3 lb	850	57	19	1650	49	3	38
Burger, Cheeseburger**	1/3 lb	620	33	13	1580	51	3	35
Burger, Double Bacon Cheese Thickburger®**	2/3 lb	1200	84	30	2450	50	3	65
Burger, Double Thickburger®**	2/3 lb	1150	78	28	2410	53	4	62
Burger, Grilled Sourdough Thickburger®**	1/2 lb	1030	77	28	1910	42	3	42
Burger, Low Carb Thickburger®**	1/3 lb	420	32	12	1010	5	2	30
Burger, Monster Thickburger®**	2/3 lb	1320	95	36	3020	46	2	70
Burger, Mushroom & Swiss Thickburger®**	1/3 lb	650	36	14	1620	47	3	39
Burger, Original Thickburger®**	1/3 lb	770	48	16	1560	53	4	35
Burger, Six Dollar Burger**	1/2 lb	930	59	21	1960	57	4	46
Cheeseburger	sm	350	19	4	730	32	1	16
Chicken Club Sandwich, Charbroiled	1	630	32	8	1730	54	4	32
Chicken Club Sandwich, Low Carb Charbroiled	1	360	23	7	1290	14	1	24
Chicken Fillet Sandwich	1	710	38	7	1610	62	5	33
Chicken Sandwich, Barbecue	1	400	6	1	1370	62	5	27
Chicken Sandwich, Spicy	1	440	21	5	1140	41	3	11
Chicken Strips	3 pcs	370	26	6	620	19	1	14
Chicken Strips	5 pcs	610	43	9	1030	32	3	23
Hamburger	sm	310	12	4	500	32	6	14
Hot Dog	1	420	30	12	1200	22	1	16
Hot Ham 'N' Cheese™	1	420	18	10	1600	39	2	30
Roast Beef	reg	310	15	5	840	28	1	17
Roast Beef	lg	400	21	7	1180	28	1	25

ITEM DESCRIPTION

ITEM DESCRIPTION	Serving Size	Calories	Total Fat (g)	Saturated Fat (g)	Sodium (mg)	Carbohydrates (g)	Fiber (g)	Protein (g)
SIDES AND SNACKS								
Chicken Breast, Fried	1	370	15	4	1190	29	0	29
Chicken Leg, Fried	1	170	7	2	570	15	0	13
Chicken Thigh, Fried	1	330	15	4	1000	30	0	19
Chicken Wing, Fried	1	200	8	2	740	23	0	10
Cole Slaw	sm	170	10	2	140	20	2	1
Crispy Curls™	med	410	20	5	1020	52	4	5
French Fries	med	430	19	4	960	60	4	5
Mashed Potatoes	sm	90	2	0	410	17	0	1
Salad, no Dressing	sm	120	7	5	160	7	2	7

* Served w/ syrup, jam & butter (Not included in nutrition above)
** Weight before cooking
† Nutrient amounts may vary slightly by flavor. Items may vary by restaurant.
For additional information visit www.hardees.com.

JACK IN THE BOX

BEVERAGES

Item	Serving Size	Calories	Total Fat (g)	Saturated Fat (g)	Sodium (mg)	Carbohydrates (g)	Fiber (g)	Protein (g)
Coca-Cola Classic®	20 oz	230	0	0	5	62	0	0
Coffee	12 oz	5	0	0	5	1	0	0
Diet Coke®	20 oz	0	0	0	25	0	0	0
Dr Pepper®	20 oz	230	0	0	85	62	0	0
Fanta® Orange	20 oz	210	0	0	65	55	0	0
Fanta® Strawberry	20 oz	210	0	0	15	56	0	0
Iced Coffee, Caramel	24 oz	150	3	2	95	25	0	7
Iced Coffee, Original	24 oz	160	3	2	95	26	0	7
Iced Coffee, Vanilla	24 oz	160	3	2	95	27	0	7
Iced Tea, Fresh Brewed	20 oz	5	0	0	15	2	0	0
Iced Tea, Mango	24 oz	80	0	0	15	21	0	0
Iced Tea, Peach	24 oz	80	0	0	15	21	0	0
Iced Tea, Raspberry	24 oz	80	0	0	10	20	0	0
Lemonade, Minute Maid®	20 oz	220	0	0	90	57	0	0
Orange Juice	10 oz	140	0	0	20	33	0	2

ITEM DESCRIPTION	Serving Size	Calories	Total Fat (g)	Saturated Fat (g)	Sodium (mg)	Carbohydrates (g)	Fiber (g)	Protein (g)
Root Beer, Barq's®	20 oz	250	0	0	50	68	0	0
Smoothie, Mango	16 oz	290	0	0	75	72	0	2
Smoothie, Strawberry	16 oz	270	0	0	70	67	1	2
Smoothie, Strawberry Banana	16 oz	290	0	0	70	73	1	2
Smoothie, Tropical	16 oz	330	0	0	85	81	1	3
Sprite®	20 oz	220	0	0	50	57	0	0
BREAKFAST ITEMS								
Bacon Breakfast Jack®	1	300	13	5	760	30	1	16
Biscuit w/ Bacon, Egg & Cheese	1	420	24	11	1040	36	2	15
Biscuit, Sausage	1	460	30	12	870	36	2	12
Biscuit w/ Sausage, Egg & Cheese	1	570	39	16	1150	37	2	19
Biscuit, Spicy Chicken	1	570	29	9	1010	54	2	25
Breakfast Bowl, Denver	1	790	57	16	1350	44	4	26
Breakfast Bowl, Hearty	1	850	65	18	1390	41	4	27
Breakfast Burrito w/ Meat, no Salsa	1	600	37	15	1500	38	4	32
Breakfast Burrito w/ Meat, w/ Salsa	1	610	37	15	1620	40	4	33
Breakfast Jack®	1	280	11	4.5	790	30	1	16
Burrito, Chorizo Sausage, no Salsa	1	720	41	12	1380	59	6	29
Burrito, Chorizo Sausage, w/ Salsa	1	730	41	12	1500	61	6	29
Croissant Supreme	1	440	26	11	870	32	2	18
Croissant w/ Sausage	1	570	40	16	780	32	2	20
Extreme Sausage® Sandwich	1	660	47	17	1360	32	2	29
French Toast Sticks	4 pcs	600	33	3.5	530	68	3	9
Hash Brown Sticks	5 pcs	280	19	2	400	26	2	3
Sausage Breakfast Jack®	1	440	27	9	870	31	1	20
Sourdough Breakfast Sandwich	1	410	21	8	1020	34	2	20
Steak & Egg Burrito, no Salsa	1	810	50	15	1500	55	5	37
Steak & Egg Burrito, w/ Salsa	1	820	50	15	1620	57	5	37
Ultimate Breakfast Sandwich	1	510	24	9	1650	41	2	31
DESSERTS								
Cake, Chocolate Overload™	1 pc	300	7	1.5	350	57	2	4
Cheesecake	1 pc	310	17	9	260	32	1	7
Churros, Mini	5 pcs	350	18	3.5	280	42	2	4
Shake, Chocolate w/ Whipped Topping	16 oz	800	38	26	300	101	1	13

ITEM DESCRIPTION	Serving Size	Calories	Total Fat (g)	Saturated Fat (g)	Sodium (mg)	Carbohydrates (g)	Fiber (g)	Protein (g)
Shake, Oreo® Cookie w/ Whipped Topping	16 oz	810	43	27	380	92	1	13
Shake, Strawberry w/ Whipped Topping	16 oz	780	38	26	260	95	0	12
Shake, Vanilla w/ Whipped Topping	16 oz	700	38	26	250	76	0	12
DRESSINGS AND SPREADS								
Chipotle Sauce	1 serv	110	12	2	230	1	0	0
Dipping Sauce, Barbecue	1 pkg	40	0	0	360	10	0	0
Dipping Sauce, Buttermilk House	1 pkg	130	13	2	210	3	0	0
Dipping Sauce, Franks® Red Hot®	1 pkg	10	0	0	840	2	0	0
Dipping Sauce, Honey Mustard	1 pkg	60	2	0	220	11	0	0
Dipping Sauce, Sweet & Sour	1 pkg	45	0	0	160	11	0	0
Dipping Sauce, Teriyaki	1 pkg	60	1	0	530	11	0	1
Dressing, Bacon Ranch	1 serv	260	26	4	700	3	0	2
Dressing, Creamy Southwest	1 serv	220	22	3.5	850	3	0	1
Dressing, Lite Ranch	1 serv	150	15	2.5	560	3	0	1
Dressing, Low Fat Balsamic	1 serv	35	1.5	0	480	5	0	0
Jelly, Grape	1 pkg	35	0	0	10	9	0	0
Jelly, Strawberry	1 pkg	35	0	0	5	9	0	0
Ketchup	1 pkg	20	0	0	180	4	0	0
Margarine Spread, Pride	1 serv	20	2.5	0.5	45	0	0	0
Mayo, Peppercorn	1 serv	190	20	3.5	250	1	0	0
Mayonnaise	1 pkg	80	9	1.5	40	0	0	0
Mayo-Onion Sauce	1 serv	90	10	1.5	90	1	0	0
Mustard	1 pkg	5	0	0	75	0	0	0
Salsa, Fire Roasted	1 pkg	5	0	0	105	1	0	0
Sauce, Creamy Ranch	1 serv	80	9	1.5	160	1	0	0
Sauce, Zesty Marinara	1 pkg	15	0	0	200	4	0	0
Sour Cream	1 pkg	60	5	3	25	2	1	1
Soy Sauce	1 pkg	5	0	0	480	1	0	1
Syrup, Log Cabin®	1 pkg	190	0	0	35	49	0	0
Taco Sauce	1 pkg	0	0	0	80	0	0	0
Tartar Sauce	1 pkg	210	22	3.5	370	2	0	0

ITEM DESCRIPTION	Serving Size	Calories	Total Fat (g)	Saturated Fat (g)	Sodium (mg)	Carbohydrates (g)	Fiber (g)	Protein (g)
Vinegar, Malt	1 pkg	0	0	0	20	0	0	0
KIDS MENU								
Breakfast Jack®	1	280	11	4.5	790	30	1	16
Chicken Strips, Crispy	2 pcs	280	12	1.5	790	26	1	17
Chicken Strips, Grilled	2 pcs	120	3	0.5	530	2	0	22
French Fries	kid	180	8	0.5	320	24	2	2
French Toast Sticks	2 pcs	300	16	1.5	260	34	2	4
Grilled Cheese Sandwich	1	330	16	6	800	34	2	11
Hamburger	1	290	12	4.5	570	32	1	14
Milk, 1% Chocolate Low Fat Chug	8 oz	180	2.5	1.5	200	30	n/a	10
Milk, 2% Chug**	8 oz	120	4.5	2.5	120	12	n/a	9
MAIN MENU								
Cheeseburger, Bacon Ultimate	1	940	66	27	1840	45	2	41
Cheeseburger, Big	1	610	38	15	1110	44	2	23
Cheeseburger, Ultimate	1	870	61	26	1490	44	2	36
Chicken Club w/ Homestyle Ranch	1	700	33	7	1940	65	3	36
Chicken Fajita Pita Made w/ Whole Grain, no Salsa	1	320	11	5	870	33	4	24
Chicken Fajita Pita Made w/ Whole Grain, w/ Salsa	1	330	11	5	990	35	4	24
Chicken Sandwich	1	440	23	4	910	42	2	15
Chicken Sandwich w/ Bacon	1	480	26	5	1140	42	2	19
Chicken Sandwiches, Mini Buffalo Ranch	1 serv	740	28	4.5	1950	90	5	32
Chicken Strips, Crispy	4 pcs	560	24	3	1580	53	3	33
Chicken Strips, Grilled w/ Teriyaki Dipping Sauce	1 serv	300	6	1	1510	18	0	45
Chicken Teriyaki Bowl	1	690	6	1	1700	133	5	27
Deli Trio Grilled Sandwich	1	630	29	10	2460	53	5	37
Fish & Chips	sm	670	35	3	1390	68	4	19
Fish Sandwich	1	470	18	2	1030	59	3	18
Fruit Cup	1	50	0	0	10	14	1	1
Hamburger	1	290	12	4.5	570	32	1	14
Hamburger w/ Cheese	1	330	15	7	770	32	1	17

ITEM DESCRIPTION	Serving Size	Calories	Total Fat (g)	Saturated Fat (g)	Sodium (mg)	Carbohydrates (g)	Fiber (g)	Protein (g)
Hamburger Deluxe	1	360	19	6	580	33	2	15
Hamburger Deluxe w/ Cheese	1	440	26	10	990	34	2	19
Jack's Spicy Chicken®	1	570	25	4	950	60	3	28
Jack's Spicy Chicken® w/ Cheese	1	650	31	8	1240	62	3	32
Jumbo Jack®	1	540	32	11	850	45	2	19
Jumbo Jack® w/ Cheese	1	620	39	15	1250	45	2	23
Junior Bacon Cheeseburger	1	420	24	8	860	32	1	18
Sirloin Burger w/ Bacon, Swiss & Grilled Onions	1	950	63	19	1900	52	3	45
Sirloin Burger w/ Swiss & Grilled Onions	1	880	59	18	1550	52	3	40
Sirloin Burgers, Mini	1 serv (3)	750	30	13	1410	77	4	43
Sirloin Cheeseburger	1	900	60	19	1870	52	3	40
Sirloin Cheeseburger w/ Bacon	1	960	64	20	2220	52	3	44
Sourdough Grilled Chicken Club	1	550	29	7	1490	38	3	37
Sourdough Jack®	1	680	46	17	1220	40	3	27
Sourdough Steak Melt	1	650	38	13	1300	38	3	37
Sourdough Ultimate Cheeseburger	1	900	67	27	1430	38	3	37
Steak Teriyaki Bowl	1	750	11	3	1750	133	5	31
Turkey, Bacon & Cheddar Grilled Sandwich	1	650	30	11	2130	54	5	39
SALADS								
Chicken Club Salad, Crispy*	1	510	27	8	700	37	5	32
Chicken Club Salad, Grilled*	1	350	18	7	1210	13	4	37
Chicken Salad, Grilled	1	240	8	3.5	650	15	5	28
Side Salad*	1	20	0	0	10	4	2	1
Southwest Chicken Salad, Crispy*	1	500	23	7	1260	53	8	29
Southwest Chicken Salad, Grilled*	1	340	14	6	1000	29	7	34
SIDES AND SNACKS								
Egg Roll	1 pc	150	7	1.5	320	15	2	5
French Fries	med	410	19	1.5	750	56	4	5
Mozzarella Sticks	3 pcs	280	16	6	590	22	2	12
Onion Rings	1 serv	450	28	2	620	45	3	6
Pita Snack, Crispy Chicken	1	410	19	4	860	43	3	16

ITEM DESCRIPTION	Serving Size	Calories	Total Fat (g)	Saturated Fat (g)	Sodium (mg)	Carbohydrates (g)	Fiber (g)	Protein (g)
Pita Snack, Fish	1	390	20	4	760	40	3	13
Pita Snack, Grilled Chicken	1	330	14	3.5	730	31	3	19
Pita Snack, Steak	1	350	16	4.5	640	31	3	19
Potato Wedges, Bacon Cheddar	1 serv	710	45	12	910	58	5	20
Sampler Trio	1	790	43	13	1950	73	7	28
Seasoned Curly Fries	med	430	25	2	940	46	4	5
Stuffed Jalapeños	3 pcs	220	12	4.5	730	21	1	6
Stuffed Jalapeños	7 pcs	510	29	10	1690	49	3	14
Taco, Beef	1	180	10	2.5	270	17	2	6
TOPPINGS AND EXTRAS								
Cheese, American	1 pc	40	3.5	2	200	0	0	2
Cheese, Real Swiss	1 pc	70	6	3.5	80	0	n/a	5
Cheese, Swiss-Style	1 pc	40	3	2	140	0	n/a	2
Corn Sticks, Spicy	1 serv	140	7	1	140	18	1	2
Croutons, Gourmet Seasoned	1 serv	100	6	1	310	17	1	3
Onions, Red	1 serv	5	0	0	0	1	0	0
Onions, Grilled	1 serv	10	0	0	0	2	0	0

* Nutritional data does not include dressing or condiments.

** 37% fat reduction compared to whole milk.

All data displayed follows the federal regulations regarding the rounding on nutritional data. Information may vary slightly from actual due to rounding of nutritional data.

Variations within the nutritional values may occur due to the use of regional suppliers, seasonal influences, manufacturing tolerances, minor differences in product assembly at the restaurant level, recipe revisions, and other factors.

Serving size designation for beverages refers to total cup capacity. The actual fill might be slightly different.

Sodium and potassium values in drinks may vary due to local water supplies.

To help our customers make better informed decisions about their menu choices at our restaurants, we have developed a Build Your Meal calculator on our website. You can combine menu items into a meal and view the complete nutritional information of each item. Once you have assembled your meal, you will be able to add or remove ingredients and choose from a list of common substitutes for each item. Jack in the Box invites you to go to www.jackinthebox.com/ourfood/ to build a meal of your favorite menu items.

KENTUCKY FRIED CHICKEN

BEVERAGES

7UP®**	16 oz	180	0	0	55	46	0	0
Capri Sun® Roarin' Waters Tropical Fruit	1	30	0	0	15	8	0	0
Code Red Mountain Dew®*	16 oz	190	0	0	60	54	0	0
Diet Dr Pepper®**	16 oz	0	0	0	60	0	0	0
Diet Mountain Dew®*	16 oz	0	0	0	70	0	0	0
Diet Pepsi®*	16 oz	0	0	0	45	0	0	0
Diet Sierra Mist®*	16 oz	0	0	0	45	0	0	0
Dr Pepper®**	16 oz	180	0	0	60	47	0	0

ITEM DESCRIPTION	Serving Size	Calories	Total Fat (g)	Saturated Fat (g)	Sodium (mg)	Carbohydrates (g)	Fiber (g)	Protein (g)
Fruit Punch*, Tropicana®	16 oz	190	0	0	45	53	0	0
Lemonade*, Tropicana®	16 oz	180	0	0	185	47	0	0
Lemonade*, Tropicana® Pink	16 oz	180	0	0	185	47	0	0
Lemonade*, Tropicana® Sugar Free	16 oz	10	0	0	165	4	0	0
Lipton® Brisk® Green w/ Peach Tea*	16 oz	0	0	0	125	0	0	0
Lipton® Brisk® Lemon Tea*	16 oz	120	0	0	25	35	0	0
Lipton® Brisk® Peach Tea*	16 oz	140	0	0	45	37	0	0
Lipton® Brisk® Raspberry Tea*	16 oz	140	0	0	45	37	0	0
Lipton® Brisk® Tea*	16 oz	0	0	0	55	0	0	0
Manzanita Sol®*	16 oz	190	0	0	45	51	0	0
Milk, 2%	16 oz	170	6	4	180	17	0	12
Miranda® Strawberry*	16 oz	190	0	0	90	51	0	0
Mountain Dew®*	16 oz	190	0	0	60	51	0	0
Pepsi®*	16 oz	180	0	0	35	49	0	0
Root Beer®*, Mug	16 oz	180	0	0	25	46	0	0
Sierra Mist®*	16 oz	180	0	0	35	47	0	0
Twister® Orange* Tropicana®	16 oz	190	0	0	45	54	0	0
Wild Cherry Pepsi®*	16 oz	180	0	0	35	49	0	0
DESSERTS								
Apple Turnover	1	250	12	3	160	33	2	2
Cake, Café Valley Bakery® Chocolate Chip	1 pc	300	15	3	260	39	1	4
Cookie, Sweet Life® Chocolate Chip	1	160	8	4	85	21	1	2
Cookie, Sweet Life® Oatmeal Raisin	1	150	6	2.5	90	22	1	2
Parfait Cup, Lil' Bucket™ Chocolate Crème	1	280	13	8	240	37	1	2
Parfait Cup, Lil' Bucket™ Lemon Crème	1	400	13	7	220	65	2	7
Parfait Cup, Lil' Bucket™ Strawberry Shortcake	1	200	7	3.5	140	35	2	2
Pie, Oreo® Cookies and Creme	1 pc	290	16	10	210	34	1	3
Pie, Reese's® Peanut Butter	1 pc	310	19	10	200	31	1	5
DRESSINGS AND SPREADS								
Buttery Spread	1 serv	30	3.5	0.5	30	0	0	0
Dipping Sauce, Creamy Ranch	1 serv	140	15	2.5	230	1	0	0
Dipping Sauce, Honey BBQ	1 serv	40	0	0	310	9	0	0

ITEM DESCRIPTION	Serving Size	Calories	Total Fat (g)	Saturated Fat (g)	Sodium (mg)	Carbohydrates (g)	Fiber (g)	Protein (g)
Dipping Sauce, Honey Mustard	1 serv	120	10	1.5	110	6	0	0
Dipping Sauce, KFC Signature	1 serv	70	5	1	135	5	0	0
Dipping Sauce, Spicy Chipotle	1 serv	70	3.5	1	220	8	1	0
Dipping Sauce, Sweet & Sour	1 serv	45	0	0	95	12	0	0
Dressing, Heinz Buttermilk Ranch	1 serv	160	17	2	220	1	0	0
Dressing, Hidden Valley® The Original Ranch® Fat Free	1 serv	35	0	0	410	8	0	1
Dressing, KFC® Creamy Parmesan Caesar	1 serv	260	26	5	540	4	0	2
Dressing, Marzetti Light Italian	1 serv	15	0.5	0	510	2	0	0
Honey Sauce	1 pkg	30	0	0	0	8	0	0
MAIN MENU								
Crispy Strips	3 pcs	340	11	4	1280	27	3	33
Crispy Strips	2 pcs	230	7	2.5	850	18	2	22
EC Chicken, Breast	1	510	33	7	1010	16	0	39
EC Chicken, Drumstick	1	150	10	2	360	5	0	12
EC Chicken, Drumstick Value Box	1	500	31	6	1360	41	4	17
EC Chicken, Thigh	1	340	24	5	780	10	0	20
EC Chicken, Thigh Value Box	1	690	45	9	1770	46	4	24
EC Chicken, Whole Wing	1	190	13	2.5	410	6	0	12
Gizzards	1 serv	200	11	2	800	15	1	11
Grilled Chicken, Breast	1	210	8	2.5	460	0	0	34
Grilled Chicken, Drumstick	1	80	4	1	230	0	0	11
Grilled Chicken, Drumstick Value Box	1	420	24	4.5	1240	36	4	15
Grilled Chicken, Thigh	1	160	11	3	420	0	0	16
Grilled Chicken, Thigh Value Box	1	500	30	6	1340	36	4	22
Grilled Chicken, Whole Wing	1	80	5	1.5	250	1	0	9
KFC® Grilled Filet	1	140	3	1	560	1	0	26
KFC® OR Filet	1	200	9	1.5	670	8	1	22
Livers	1 serv	180	10	2	620	11	0	11
OR Chicken, Breast	1	360	21	5	1080	11	0	34
OR Chicken, Breast, no Skin or Breading	1	160	3.5	1	580	2	0	31
OR Chicken, Drumstick	1	120	7	1.5	310	3	0	11
OR Chicken, Drumstick Value Box	1	420	25	4.5	1180	34	4	15

ITEM DESCRIPTION	Serving Size	Calories	Total Fat (g)	Saturated Fat (g)	Sodium (mg)	Carbohydrates (g)	Fiber (g)	Protein (g)
OR Chicken, Thigh	1	250	17	4.5	730	7	0	17
OR Chicken, Thigh Value Box	1	560	36	8	1610	39	4	21
OR Chicken, Whole Wing	1	120	7	1.5	380	3	0	11
Spicy Crispy, Breast	1	420	25	5	1250	12	1	38
Spicy Crispy, Drumstick	1	160	10	2	440	5	0	11
Spicy Crispy, Thigh	1	360	27	6	1010	13	1	17
Spicy Crispy, Whole Wing	1	170	12	2.5	470	6	0	11
Steak, Country Fried w/ Peppered White Gravy	1	420	29	9	1130	25	2	16
Steak, Country Fried, no Gravy	1	390	27	9	960	21	2	15
SALADS								
Caesar, no Dressing or Croutons	side	40	2	1	90	2	1	3
Chicken BLT Salad, Crispy, no Dressing	1	320	12	4	1220	25	5	31
Chicken BLT Salad, Grilled, no Dressing	1	230	8	2.5	920	8	4	35
Chicken Caesar Salad, Crispy, no Dressing & Croutons	1	310	11	5	1030	23	5	29
Chicken Caesar Salad, Grilled, no Dressing & Croutons	1	220	7	3.5	740	6	3	33
House Salad, no Dressing	side	15	0	0	10	3	1	1
SANDWICHES								
Double Down, w/ Grilled Filet	1	480	25	9	1770	4	0	60
Double Down, w/ OR Filet	1	610	37	11	1990	18	1	52
Doublicious w/ Grilled Filet	1	380	11	4	950	35	2	35
Doublicious w/ Grilled Filet, no Sauce	1	340	8	3.5	880	32	2	35
Doublicious w/ OR Filet	1	520	25	7	1300	40	2	32
Honey BBQ Sandwich	1	320	3.5	1	770	47	3	24
KFC Snacker® w/ Crispy Strip	1	290	11	2.5	730	33	3	15
KFC Snacker® w/ Crispy Strip, Buffalo	1	250	6	1.5	770	35	3	15
KFC Snacker® w/ Crispy Strip, no Sauce	1	240	6	1.5	600	33	2	15
KFC Snacker® w/ Crispy Strip, Ultimate Cheese	1	270	8	2.5	750	34	2	16
KFC Snacker®, Honey Barbecue	1	210	3	1	470	32	2	13
SIDES AND SNACKS								
Beans, Barbecue Baked	1 serv	210	1.5	0	780	41	8	8

ITEM DESCRIPTION	Serving Size	Calories	Total Fat (g)	Saturated Fat (g)	Sodium (mg)	Carbohydrates (g)	Fiber (g)	Protein (g)
Biscuit	1	180	8	6	530	23	1	4
Cheese, Sargento® Light String	1	50	2.5	1.5	160	1	0	6
Chicken Pot Pie	1	790	45	37	1970	66	3	29
Cole Slaw	1 serv	180	10	1.5	150	20	2	1
Corn on the Cob	3 in	70	0.5	0	0	16	2	2
Corn on the Cob	5.5 in	140	1	0	5	33	4	5
Corn, Sweet Kernel	1 serv	100	0.5	0	0	21	2	3
Cornbread Muffin	1	210	9	1.5	240	28	0	3
Croutons, Parmesan Garlic	1 pkg	70	3	0	160	8	0	1
Famous Bowls® w/ Mashed Potato w/ Gravy	1	680	31	8	2130	74	6	26
Green Beans	1 serv	20	0	0	290	3	1	1
Jalapeño Peppers	1 serv	20	1.5	0	480	1	1	0
Macaroni & Cheese	1 serv	160	7	2.5	720	19	1	5
Macaroni Salad	1 serv	190	10	2	430	22	1	4
Mashed Potatoes w/ Gravy	1 serv	120	4	1	530	19	1	2
Mashed Potatoes, no Gravy	1 serv	90	3	0.5	320	15	1	2
Popcorn Chicken, Individual	1 serv	400	26	6	1040	18	1	22
Popcorn Chicken Value Box	1	700	44	9	1920	50	5	26
Potato Salad	1 serv	210	11	2.5	560	26	3	2
Potato Wedges	1 serv	310	18	3	870	32	4	4
Snack Bowl	1 serv	310	14	4	930	33	3	12
Wings, Fiery Buffalo Hot™	1	70	4	.5	270	5	0	4
Wings, Fiery Buffalo Hot™ Value Box	1	560	31	5	1600	55	5	16
Wings, Honey BBQ Hot™	1	80	4	.5	240	8	0	4
Wings, Honey BBQ Hot™ Value Box	1	560	31	5	1600	55	5	16
Wings, Hot™	1	70	4	.5	140	4	0	4
Wings, Hot™ Value Box	1	510	31	5	1290	43	4	15

The Dietary Guidelines for Americans recommend limiting saturated fat to 20 grams and sodium to 2,300 milligrams for a typical adult eating 2,000 calories daily. Recommended limits may be higher or lower depending upon daily calorie consumption.

Substitution of ingredients may alter nutritional values. Menu items and hours of availability may vary at participating locations. Although this data is based on standard portion product guidelines, variation can be expected due to seasonal influences, minor differences in product assembly per restaurant, and other factors. Except for limited time offerings or test market items, menu products as of this printing are included in this brochure. Product data is based on current formulation as of date of publication. If you have any questions about KFC® and nutrition or are particularly sensitive to specific ingredients or foods, please contact us at 1-800-CALL-KFC. Nutrition values for fountain beverages do not account for ice. Depending on the sodium content of the water where the beverage is dispensed, the actual sodium content may be higher or lower than the listed values.

Please visit www.MyPyramid.gov for more information.
 * Registered Trademark of PepsiCo, Inc.
 ** Registered Trademark of Dr Pepper/Seven Up, Inc

LONG JOHN SILVER'S

ITEM DESCRIPTION	Serving Size	Calories	Total Fat (g)	Saturated Fat (g)	Sodium (mg)	Carbohydrates (g)	Fiber (g)	Protein (g)
BEVERAGES								
Diet Mountain Dew®	sm (20 oz)	0	0	0	100	0	0	0
Diet Pepsi®	sm (20 oz)	0	0	0	60	0	0	0
Dr Pepper®	sm (20 oz)	250	0	0	85	67	0	0
Fruit Punch, Tropicana®	sm (20 oz)	270	0	0	60	75	0	0
Iced Tea, Unsweetened	sm (20 oz)	0	0	0	0	0	0	0
Iceflow Lemonade	16 oz	190	0	0	15	47	0	0
Iceflow Strawberry Lemonade	16 oz	240	0	0	15	60	0	0
Lemonade, Tropicana®	sm (20 oz)	250	0	0	265	68	0	0
Mountain Dew®	sm (20 oz)	270	0	0	85	72	0	0
Pepsi®	sm (20 oz)	250	0	0	60	70	0	0
Raspberry Tea, Lipton®	sm (20 oz)	200	0	0	60	52	0	0
Sierra Mist®	sm (20 oz)	250	0	0	50	67	0	0
Twister® Orange, Tropicana®	sm (20 oz)	280	0	0	65	78	0	0
Wild Cherry Pepsi®	sm (20 oz)	250	0	0	50	70	0	0
DESSERTS								
Pie, Chocolate Cream	1 pc	280	17	10	230	28	1	3
Pie, Pineapple Cream	1 pc	300	17	11	250	35	0	3
DRESSINGS AND SPREADS								
BBQ	1 pkg	40	0	0	230	10	0	0
Cocktail Sauce	1 serv	25	0	0	250	6	0	0
Honey Mustard	1 pkg	100	6	1.5	170	12	0	0
Ketchup	1 pkg	10	0	0	100	2	0	0
Lemon Juice	1 pkg	0	0	0	0	0	0	0
Louisiana Hot Sauce	1 pkg	0	0	0	140	0	0	0
Malt Vinegar	1 serv	0	0	0	35	0	0	0
Marinara	1 pkg	15	0	0	125	4	1	1
Ranch	1 pkg	160	17	2.5	240	2	0	0
Sweet & Sour	1 pkg	45	0	0	120	12	0	0
Tartar Sauce	1 serv	100	9	1.5	250	4	0	0
MAIN MENU								
Alaskan Pollock, Battered	1 pc	260	16	4	790	17	0	12

ITEM DESCRIPTION	Serving Size	Calories	Total Fat (g)	Saturated Fat (g)	Sodium (mg)	Carbohydrates (g)	Fiber (g)	Protein (g)
Alaskan Pollock Sandwich	1	470	23	5	1180	49	3	18
Alaskan Pollock Sandwich, Ultimate	1	530	27	8	1500	50	3	21
Chicken Strip Sandwich	1	440	30	6	1350	47	4	22
Chicken Strips	1 pc	140	8	2	480	9	0	8
Clam Strips, Breaded	1 serv	320	19	4.5	1190	29	2	9
Crab Cake, Lobster Stuffed	1 pc	170	9	2	390	16	1	6
Fish Sandwich	1	470	23	5	1180	49	3	18
Fish Sandwich, Ultimate®	1	530	27	8	1500	50	3	21
Fish, Battered	1 pc	260	16	4	790	17	0	12
Freshside Grille® Salmon	1 serv	280	7	2	1010	27	3	27
Freshside Grille® Shrimp Scampi	1 serv	330	15	3.5	1230	29	3	20
Freshside Grille® Tilapia	1 serv	250	4.5	2	820	27	3	25
Lobster Bites, Buttered	1 serv	230	9	3	520	24	2	13
Pacific Salmon, Grilled	2 pcs	150	5	1	440	2	0	24
Shrimp Scampi	8 pcs	200	13	2.5	650	3	0	17
Shrimp, Battered	3 pcs	130	9	2.5	480	8	0	5
Shrimp, Popcorn	1 serv	270	16	4	570	23	1	9
Tilapia, Grilled	1 pc	110	2.5	1	250	1	0	22
SIDES AND SNACKS								
Breadstick	1	170	3.5	1	290	29	1	6
Broccoli Cheese Bites	5 pcs	230	12	4.5	550	25	2	5
Broccoli Cheese Soup	1	220	18	8	650	8	1	5
Chicken Sandwich, Zesty	1	380	19	4	880	39	3	14
Cole Slaw	1	200	15	2.5	340	15	3	1
Corn Cobbette w/ Butter Oil	1	150	10	2	30	14	3	3
Corn Cobbette, no Butter Oil	1	90	3	0.5	0	14	3	3
Crumblies®	1 serv	170	12	2.5	410	14	1	1
French Fries Basket	1	310	14	3.5	460	45	4	3
French Fries Platter	1	230	10	2.5	350	34	3	3
Hushpuppy	1 pc	60	2.5	0.5	200	9	1	1
Jalapeño Cheddar Bites	5 pcs	240	14	5	730	23	2	6
Jalapeño Peppers	1 pc	15	0	0	190	2	0	1
Mozzarella Sticks	3 pcs	150	9	3.5	350	13	1	5
Rice	1 serv	180	1	0.5	470	37	2	4

ITEM DESCRIPTION	Serving Size	Calories	Total Fat (g)	Saturated Fat (g)	Sodium (mg)	Carbohydrates (g)	Fiber (g)	Protein (g)
Taco, Baja Chicken Strip	1	370	23	5	890	31	3	11
Taco, Baja Fish	1	360	23	4.5	810	30	3	9
Vegetable Medley	1 serv	50	2	0.5	360	8	3	1

Recommended limits for a 2,000 calorie daily diet are 20 grams of saturated fat and 2,300 milligrams of sodium.

Substitution of ingredients may alter nutritional values. Menu items and hours of availability may vary at participating locations. Although this data is based on standard portion product guidelines, variation can be expected due to seasonal influences, minor differences in product assembly per restaurant, and other factors. Except for limited time offerings, optional, or test market items, menu products as of this printing are included in this brochure.

Please visit www.MyPyramid.gov for more information.

Data Revised: April 2010

McDONALD'S

BEVERAGES

Apple Juice	1	100	0	0	15	23	0	0
Cappuccino w/ Sugar Free Vanilla Syrup§	med (16 oz)	120	6	3.5	130	18	0	6
Cappuccino§	med (16 oz)	140	8	4.5	105	11	0	8
Cappuccino§, Caramel	med (16 oz)	240	6	3.5	150	41	0	6
Cappuccino§, Hazelnut	med (16 oz)	240	6	3.5	85	42	0	6
Cappuccino§, Vanilla	med (16 oz)	240	6	3.5	85	42	0	6
Coca-Cola® Classic§	sm (16 oz)	150	0	0	10	40	0	0
Coffee Cream	1 pkg	20	2	1.5	15	0	0	0
Coffee§	sm (12 oz)	0	0	0	0	0	0	0
Diet Coke®§	sm (16 oz)	0	0	0	20	0	0	0
Equal® 0 Calorie Sweetener	1 pkg	0	0	0	0	1	0	0
Frappe Caramel	med (16 oz)	550	24	15	160	76	0	8
Frappe Mocha	med (16 oz)	560	24	15	160	78	1	8
Hi-C® Orange Lavaburst§	sm (16 oz)	160	0	0	5	44	0	0
Hot Chocolate w/ Nonfat Milk§	med (16 oz)	310	6	3.5	190	55	0	11
Hot Chocolate§	med (16 oz)	380	15	9	170	53	0	10
Iced Coffee w/ Sugar Free Vanilla Syrup§	med (11.5 oz)	90	8	5	100	11	0	2
Iced Coffee, Caramel§	med (11.5 oz)	190	8	5	115	27	0	2
Iced Coffee, Hazelnut§	med (11.5 oz)	190	8	5	60	29	0	2
Iced Coffee, Vanilla§	med (11.5 oz)	190	8	5	60	29	0	2
Iced Coffee§	med (11.5 oz)	200	8	5	60	30	0	2
Iced Latte w/ Sugar Free Vanilla Syrup§	med (16 oz)	90	5	3	105	14	0	5

ITEM DESCRIPTION	Serving Size	Calories	Total Fat (g)	Saturated Fat (g)	Sodium (mg)	Carbohydrates (g)	Fiber (g)	Protein (g)
Iced Latte§	med (16 oz)	100	6	3.5	80	8	0	6
Iced Latte§, Caramel	med (16 oz)	180	4.5	2.5	120	31	0	4
Iced Latte§, Hazelnut	med (16 oz)	180	4.5	2.5	65	33	0	4
Iced Latte§, Vanilla	med (16 oz)	190	4.5	2.5	70	33	0	5
Iced Mocha w/ Nonfat Milk§	med (16 oz)	270	8	4.5	140	43	0	7
Iced Mocha§	med (16 oz)	310	13	8	140	42	0	7
Iced Mocha§, Caramel	med (16 oz)	300	14	8	160	36	0	8
Iced Nonfat Latte w/ Sugar Free Vanilla Syrup§	med (16 oz)	50	0	0	100	14	0	5
Iced Nonfat Latte§	med (16 oz)	60	0	0	90	9	0	6
Iced Nonfat Latte§, Caramel	med (16 oz)	150	0	0	120	32	0	5
Iced Nonfat Latte§, Hazelnut	med (16 oz)	150	0	0	70	33	0	5
Iced Nonfat Latte§, Vanilla	med (16 oz)	150	0	0	70	33	0	5
Iced Nonfat Mocha§, Caramel	med (16 oz)	240	6	4	190	37	0	9
Iced Tea§	sm (16 oz)	0	0	0	10	0	0	0
Latte w/ Sugar Free Vanilla Syrup§	med (16 oz)	160	8	5	150	21	0	8
Latte§	med (16 oz)	180	10	6	130	13	0	10
Latte§, Caramel	med (16 oz)	280	8	4.5	170	43	0	8
Latte§, Hazelnut	med (16 oz)	280	8	4.5	110	45	0	8
Latte§, Vanilla	med (16 oz)	280	8	4.5	110	44	0	8
Milk, 1% Low Fat Chocolate	1	170	3	1.5	150	26	1	9
Milk, 1% Low Fat	1	100	2.5	1.5	125	12	0	8
Mocha w/ Nonfat Milk§	med (16 oz)	280	6	3.5	160	50	0	8
Mocha§	med (16 oz)	330	12	7	150	48	0	7
Mocha§, Caramel	med (16 oz)	290	12	7	180	39	0	8
Nonfat Cappuccino w/ Sugar Free Vanilla Syrup§	med (16 oz)	70	0	0	130	19	0	7
Nonfat Cappuccino§	med (16 oz)	80	0	0	110	12	0	8
Nonfat Cappuccino§, Caramel	med (16 oz)	190	0	0	150	41	0	6
Nonfat Cappuccino§, Hazelnut	med (16 oz)	190	0	0	90	43	0	6
Nonfat Cappuccino§, Vanilla	med (16 oz)	190	0	0	90	42	0	6
Nonfat Latte w/ Sugar Free Vanilla Syrup§	med (16 oz)	90	0	0	160	22	0	9
Nonfat Latte§	med (16 oz)	110	0	0	140	15	0	10

ITEM DESCRIPTION	Serving Size	Calories	Total Fat (g)	Saturated Fat (g)	Sodium (mg)	Carbohydrates (g)	Fiber (g)	Protein (g)
Nonfat Latte§, Caramel	med (16 oz)	220	0	0	180	45	0	9
Nonfat Latte§, Hazelnut	med (16 oz)	220	0	0	115	46	0	9
Nonfat Latte§, Vanilla	med (16 oz)	220	0	0	115	46	0	9
Nonfat Mocha§, Caramel	med (16 oz)	240	4	2.5	200	41	0	9
Orange Juice§	med (16 oz)	190	0	0	0	39	0	3
Powerade® Mountain Blast§	sm (16 oz)	100	0	0	85	27	0	0
Splenda® No Calorie Sweetener	1 pkg	0	0	0	0	1	0	0
Sprite®§	sm (16 oz)	150	0	0	40	39	0	0
Sugar Packet	1 pkg	15	0	0	0	4	0	0
Sweet Tea†	sm (16 oz)	150	0	0	10	36	0	1
BREAKFAST ITEMS								
Bagel w/ Bacon, Egg & Cheese	1	560	27	9	1300	56	3	24
Bagel w/ Steak, Egg & Cheese	1	660	33	12	1580	56	3	33
Big Breakfast®	reg	740	48	17	1560	51	3	28
Big Breakfast w/ Hotcakes	reg	1090	56	19	2150	111	6	36
Biscuit w/ Bacon, Egg & Cheese	reg	420	23	12	1160	37	2	15
Biscuit w/ Egg, Sausage	reg	510	33	14	1170	36	2	18
Biscuit, Sausage	reg	430	27	12	1080	34	2	11
Biscuit, Southern Style Chicken	reg	410	20	8	1180	41	2	17
Burrito w/ Sausage	1	300	16	7	830	26	1	12
English Muffin	1	160	3	0.5	280	27	2	5
Hash Brown	1	150	9	1.5	310	15	2	1
Hotcakes & Sausage, no Syrup or Margarine	1 serv	520	24	7	930	61	3	15
Hotcakes, no Syrup or Margarine	1 serv	350	9	2	590	60	3	8
McGriddles® w/ Bacon, Egg & Cheese	1	420	18	8	1110	48	2	15
McGriddles® w/ Sausage, Egg & Cheese	1	560	32	12	1360	48	2	20
McGriddles®, Sausage	1	420	22	8	1030	44	2	11
McMuffin® w/ Egg	1	300	12	5	820	30	2	18
McMuffin® w/ Egg, Sausage	1	450	27	10	920	30	2	21
McMuffin® w/ Sausage	1	370	22	8	850	29	2	14
McSkillet™ Burrito w/ Sausage	1 serv	610	36	14	1390	44	3	27
Oatmeal, Fruit & Maple	1	290	4.5	1.5	160	57	5	5
Oatmeal, Fruit & Maple, no Brown Sugar	1	260	4.5	2	115	48	5	5

ITEM DESCRIPTION

	Serving Size	Calories	Total Fat (g)	Saturated Fat (g)	Sodium (mg)	Carbohydrates (g)	Fiber (g)	Protein (g)
DESSERTS								
Apple Dippers / Low Fat Caramel Dip	1 pkg	100	0.5	0	35	23	0	0
Caramel Dip, Low Fat	1 serv	70	0.5	0	35	15	0	0
Cinnamon Melts	1 serv	460	19	9	370	66	3	6
Cookie, Chocolate Chip	1	160	8	3.5	90	21	1	2
Cookie, Oatmeal Raisin	1	150	6	2.5	135	22	1	2
Cookie, Sugar	1	160	7	3	120	21	0	2
Cookies, McDonaldland®	1 pkg	260	8	2.5	300	43	1	4
Fruit 'n Yogurt Parfait	1 serv	160	2	1	85	31	1	4
Ice Cream Cone, Reduced Fat Vanilla	1	150	3.5	2	60	24	0	4
Kiddie Cone	1	45	1	0.5	20	8	0	1
McFlurry® w/ M&M'S® Candies	12 oz	710	25	16	220	105	4	15
McFlurry® w/ M&M'S® Candies	snack	430	16	10	130	64	2	9
McFlurry® w/ Oreo® Cookies	12 oz	580	19	10	320	89	3	13
McFlurry® w/ Oreo® Cookies	snack	340	12	6	200	53	2	8
Peanuts	1 serv	45	3.5	0.5	0	2	1	2
Pie, Baked Hot Apple	1	250	13	7	170	32	4	2
Shake, Chocolate McCafe®	16 oz	720	20	12	300	119	1	15
Shake, Chocolate Triple Thick®	16 oz	580	14	8	250	102	1	13
Shake, Strawberry McCafe®	16 oz	710	20	12	210	116	0	14
Shake, Strawberry Triple Thick®	16 oz	560	13	8	170	97	0	13
Shake, Vanilla McCafe®	16 oz	680	20	12	220	111	0	14
Shake, Vanilla Triple Thick®	16 oz	550	13	8	190	96	0	13
Smoothie, Strawberry Banana	16 oz	260	1	0	40	60	3	2
Smoothie, Wild Berry	16 oz	260	1	0	35	60	4	3
Sundae, Hot Caramel	1	340	8	5	160	60	1	7
Sundae, Hot Fudge	1	330	10	7	180	54	2	8
Sundae, Strawberry	1	280	6	4	95	49	1	6
DRESSINGS AND SPREADS								
Barbecue Sauce	1 pkg	50	0	0	260	12	0	0
Barbecue Sauce, Southwestern Chipotle	1 pkg	60	0	0	210	15	1	0
Buffalo Sauce, Spicy	1 pkg	60	6	1	800	1	0	0
Dressing, Newman's Own® Creamy Caesar	1 pkg	190	18	3.5	500	4	0	2

ITEM DESCRIPTION	Serving Size	Calories	Total Fat (g)	Saturated Fat (g)	Sodium (mg)	Carbohydrates (g)	Fiber (g)	Protein (g)
Dressing, Newman's Own® Creamy Southwest	1 pkg	100	6	1	340	11	0	1
Dressing, Newman's Own® Low Fat Balsamic Vinaigrette	1 pkg	40	3	0	730	4	0	0
Dressing, Newman's Own® Low Fat Family Recipe Italian	1 pkg	60	2.5	0	730	8	0	1
Dressing, Newman's Own® Ranch	1 pkg	170	15	2.5	530	9	0	1
Honey	1 pkg	50	0	0	0	12	0	0
Honey Mustard Sauce, Tangy	1 pkg	60	2	0	140	10	0	1
Jam, Grape	1 pkg	35	0	0	0	9	0	0
Margarine, Whipped	1 pkg	40	4.5	1.5	55	0	0	0
Mustard Sauce, Hot	1 pkg	60	2.5	0	250	9	2	1
Ranch Sauce, Creamy	1 pkg	170	18	3	270	2	0	0
Strawberry Preserves	1 pkg	35	0	0	0	9	0	0
Sweet 'N Sour Sauce	1 pkg	50	0	0	150	12	0	0
Syrup	1 pkg	180	0	0	20	45	0	0
MAIN MENU								
Angus Bacon & Cheese	1	790	39	17	2070	63	4	45
Angus Chipotle BBQ Bacon	1	800	39	18	2020	66	4	45
Angus Deluxe	1	750	39	16	1700	61	4	40
Angus Mushroom & Swiss	1	770	40	17	1170	59	4	44
Big Mac®	1	540	29	10	1040	45	3	25
Big N' Tasty®	1	460	24	8	720	37	3	24
Big N' Tasty® w/ Cheese	1	510	28	11	960	38	3	27
Cheeseburger	1	300	12	6	750	33	2	15
Chicken Classic Sandwich, Premium Crispy	1	530	20	3.5	1150	59	3	28
Chicken Classic Sandwich, Premium Grilled	1	420	10	2	1190	51	3	32
Chicken Club Sandwich, Premium Crispy	1	630	28	7	1360	60	4	35
Chicken Club Sandwich, Premium Grilled	1	530	17	6	1410	52	4	39
Chicken McNuggets®	4 pcs	190	12	2	400	11	0	10
Chicken McNuggets®	6 pcs	280	17	3	600	16	0	14
Chicken McNuggets®	10 pcs	460	29	5	1000	27	0	24
Chicken Ranch BLT Sandwich, Premium Crispy	1	580	23	4.5	1400	62	3	31

ITEM DESCRIPTION	Serving Size	Calories	Total Fat (g)	Saturated Fat (g)	Sodium (mg)	Carbohydrates (g)	Fiber (g)	Protein (g)
Chicken Ranch BLT Sandwich, Premium Grilled	1	470	12	3	1440	54	3	36
Chicken Sandwich, Southern Style Crispy	1	400	17	3	1030	39	1	24
Chicken Selects® Premium Breast Strips	3 pcs	400	24	3.5	1010	23	0	23
Chicken Selects® Premium Breast Strips	5 pcs	660	40	6	1680	39	0	38
Double Cheeseburger	1	440	23	11	1150	34	2	25
Double Quarter Pounder® w/ Cheese++	1	740	42	19	1380	40	3	48
Filet-O-Fish®	1	380	18	3.5	640	38	2	15
Hamburger	1	250	9	3.5	520	31	2	12
Mac Snack Wrap†	1	330	19	7	690	26	1	15
McChicken®	1	360	16	3	830	40	2	14
McDouble	1	390	19	8	920	33	2	22
McRib®†	1	500	26	10	980	44	3	22
Quarter Pounder® w/ Cheese+	1	510	26	12	1190	40	3	29
Snack Wrap®, Angus Bacon & Cheese	1	390	21	9	1080	28	1	21
Snack Wrap®, Angus Chipotle BBQ Bacon	1	400	22	10	1060	30	1	21
Snack Wrap®, Angus Deluxe	1	410	25	10	990	27	2	20
Snack Wrap®, Angus Mushroom& Swiss	1	430	26	10	730	27	2	22
Snack Wrap® Chipotle Barbecue, Crispy	1	330	15	4.5	810	35	1	14
Snack Wrap® Chipotle Barbecue, Grilled	1	260	9	3.5	830	28	1	18
Snack Wrap® Honey Mustard, Crispy	1	330	16	4.5	780	34	1	14
Snack Wrap® Honey Mustard, Grilled	1	260	9	3.5	800	27	1	18
Snack Wrap® Ranch, Crispy	1	340	17	4.5	810	33	1	14
Snack Wrap® Ranch, Grilled	1	270	10	4	830	26	1	18
SALADS								
Bacon Ranch Salad w/ Crispy Chicken	1	370	20	6	970	20	3	29
Bacon Ranch Salad w/ Grilled Chicken	1	260	9	4	1010	12	3	33
Bacon Ranch Salad, no Chicken	1	140	7	3.5	300	10	3	9
Butter Garlic Croutons	1 serv	60	1.5	0	140	10	1	2
Caesar Salad w/ Crispy Chicken	1	330	17	4.5	840	20	3	26
Caesar Salad w/ Grilled Chicken	1	220	6	3	890	12	3	30
Caesar Salad, no Chicken	1	90	4	2.5	180	9	3	7
Fruit & Walnut Salad	snack	210	8	1.5	60	31	2	4
Side Salad	1	20	0	0	10	4	1	1

ITEM DESCRIPTION	Serving Size	Calories	Total Fat (g)	Saturated Fat (g)	Sodium (mg)	Carbohydrates (g)	Fiber (g)	Protein (g)
Southwest Salad w/ Crispy Chicken	1	430	20	4	920	38	6	26
Southwest Salad w/ Grilled Chicken	1	320	9	3	960	30	6	30
Southwest Salad, no Chicken	1	140	4.5	2	150	20	6	6
SIDES AND SNACKS								
French Fries	med	380	19	2.5	270	48	5	4
Ketchup	1 pkg	15	0	0	110	3	0	0
Salt	1 pkg	0	0	0	270	0	0	0

Note: Nutrient contributions from individual components may not equal the total due to federal rounding regulations. Percent Daily Values (DV) and RDIs are based on unrounded values.

This list is effective 06-03-2010.

* Contains less than 2% of the Daily Value of these nutrients

† Available at participating McDonald's

+ Based on the weight before cooking 4 oz (113.4 g)

++ Based on the weight before cooking 8 oz (226.8 g)

§ The values represent the sodium derived from ingredients plus water. Sodium content of the water is based on the value listed for municipal water in the USDA National Nutrient Database. The actual amount of sodium may be higher or lower depending upon the sodium content of the water where the beverage is dispensed.

= Made with low fat yogurt

** Percent Daily Values (DV) are based on a 2,000 calorie diet. Your daily values may be higher or lower depending on your calorie needs.

The nutrition information on this website is derived from testing conducted in accredited laboratories, published resources, or from information provided from McDonald's suppliers. The nutrition information is based on standard product formulations and serving sizes. All nutrition information is based on average values for ingredients from McDonald's suppliers throughout the U.S. and is rounded to meet current U.S. FDA NLEA guidelines. Variation in serving sizes, preparation techniques, product testing, and sources of supply, as well as regional and seasonal differences may affect the nutrition values for each product. In addition, product formulations change periodically. You should expect some variation in the nutrient content of the products purchased in our restaurants. None of our products is certified as vegetarian. This information is correct as of January 2007, unless stated otherwise.

SPLENDA® No Calorie Sweetener is the registered trademark of McNeil Nutritionals, LLC

EQUAL® 0 Calorie Sweetener is a registered trademark of Merisant Company

NATHAN'S FAMOUS

BEVERAGES

	Serving Size	Calories	Total Fat (g)	Saturated Fat (g)	Sodium (mg)	Carbohydrates (g)	Fiber (g)	Protein (g)
Coca-Cola	16 oz	130	0	0	10	36	0	0
Coffee	16 oz	7	0	0	7	0	0	0
Lemonade	16 oz	197	0	0	0	47	0	0
MAIN MENU								
Cheese Dog, Nathan's Famous All Beef	1	390	25	8	1440	30	1	12
Cheeseburger w/ Bacon	1	783	50	20	1365	45	2	36
Cheeseburger, Super	1	987	72	23	1349	47	3	35
Cheesesteak Sandwich	1	849	45	21	1554	70	2	44
Cheesesteak Supreme	1	879	45	20	1625	76	3	46
Chicken Cheesesteak Supreme	1	601	19	9	1719	70	3	40
Chicken Tender Pita	1	823	52	8	1462	66	5	22
Chicken Tender Platter	1 serv	1245	90	14	1352	80	10	26
Chicken Tender Sandwich	1	706	43	6	1165	58	5	22
Chicken Tenders	3 pcs	526	39	6	900	24	3	21
Chicken Wings	5 pcs	400	27	7	650	12	0	27

ITEM DESCRIPTION	Serving Size	Calories	Total Fat (g)	Saturated Fat (g)	Sodium (mg)	Carbohydrates (g)	Fiber (g)	Protein (g)
Chili Dog, Nathan's Famous All Beef	1	400	23	6	1000	33	2	16
Corn Dog on a Stick	1	380	21	5	730	39	1	7
Corn on the Cob	1	140	1.5	0	20	34	2	5
Fish & Chips Platter	2 pcs	1516	95	15	2732	156	10	34
Fish Sandwich	1	437	18	3	715	50	3	18
French Fries	reg	464	34	5	55	35	4	4
French Fries w/ Cheese	reg	564	42	7	785	41	4	5
Funnel Cake	1	580	29	5	360	73	1	5
Grilled Chicken Platter	1	839	56	9	1134	58	7	24
Grilled Chicken Sandwich	1	554	32	5	1158	40	3	27
Hamburger w/ Cheese	1	705	43	16	1071	45	2	33
Hamburger, Double w/ Cheese	1	1178	84	32	1299	45	2	57
Hot Dog Nuggets	6 pcs	348	28	6	400	20	0	5
Hot Dog, Nathan's Famous All Beef	1	297	18	7	692	24	1	11
Mozzarella Sticks	3 pcs	390	28	8	941	20	1	14
Onion Rings	sm	544	45	6	580	36	1.5	3
Pie, Apple	1 pc	314	19	4	310	33	0	3
Pretzel Dog	1	390	16	6	970	49	1	12
Pretzel, King-Size	1	180	1	0	940	38	1	6
Seafood Sampler	1 pc	1965	123	20	2893	196	16	47
Shrimp & Chips Platter	15 pcs	1834	120	22	3395	178	12	32
Wrap, Grilled Chicken Caesar	1	700	34	11	1340	60	1	38
Wrap, Krispy Southwest Chipotle	1	750	39	13	1160	62	1	68

OLIVE GARDEN

BEVERAGES

Beer, Light Bottle	1	110	0	0	15	6	n/a	n/a
Beer, Light Draft	14 oz	130	0	0	20	8	n/a	n/a
Beer, Light Draft	20 oz	190	0	0	25	11	n/a	n/a
Beer, Non-Alcoholic Bottle	1	60	0	0	5	13	n/a	n/a
Beer, Regular Bottle	1	160	0	0	15	12	n/a	n/a
Beer, Regular Draft	14 oz	170	0	0	15	13	n/a	n/a
Beer, Regular Draft	20 oz	250	0	0	25	19	n/a	n/a
Bellini, Peach	1	170	0	0	0	33	n/a	n/a

ITEM DESCRIPTION	Serving Size	Calories	Total Fat (g)	Saturated Fat (g)	Sodium (mg)	Carbohydrates (g)	Fiber (g)	Protein (g)
Bellini, Peach-Raspberry Iced Tea	1	70	0	0	0	16	n/a	n/a
Bellini, Strawberry	1	220	0	0	0	46	n/a	n/a
Bellini, Wild Berry	1	160	0	0	10	31	n/a	n/a
Caffè la Toscana Coffee	1	0	0	0	5	0	n/a	n/a
Caffè Latte	1	130	4	2	85	15	n/a	n/a
Caffè Mocha	1	180	4	2.5	75	30	n/a	n/a
Cappuccino	1	150	8	4	65	14	n/a	n/a
Caramel Hazelnut Macchiato	1	220	4.5	2.5	40	43	n/a	n/a
Coca-Cola Classic	1	100	0	0	5	27	n/a	n/a
Cream Soda	1	190	5	3	40	35	n/a	n/a
Daiquiri, Mango	1	240	0	0	10	43	n/a	n/a
Daiquiri, Peach	1	270	0	0	10	51	n/a	n/a
Daiquiri, Strawberry	1	250	0	0	15	47	n/a	n/a
Daiquiri, Wild Berry	1	270	0	0	5	49	n/a	n/a
Diet Coke	1	0	0	0	10	0	n/a	n/a
Dr Pepper	1	100	0	0	35	27	n/a	n/a
Espresso, Lavazza	1	0	0	0	10	0	n/a	n/a
Fresca, Berry Acqua	1	390	1.5	1	40	94	n/a	n/a
Fresco, Strawberry	1	230	0	0	5	31	n/a	n/a
Frozen Cappuccino	1	320	10	6	60	52	n/a	n/a
Frozen Margarita, Strawberry	1	340	0	0	25	67	n/a	n/a
Frozen Margarita, Strawberry-Mango	1	350	0	0	20	68	n/a	n/a
Frozen Margarita, Wild Berry	1	290	0	0	20	55	n/a	n/a
Iced Tea, Fresh Brewed	1	0	0	0	0	0	n/a	n/a
Italian Soda	1	120	0	0	5	29	n/a	n/a
Juice	1	270	0	0	50	60	n/a	n/a
Lemonade, Limoncello	1	260	0	0	5	42	n/a	n/a
Lemonade, Raspberry	1	110	0	0	15	29	n/a	n/a
Limonata, Bella	1	190	0	0	35	48	n/a	n/a
Limonata, Strawberry-Mango	1	200	0	0	30	50	n/a	n/a
Margarita, Italian	1	240	0	0	10	32	n/a	n/a
Martini, Chocolate	1	260	3.5	2	45	36	n/a	n/a
Martini, Mango	1	180	0	0	0	31	n/a	n/a
Martini, Pomegranate Margarita	1	290	0	0	5	44	n/a	n/a

ITEM DESCRIPTION	Serving Size	Calories	Total Fat (g)	Saturated Fat (g)	Sodium (mg)	Carbohydrates (g)	Fiber (g)	Protein (g)
Martini, Strawberry-Limoncello	1	300	0	0	15	42	n/a	n/a
Milk, 2% Reduced Fat	1	260	10	6	250	26	n/a	n/a
Sangria, Berry	1	230	0	0	15	35	n/a	n/a
Sangria, Berry Pitcher	1	910	0	0	50	138	n/a	n/a
Sangria, Peach	1	250	0	0	50	40	n/a	n/a
Sangria, Peach Pitcher	1	1010	0	0	200	158	n/a	n/a
Sangria, Tropical	1	220	0	0	10	31	n/a	n/a
Sangria, Tropical Pitcher	1	870	0	0	45	126	n/a	n/a
Sprite	1	100	0	0	20	26	n/a	n/a
Teas, Herbal & Flavored, Hot	1	0	0	0	0	0	n/a	n/a
Venetian Sunset	1	190	0	0	10	38	n/a	n/a
Wine, Red, White, or Blush	1	150	0	0	20	8	n/a	n/a
Wine, Red, White, or Blush Bottle	1	640	0	0	90	35	n/a	n/a
Wine, Red, White, or Blush Magnum Bottle	1	1360	0	0	190	74	n/a	n/a
Wine, Sparkling	1	130	0	0	20	8	n/a	n/a
Wine, Sparkling Bottle	1	550	0	0	90	35	n/a	n/a
DESSERTS								
Apple Crostata	1	730	32	15	240	104	6	n/a
Cake, Black Tie Mousse	1	760	48	27	270	73	8	n/a
Cake, Dark Chocolate w/ Chocolate Mousse & Caramel Cream	1	270	18	8	140	25	0	n/a
Cake, Lemon Cream	1	610	35	16	430	69	2	n/a
Cake, Strawberry & White Chocolate Cream	1	210	11	6	70	27	0	n/a
Cheesecake, White Chocolate Raspberry	1	890	62	36	490	70	6	n/a
Chocolate Mousse w/ Dark Chocolate Cookie Crust	1	290	21	10	120	23	2	n/a
Chocolate Sauce	1 serv	210	2.5	1.5	75	44	2	n/a
Limoncello Mousse w/ Vanilla Cookie Crust	1	230	13	8	70	28	0	n/a
Strata, Triple Chocolate	1	700	41	20	390	73	6	n/a
Tiramisu	1	510	32	19	75	48	2	n/a
Tiramisu, Amaretto w/ Almond Cookie Crumble	1	240	17	9	50	16	0	n/a
Zeppoli	1	920	35	3.5	590	131	4	n/a

ITEM DESCRIPTION	Serving Size	Calories	Total Fat (g)	Saturated Fat (g)	Sodium (mg)	Carbohydrates (g)	Fiber (g)	Protein (g)
DRESSINGS AND SPREADS								
Dipping Sauce, Alfredo	1 serv	380	35	22	510	9	1	n/a
Dipping Sauce, Marinara	1 serv	70	2.5	0	540	10	3	n/a
Parmesan-Peppercorn Sauce	1 serv	300	30	5	340	6	1	n/a
Sauce, Tomato	1 serv	45	1.5	0	270	6	1	n/a
GLUTEN FREE								
Children's Chicken, Grilled	1	230	6	1.5	490	13	4	n/a
Mixed Grill	1	750	23	6	1760	24	4	n/a
Mixed Grill, All Chicken	1	640	19	4	1260	27	7	n/a
Pennine Rigate, w/ Marinara	1	560	19	4.5	690	90	8	n/a
Salad, Caesar, no Croutons	1	560	54	12	820	10	4	n/a
Salad, Garden-Fresh, no Croutons	1	260	20	3	1500	19	6	n/a
Salmon, Herb-Grilled	1	510	26	6	760	5	4	n/a
Steak Toscano	1	760	43	19	1280	8	4	n/a
KIDS MENU								
Broccoli	1	25	0	0	10	4	2	n/a
Chicken Fingers	1	330	16	1.5	930	22	0	n/a
Chicken, Grilled w/ Pasta & Broccoli	1	310	5	1	680	33	6	n/a
Fettuccine Alfredo	1	800	48	30	810	69	4	n/a
French Fries	1	400	21	2	880	47	4	n/a
Macaroni & Cheese	1	340	6	2.5	1000	58	3	n/a
Milkshake, Chocolate	1	520	22	14	230	72	7	n/a
Milkshake, Strawberry	1	500	24	15	160	62	10	n/a
Milkshake, Vanilla	1	530	23	14	170	73	16	n/a
Pizza, Cheese	1	470	14	6	1170	66	4	n/a
Ravioli w/ Tomato Sauce	1	300	8	4	440	43	4	n/a
Spaghetti & Tomato Sauce	1	250	3	0.5	370	45	4	n/a
Sundae	1	180	9	6	45	21	0	n/a
LUNCH MENU								
Beef & Tortelloni, Braised	1	740	41	17	1280	60	5	n/a
Capellini Pomodoro	1	480	11	2	970	78	11	n/a
Chicken Alfredo	1	910	52	30	1150	71	4	n/a
Chicken Parmigiana	1	570	18	5	1720	67	18	n/a
Chicken Scampi	1	740	38	14	1350	57	7	n/a

ITEM DESCRIPTION	Serving Size	Calories	Total Fat (g)	Saturated Fat (g)	Sodium (mg)	Carbohydrates (g)	Fiber (g)	Protein (g)
Chicken Spiedini, Grilled	1	460	13	2.5	1180	26	7	n/a
Chicken, Venetian Apricot	1	280	3	1	1180	32	8	n/a
Eggplant Parmigiana	1	620	26	8	1540	70	11	n/a
Fettuccine Alfredo	1	800	48	30	810	69	4	n/a
Five Cheese Ziti Al Forno	1	770	32	17	1450	89	5	n/a
Lasagna Classico	1	580	32	18	1930	35	7	n/a
Lasagna Rollata al Forno	1	840	49	28	1830	65	8	n/a
Ravioli di Portobello	1	450	19	11	960	53	8	n/a
Ravioli w/ Marinara Sauce	1	530	18	9	1160	64	6	n/a
Ravioli w/ Meat Sauce	1	600	22	12	1210	65	8	n/a
Seafood Alfredo	1	670	36	21	1320	59	5	n/a
Shrimp Caprese, Grilled	1	820	39	17	2800	81	0	n/a
Shrimp Primavera	1	510	9	1.5	1130	79	12	n/a
Spaghetti & Italian Sausage	1	830	44	16	1920	61	9	n/a
Spaghetti & Meatballs	1	820	40	16	1600	66	6	n/a
Spaghetti w/ Meat Sauce	1	550	21	8	1040	59	6	n/a
Tour of Italy	1	1450	74	33	3830	97	10	n/a
MAIN MENU								
Beef & Tortelloni, Braised	1	1020	53	22	2060	82	10	n/a
Bistecca, Parmesan Crusted	1	690	35	19	1480	40	7	n/a
Capellini di Mare	1	650	18	5	1830	82	7	n/a
Capellini Pomodoro	1	840	17	3	1250	141	19	n/a
Chicken & Shrimp Carbonara	1	1440	88	38	3000	80	9	n/a
Chicken Alfredo	1	1440	82	48	2070	103	5	n/a
Chicken con Broccoli, Garlic-Herb	1	960	41	18	2180	90	12	n/a
Chicken Marsala	1	770	37	5	1800	59	16	n/a
Chicken Marsala, Stuffed	1	800	36	16	2830	40	6	n/a
Chicken Parmigiana	1	1090	49	18	3380	79	27	n/a
Chicken Scampi	1	1070	53	20	2220	88	8	n/a
Chicken, Venetian Apricot	1	380	4	1.5	1420	32	8	n/a
Eggplant Parmigiana	1	850	35	10	1900	98	19	n/a
Fettuccine Alfredo	1	1220	75	47	1350	99	5	n/a
Five Cheese Ziti al Forno	1	1050	48	26	2370	112	9	n/a
Lasagna Classico	1	850	47	25	2830	39	19	n/a

ITEM DESCRIPTION	Serving Size	Calories	Total Fat (g)	Saturated Fat (g)	Sodium (mg)	Carbohydrates (g)	Fiber (g)	Protein (g)
Lasagna Rollata al Forno	1	1170	68	39	2510	90	11	n/a
Mixed Grill	1	830	28	5	1840	72	10	n/a
Pizza w/ Cheese & Sauce	1	910	28	12	2970	129	8	n/a
Pizza w/ Chicken Alfredo	1	1180	40	17	3330	144	11	n/a
Pork Milanese	1	1510	87	37	3100	118	11	n/a
Ravioli di Portobello	1	670	30	17	1400	74	15	n/a
Ravioli w/ Marinara Sauce	1	660	22	11	1440	84	7	n/a
Ravioli w/ Meat Sauce	1	790	28	14	1510	88	12	n/a
Salmon, Herb-Grilled	1	510	26	6	760	5	2	n/a
Seafood Alfredo	1	1020	52	31	2430	88	9	n/a
Seafood Brodetto	1	480	16	3	2250	35	7	n/a
Seafood Portofino	1	800	33	14	1880	85	16	n/a
Short Ribs, Chianti Braised	1	1060	58	26	2970	71	17	n/a
Shrimp Caprese, Grilled	1	900	40	17	3490	82	0	n/a
Shrimp & Crab Tortelli Romana	1	840	42	24	1710	67	4	n/a
Shrimp Primavera	1	730	12	2	1620	110	14	n/a
Spaghetti & Italian Sausage	1	1270	67	24	3090	97	15	n/a
Spaghetti & Meatballs	1	1110	50	20	2180	103	9	n/a
Spaghetti w/ Meat Sauce	1	710	22	8	1340	94	9	n/a
Steak Gorgonzola-Alfredo	1	1310	73	41	2190	82	9	n/a
Steak Toscano	1	810	35	8	1690	62	11	n/a
Tilapia, Parmesan Crusted	1	590	25	10	910	42	6	n/a
Tour of Italy	1	1450	74	33	3830	97	10	n/a
SALADS								
Chicken Caesar, Grilled	1	850	64	13	1880	14	4	n/a
Garden-Fresh	1	120	3.5	0.5	550	17	3	n/a
Garden-Fresh w/ Dressing	1	350	26	4.5	1930	22	3	n/a
SIDES AND SNACKS								
Artichoke-Spinach Dip	1 serv	650	31	15	1430	68	6	n/a
Breadstick w/ Garlic-Butter Spread	1 pc	150	2	0	400	28	2	n/a
Bruschetta	1 serv	610	13	2.5	1760	100	10	n/a
Calamari	1 serv	890	54	5	2340	64	2	n/a
Calamari in Sampler Italiano	1 serv	440	27	2.5	1160	32	0	n/a
Caprese Flatbread	1 serv	600	36	11	1520	46	5	n/a

ITEM DESCRIPTION	Serving Size	Calories	Total Fat (g)	Saturated Fat (g)	Sodium (mg)	Carbohydrates (g)	Fiber (g)	Protein (g)
Chicken Fingers in Sampler Italiano	1 serv	330	16	1.5	930	22	0	n/a
Chicken Flatbread, Grilled	1 serv	760	44	15	1500	47	5	n/a
Fried Mozzarella in Sampler Italiano	1 serv	370	22	9	800	26	2	n/a
Fried Zucchini in Sampler Italiano	1 serv	370	20	1.5	630	42	4	n/a
Lasagna Fritta	1 serv	1030	63	21	1590	82	9	n/a
Mozzarella Fonduta, Smoked	1 serv	940	48	28	1940	72	7	n/a
Mushrooms, Stuffed	1 serv	280	19	5	720	15	3	n/a
Mushrooms, Stuffed in Sampler Italiano	1 serv	280	19	5	720	15	3	n/a
Mussels di Napoli	1 serv	180	8	4	1770	13	0	n/a
Ravioli, Toasted Beef & Pork in Sampler Italiano	1 serv	360	16	2.5	780	39	2	n/a
Sicilian Scampi	1 serv	500	22	10	1850	43	7	n/a
SOUPS								
Chicken & Gnocchi	1	250	8	3	1180	29	2	n/a
Minestrone	1	100	1	0	1020	18	3	n/a
Pasta E Fagioli	1	130	2.5	1	680	17	6	n/a
Zuppa Toscana	1	170	4	2	960	24	2	n/a
TOPPINGS AND EXTRAS								
Bell Peppers Pizza Topping	1	10	0	0	0	2	1	n/a
Black Olives Pizza Topping	1	45	4	0.5	350	3	1	n/a
Italian Sausage Pizza Topping	1	130	11	4	360	1	0	n/a
Mushrooms Pizza Topping	1	5	0	0	0	1	0	n/a
Onions Pizza Topping	1	15	0	0	0	4	1	n/a
Pepperoni Pizza Topping	1	120	11	4	460	0	0	n/a
Tomatoes Pizza Topping	1	10	0	0	0	2	1	n/a

Olive Garden has made an effort to provide complete and current nutrition information, but the handcrafted nature of our menu items and changes in recipes, ingredients, offerings, and kitchen procedures can cause variations from these values to occur. Therefore, the values shown here should be considered approximations. For more current information, please visit our website at www.olivegarden.com.

ITEM DESCRIPTION	Serving Size	Calories	Total Fat (g)	Saturated Fat (g)	Sodium (mg)	Carbohydrates (g)	Fiber (g)	Protein (g)

P.F. CHANG'S CHINA BISTRO

DESSERTS

ITEM DESCRIPTION	Serving Size	Calories	Total Fat (g)	Saturated Fat (g)	Sodium (mg)	Carbohydrates (g)	Fiber (g)	Protein (g)
Banana Spring Rolls	1 serv	235	10	4	128	34	1	4
Cheesecake, New York-Style	1	460	28	18	310	46	1	9
Flourless Chocolate Dome	1	235	4	2	85	55	3	5
Mini Apple Pie	1	150	4	1	85	29	0	1
Mini Carrot Cake	1	130	6	2	85	19	0	1
Mini Cheesecake	1	220	18	10	80	15	1	2
Mini Great Wall	1	100	4	1	115	18	0	1
Mini Lemon Dream	1	190	4	2	30	30	0	4
Mini Red Velvet Cake	1	130	7	2	85	18	0	1
Mini Tiramisu	1	100	11	5	50	10	0	2
Mini Triple Chocolate Mousse	1	300	22	14	50	25	1	3
The Great Wall of Chocolate™	1 serv	383	18	6	355	61	3	4

DRESSINGS AND SPREADS

ITEM DESCRIPTION	Serving Size	Calories	Total Fat (g)	Saturated Fat (g)	Sodium (mg)	Carbohydrates (g)	Fiber (g)	Protein (g)
Calamari Sauce	1 serv	50	2	0	610	7	0	1
Chili Honey Sauce	1 serv	130	0	0	350	31	0	0
Citrus Dressing	1 serv	200	20	3	140	6	0	0
Green Beans Sauce	1 serv	310	32	5	520	2	0	0
Hoisin Sauce	1 serv	210	12	0	1150	23	0	2
Honey Sauce	1 serv	140	0	0	360	33	0	0
Plum Sauce, Spicy	1 serv	200	0	0	1460	50	0	0
Potsticker Sauce	1 serv	50	2	0	610	7	0	1
Shrimp Dumpling Sauce	1 serv	15	0	0	1250	2	0	2
Sweet & Sour Sauce	1 serv	80	0	0	210	21	0	0
Sweet & Sour Sauce, Mustard	1 serv	90	2	0	140	17	1	1

GLUTEN FREE

ITEM DESCRIPTION	Serving Size	Calories	Total Fat (g)	Saturated Fat (g)	Sodium (mg)	Carbohydrates (g)	Fiber (g)	Protein (g)
Beef a la Sichuan	1	293	11	3	910	26	1	23
Beef & Broccoli	1 bowl	420	13	3	1435	52	5	24
Beef & Broccoli	1	290	12	3	1300	21	2	24
Beef, Hong Kong w/ Snow Peas	1	335	14	3	1480	28	3	25
Beef, Mongolian	1	337	15	4	1123	21	1	30
Buddha's Feast, Steamed	1 bowl	210	2	0	80	39	5	10

ITEM DESCRIPTION	Serving Size	Calories	Total Fat (g)	Saturated Fat (g)	Sodium (mg)	Carbohydrates (g)	Fiber (g)	Protein (g)
Buddha's Feast, Steamed	1	55	0	0	40	11	4	4
Chicken, Chang's Spicy	1	323	13	2	550	23	0	28
Chicken, Dali	1	280	12	2	370	16	1	27
Chicken, Ginger w/ Broccoli	1	270	11	2	990	17	2	28
Chicken, Philip's Better Lemon	1	350	13	2	207	31	1	29
Cucumbers, Shanghai	sm	40	2	0	743	3	1	2
Fried Rice Combo	1	353	13	3	900	40	1	19
Fried Rice w/ Beef	1	293	9	2	640	41	1	13
Fried Rice w/ Chicken	1	293	9	2	585	39	1	14
Fried Rice w/ Pork	1	320	13	4	953	39	1	12
Fried Rice w/ Shrimp	1	260	7	0	675	38	1	10
Moo Goo Gai Pan	1 bowl	365	12	2	1035	41	3	24
Moo Goo Gai Pan	1	223	10	2	987	9	1	23
Noodles, Singapore Street	1	300	7	1	980	41	3	11
Salmon, Steamed w/ Ginger	1	220	3	1	1160	13	2	32
Scallops, Cantonese	1	245	14	2	1000	17	2	15
Scallops, Chang's Lemon	1	233	10	3	540	27	1	11
Shrimp w/ Lobster Sauce	1 bowl	315	11	2	1120	39	3	16
Shrimp w/ Lobster Sauce	1	255	14	2	1745	13	1	23
Shrimp, Cantonese	1	215	10	2	950	10	2	21
Snap Peas, Garlic	sm	63	2	0	107	7	2	2
Soup, Egg Drop	1 cup	60	3	0	640	8	0	1
Spinach, Stir-Fried w/ Garlic	sm	53	3	1	300	5	3	4
Steak, Pepper	1 bowl	400	13	3	1045	48	3	22
Steak, Pepper	1	300	13	3	1197	19	1	25
Wraps, Chang's Chicken Lettuce	1	158	7	1	670	15	2	9
HAPPY HOUR								
Bacon & Egg Siu Mai	1 serv	70	3	1	180	8	0	3
Edamame Dumplings	1 serv	45	1	0	105	7	0	2
Edamame w/ Kosher Salt	1 serv	130	4	0	680	11	5	10
Lemongrass Chicken Dumplings	1 serv	40	1	0	85	5	0	2
Pork Dumplings	1 serv	60	2	1	125	6	0	4
Pork & Leek Dumplings	1 serv	50	2	1	70	5	1	2
Pork & Rice Siu Mai	1 serv	50	5	0	125	9	0	2

ITEM DESCRIPTION	Serving Size	Calories	Total Fat (g)	Saturated Fat (g)	Sodium (mg)	Carbohydrates (g)	Fiber (g)	Protein (g)
Shanghai Street Dumplings	1 serv	140	5	1	250	19	1	6
Shrimp Dumplings	1 serv	45	0	0	170	6	0	4
Shrimp & Pork Dumplings	1 serv	40	1	0	125	5	1	3
Taco, Beef Asian Street	1 serv	170	7	2	350	18	1	7
Taco, Mahi-Mahi Asian Street	1 serv	230	9	2	390	26	2	8
Taco, Pork Asian Street	1 serv	140	5	1	450	19	1	5
Taco, Shrimp Asian Street	1 serv	180	10	2	350	14	1	7
Tuna Tataki Crisp	1 serv	60	3	0	140	3	0	5
Vegetable Dumplings	1 serv	45	0	0	80	8	0	2
Wontons, Flaming Red	1 serv	80	5	1	280	5	0	4
KIDS MENU								
Baby Buddha's Feast, Steamed	1	30	0	0	25	6	3	2
Baby Buddha's Feast, Stir-Fried	1	90	4	1	760	12	2	3
Chicken	1	165	10	2	120	10	0	9
Fried Rice w/ Chicken	1	290	9	2	755	37	1	15
Lo Mein	1	195	8	1	720	21	1	9
MAIN MENU								
Beef a la Sichuan	1	303	12	3	1084	25	1	22
Beef & Broccoli	1	290	12	3	1573	21	2	24
Beef & Broccoli w/ Brown Rice	1 bowl	420	13	3	1760	52	4	23
Beef & Broccoli w/ White Rice	1 bowl	440	12	3	1760	58	3	23
Beef, Cantonese Chow Fun	1	745	20	4	903	94	5	27
Beef, Hong Kong w/ Snow Peas	1	310	14	3	926	24	3	24
Beef, Mongolian	1	337	15	4	1340	20	1	29
Beef, Wok-Charred	1	317	17	5	1157	16	1	25
Buddha's Feast, Steamed	1	55	0	0	40	11	4	4
Buddha's Feast, Steamed w/ Brown Rice	1 bowl	210	2	0	80	39	5	10
Buddha's Feast, Steamed w/ White Rice	1 bowl	235	1	0	575	45	3	10
Buddha's Feast, Stir-Fried	1	220	6	1	1620	29	5	14
Buddha's Feast, Stir-Fried w/ Brown Rice	1 bowl	290	6	1	1050	48	5	11
Buddha's Feast, Stir-Fried w/ White Rice	1 bowl	310	5	1	1050	54	3	11
Chicken w/ Black Bean Sauce	1	300	16	2	1850	14	0	29

ITEM DESCRIPTION	Serving Size	Calories	Total Fat (g)	Saturated Fat (g)	Sodium (mg)	Carbohydrates (g)	Fiber (g)	Protein (g)
Chicken & Mushrooms, Canton	1	550	23	4	1410	48	3	38
Chicken, Almond & Cashew	1	373	18	3	1960	24	2	29
Chicken, Almond & Cashew w/ Brown Rice	1 bowl	535	22	4	2085	59	5	25
Chicken, Almond & Cashew w/ White Rice	1 bowl	560	21	3	2085	66	3	25
Chicken, Cantonese Chow Fun	1	790	20	4	1615	88	5	32
Chicken, Chang's Spicy	1	323	13	2	550	23	0	28
Chicken, Crispy Honey	1	477	23	4	510	49	0	16
Chicken, Crispy Honey w/ Brown Rice	1 bowl	655	24	4	710	92	3	15
Chicken, Crispy Honey w/ White Rice	1 bowl	680	23	4	705	99	1	15
Chicken, Dali	1	283	13	2	707	15	1	27
Chicken, Ginger w/ Broccoli	1	273	11	2	1457	18	2	28
Chicken, Ground w/ Eggplant	1	288	20	3	1233	17	2	8
Chicken, Mandarin	1	360	15	2	1715	29	3	33
Chicken, Philip's Better Lemon	1	343	14	2	187	30	1	26
Chicken, Sesame	1	343	14	2	1020	25	2	30
Chicken, Sesame w/ Brown Rice	1 bowl	510	16	3	1320	69	5	24
Chicken, Sesame w/ White Rice	1 bowl	535	15	2	1320	76	3	24
Chicken, Sweet & Sour	1	370	19	3	367	38	0	12
Duck, VIP	1	650	29	8	1880	55	1	52
Eggplant, Stir-Fried	1	270	22	3	760	14	2	2
Fish, Hot	1	340	22	3	1043	21	1	16
Fried Rice Combo	1	363	13	3	1063	41	1	19
Fried Rice w/ Beef	1	303	9	2	803	41	1	13
Fried Rice w/ Chicken	1	303	9	2	748	39	1	15
Fried Rice w/ Pork	1	320	13	4	1115	39	1	12
Fried Rice w/ Shrimp	1	273	8	1	838	39	1	11
Fried Rice, Vegetarian	1	190	2	0	230	38	2	5
Kung Pao Chicken	1	383	23	4	940	14	2	33
Kung Pao Scallops	1	307	20	3	1126	17	2	16
Kung Pao Shrimp	1	280	17	3	1083	12	2	21
Lamb, Chengdu Spiced	1	237	12	3	740	11	1	23
Lamb, Wok-Seared	1	283	16	3	1410	9	1	25

ITEM DESCRIPTION	Serving Size	Calories	Total Fat (g)	Saturated Fat (g)	Sodium (mg)	Carbohydrates (g)	Fiber (g)	Protein (g)
Lo Mein Combo	1	347	14	0	1413	23	2	23
Lo Mein w/ Beef	1	270	9	2	1070	33	2	15
Lo Mein w/ Chicken	1	267	9	2	997	30	2	17
Lo Mein w/ Pork	1	290	13	4	1483	30	2	13
Lo Mein w/ Shrimp	1	227	6	1	1113	30	2	12
Mahi-Mahi	1	420	17	8	605	42	2	25
Moo Goo Gai Pan	1	247	13	2	823	13	1	18
Moo Goo Gai Pan w/ Brown Rice	1 bowl	380	13	2	1000	43	3	21
Moo Goo Gai Pan w/ White Rice	1 bowl	390	11	2	1035	47	1	24
Mu Shu Chicken	1	285	13	3	1540	16	3	26
Mu Shu Pancake	1 pc	90	2	0	30	14	0	2
Mu Shu Pork	1	320	19	7	2275	16	3	21
Noodles, Dan Dan	1	270	7	1	1388	30	2	13
Noodles, Double Pan-Fried Combo	1	455	21	2	1923	44	1	16
Noodles, Double Pan-Fried w/ Beef	1	395	17	1	1665	44	2	15
Noodles, Double Pan-Fried w/ Chicken	1	393	17	1	1608	43	2	16
Noodles, Double Pan-Fried w/ Pork	1	413	21	3	1975	42	2	13
Noodles, Double Pan-Fried w/ Shrimp	1	363	16	0	1698	42	2	12
Noodles, Garlic	1	178	4	1	360	31	1	5
Noodles, Singapore Street	1	300	6	1	1157	42	3	11
Orange Peel Beef	1	283	13	3	833	21	1	12
Orange Peel Chicken	1	333	15	3	770	20	1	29
Orange Peel Shrimp	1	187	14	1	937	14	1	15
Pork, Hunan	1	395	19	1	1850	38	2	16
Pork, Sweet & Sour	1	460	14	7	950	72	2	14
Prawns, Lemongrass w/ Garlic Noodles	1	485	30	10	935	32	2	24
Prawns, Salt & Pepper	1	197	11	2	1070	8	2	21
Salmon, Asian Grilled	1	345	6	2	715	38	1	32
Salmon, Asian Grilled w/ Brown Rice	1 bowl	320	6	1	575	44	3	22
Salmon, Asian Grilled w/ White Rice	1 bowl	345	5	1	570	50	1	22
Salmon, Steamed w/ Ginger	1	330	19	3	605	12	3	31
Scallops, Cantonese	1	245	14	2	1000	17	2	15
Scallops, Chang's Lemon	1	243	10	2	540	28	1	11
Sea Bass*, Oolong Marinated	1	315	19	5	1550	15	2	24

ITEM DESCRIPTION	Serving Size	Calories	Total Fat (g)	Saturated Fat (g)	Sodium (mg)	Carbohydrates (g)	Fiber (g)	Protein (g)
Shrimp w/ Candied Walnuts	1	377	24	4	654	25	1	16
Shrimp w/ Lobster Sauce	1	250	14	2	1745	11	1	23
Shrimp, Cantonese	1	215	10	2	950	10	2	21
Shrimp, Crispy Honey	1	460	22	4	805	55	1	10
Shrimp, Lemon Pepper	1	235	10	2	1080	19	3	21
Shrimp, Lobster Sauce w/ Brown Rice	1 bowl	315	11	2	1120	39	3	16
Shrimp, Lobster Sauce w/ White Rice	1 bowl	340	10	2	1120	45	1	16
Shrimp, Shanghai w/ Garlic Sauce	1	195	20	2	1050	10	3	17
Sichuan from the Sea Combo	1	215	12	2	553	14	0	12
Sichuan from the Sea, Calamari	1	348	21	4	538	28	1	12
Sichuan from the Sea, Scallops	1	295	15	3	1230	26	1	16
Sichuan from the Sea, Shrimp	1	173	7	1	747	10	0	16
Steak, Asian Marinated New York Strip	1	370	20	9	933	17	0	33
Steak, Pepper	1	297	13	3	1300	19	1	24
Steak, Pepper w/ Brown Rice	1 bowl	395	13	3	1225	47	3	22
Steak, Pepper w/ White Rice	1 bowl	415	12	3	1225	54	2	22
Tofu, Ma Po	1	350	23	5	1060	17	2	20
Vegetable Chow Fun	1	250	2	0	750	46	3	2
Vegetables, Coconut Curry	1	510	36	12	650	26	5	22
SALADS								
Chicken Chopped Salad w/ Ginger Dressing	1	365	24	4	640	13	2	23
Shrimp Salad, Asian	1	225	13	2	635	16	3	14
SIDES AND SNACKS								
Ahi Tuna*, Seared	1 serv	160	11	2	860	7	1	10
Asian Slaw	sm	237	22	3	360	7	2	2
Asparagus, Sichuan-Style	sm	100	6	1	730	10	2	3
Calamari, Salt & Pepper	1 serv	160	10	2	208	11	0	6
Crab Wontons	6 pcs	163	10	4	303	13	0	5
Cucumbers, Shanghai	sm	40	2	0	743	3	1	2
Egg Rolls	1	174	8	1	673	22	3	5
Green Beans, Crispy	1 serv	260	18	3	140	21	2	2
Green Beans, Spicy	sm	110	6	1	720	13	4	3
Mushrooms, Wok-Seared	sm	115	9	4	645	6	0	4

ITEM DESCRIPTION	Serving Size	Calories	Total Fat (g)	Saturated Fat (g)	Sodium (mg)	Carbohydrates (g)	Fiber (g)	Protein (g)
Noodles, Green Tea	sm	284	12	2	163	37	2	6
Pork Dumplings, Pan-Fried	1	70	4	1	125	6	0	4
Pork Dumplings, Steamed	1	60	2	1	125	6	0	4
Rice, Brown Steamed	1	190	2	0	0	40	3	4
Rice, White Steamed	1	220	0	0	0	49	1	4
Shrimp Dumplings, Pan-Fried	1	60	2	0	170	6	0	4
Shrimp Dumplings, Steamed	1	45	0	0	170	6	0	4
Shrimp, Dynamite	1 serv	290	12	2	285	6	0	5
Sichuan Flatbread, Chicken	1 serv	195	10	5	523	12	1	15
Snap Peas, Garlic	sm	64	2	0	107	7	2	2
Spare Ribs, Chang's	1 serv	344	24	7	336	7	1	26
Spare Ribs, Northern Style	1 serv	343	19	2	985	11	0	31
Spinach, Stir-Fried w/ Garlic	sm	53	3	1	300	5	3	4
Spring Rolls	2	156	8	1	271	17	2	4
Vegetable Dumplings, Pan-Fried	1	60	2	0	80	8	0	2
Vegetable Dumplings, Steamed	1	45	0	0	80	8	0	2
Wontons, Crispy	1 serv	45	3	0	60	4	0	2
Wraps, Chang's Chicken Lettuce	1 serv	160	7	1	650	17	2	8
Wraps, Chang's Vegetarian Lettuce	1 serv	140	7	1	530	11	2	6
SOUPS								
Chicken Noodle, Chang's	1 bowl	120	4	1	510	15	1	6
Egg Drop	1 cup	60	3	0	640	8	0	1
Hot & Sour	1 cup	80	3	1	1000	9	0	5
Wonton	1 cup	92	3	1	482	9	0	7

The Dietary Guidelines for Americans recommend limiting saturated fat to 20 grams and sodium to 2,300 milligrams for a typical adult eating 2,000 calories daily. Recommended limits may be higher or lower depending upon daily calorie consumption.

    All entrees served with a choice of steamed brown or white rice.

    * These items are cooked to order and may be served raw or undercooked. Consuming raw or undercooked meats, poultry, seafood, shellfish, or eggs may increase your risk of foodborne illness. Signature drinks or liqueurs with added ingredients may increase caloric content.

PANDA EXPRESS

DESSERTS

Fortune Cookie	1	32	0	0	8	7	0	1

DRESSINGS AND SPREADS

Mandarin Sauce	1 serv	160	0	0	340	40	0	0
Sweet & Sour Sauce	1 serv	80	0	0	160	20	0	0

ITEM DESCRIPTION

MAIN MENU

Item Description	Serving Size	Calories	Total Fat (g)	Saturated Fat (g)	Sodium (mg)	Carbohydrates (g)	Fiber (g)	Protein (g)
Beef, Beijing	1 serv	690	41	8	930	56	4	26
Beef & Broccoli	1 serv	130	4	1	740	13	3	10
Beef, Kobari	1 serv	210	7	1.5	840	20	2	15
Chicken, Black Pepper	1 serv	250	14	3	980	12	2	19
Chicken, Kung Pao	1 serv	300	19	3.5	880	13	2	19
Chicken, Mandarin	1 serv	310	16	4	740	8	0	34
Chicken, Mushroom	1 serv	220	13	3	780	9	2	17
Chicken, Orange	1 serv	400	20	3.5	640	42	0	15
Chicken, Potato	1 serv	220	11	2	810	19	3	11
Chicken Breast, String Bean	1 serv	170	7	1.5	760	13	2	15
Chicken Breast, Sweet Fire	1 serv	440	18	3.5	370	53	1	17
Chicken Breast, Sweet & Sour	1 serv	390	17	3	350	45	1	15
Chicken Potsticker	3 pcs	220	11	2.5	280	23	1	7
Chow Mein	1 serv	400	12	2	1060	61	8	12
Cream Cheese Rangoon	3 pcs	190	8	5	180	24	2	5
Egg Roll, Chicken	1	200	12	4	390	16	2	8
Eggplant & Tofu	1 serv	310	24	3	680	19	3	7
Pork, BBQ	1 serv	360	19	8	1310	13	1	34
Pork, Sweet & Sour	1 serv	450	26	5	400	40	3	14
Rice, Fried	1 serv	570	18	4	900	85	8	16
Rice, Steamed	1 serv	420	0	0	0	93	0	8
Shrimp, Crispy	6 pcs	260	13	2.5	810	26	1	9
Shrimp, Golden Treasure	1 serv	390	19	3	500	39	2	16
Shrimp, Honey Walnut	1 serv	370	23	4	470	27	2	14
Soup, Hot & Sour	1 serv	90	3.5	0.5	970	12	1	4
Veggie Spring Roll	2	160	7	1	540	22	4	4
Veggies, Mixed	reg	35	0	0	260	7	3	2
Veggies, Mixed	side	70	0.5	0	530	13	5	4

Entrées may vary by location.

The Dietary Guidelines for Americans recommend limiting saturated fat to 20 grams and sodium to 2,300 milligrams for a typical adult eating 2,000 calories daily. Recommended limits may be higher or lower depending upon daily calorie consumption. These values are based on standard product formulation. Minor acceptable variations can be expected due to sampling differences, product assembly, seasonal influences, and regional suppliers. Promotional entrées have not been included.

* Not applicable in Hawaii where Trans Fat (g) equals 1. Please contact Panda Guest Relations at (800) 877-8988 for more information.

PANERA BREAD

BAKED ITEMS

ITEM DESCRIPTION	Serving Size	Calories	Total Fat (g)	Saturated Fat (g)	Sodium (mg)	Carbohydrates (g)	Fiber (g)	Protein (g)
Bagel, Asiago Cheese	1	330	6	3.5	580	55	2	13
Bagel, Blueberry	1	330	1.5	0	490	68	2	10
Bagel, Chocolate Chip	1	370	6	4	480	69	2	10
Bagel, Cinnamon Crunch	1	430	8	5	430	80	2	9
Bagel, Cinnamon Swirl & Raisin	1	320	2.5	1	470	64	3	9
Bagel, Everything	1	300	2.5	0	640	59	2	10
Bagel, French Toast	1	350	5	2.5	620	67	2	9
Bagel, Jalapeño & Cheddar	1	310	3	1.5	740	56	2	12
Bagel, Plain	1	290	1.5	0	460	59	2	10
Bagel, Sesame	1	310	3	0	460	59	2	10
Bagel, Sweet Onion & Poppyseed	1	390	7	1	520	72	4	13
Bagel, Whole Grain	1	340	2.5	0	400	67	6	13
Baguette, French	2 oz	150	1	0	370	30	1	5
Baguette, Whole Grain	2 oz	140	1	0	310	29	3	6
Ciabatta	1	460	6	1	760	84	3	16
Demi, Asiago Cheese	2 oz	160	4	2.5	320	22	1	7
Demi, Three Cheese	2 oz	160	2	1	320	29	1	6
Demi, Three Seed	2 oz	160	3.5	0	300	27	2	6
Focaccia	2 oz	180	4.5	0.5	320	28	1	5
Focaccia w/ Asiago Cheese	2 oz	160	5	1.5	230	23	1	5
Loaf, Asiago Cheese	2 oz	160	4	2.5	320	23	1	7
Loaf, Cinnamon Raisin	2 oz	180	3	1.5	135	34	1	5
Loaf, Country	2 oz	140	0.5	0	310	27	1	5
Loaf, Honey Wheat	2 oz	170	3	1.5	240	30	2	5
Loaf, Sesame Semolina	2 oz	140	0.5	0	350	29	1	4
Loaf, Sourdough Round	2 oz	140	0.5	0	290	28	1	5
Loaf, Stone-Milled Rye	2 oz	140	0.5	0	380	28	2	5
Loaf, Three Cheese	2 oz	140	2	1	290	26	1	6
Loaf, Tomato Basil	2 oz	140	0.5	0	330	27	1	5
Loaf, White Whole Grain	2 oz	140	2.5	1	310	26	2	5
Loaf, Whole Grain	2 oz	130	1	0	290	27	3	6

ITEM DESCRIPTION	Serving Size	Calories	Total Fat (g)	Saturated Fat (g)	Sodium (mg)	Carbohydrates (g)	Fiber (g)	Protein (g)
Miche, Country	2 oz	140	0.5	0	330	28	1	5
Miche, French	2 oz	140	0.5	0	360	28	1	5
Miche, Sesame Semolina	2 oz	140	1	0	360	30	1	5
Miche, Stone-Milled Rye	2 oz	140	0.5	0	420	27	2	5
Miche, Three Cheese	2 oz	150	2	1	320	27	1	6
Miche, Whole Grain	2 oz	130	1	0	250	26	3	6
Roll, Sourdough	1	200	1	0	400	39	1	7
Soup Bowl, Sourdough	1	590	2.5	0	1210	118	4	21
BEVERAGES								
Apple Juice, Organic	1	120	0	0	25	29	0	0
Caffe Latte	1	120	4.5	3	95	11	0	8
Caffe Mocha	1	380	16	11	160	50	2	11
Cappuccino	1	120	4.5	3	95	11	0	8
Frozen Drink, Caramel	16 oz	600	22	15	190	97	0	5
Frozen Drink, Mango	16 oz	330	10	7	20	61	2	2
Frozen Drink, Mocha	16 oz	570	20	14	140	94	2	6
Hot Chocolate	1	380	16	11	160	50	2	11
Iced Green Tea	16 oz	90	0	0	10	23	0	0
Iced Latte, Chai Tea	1	160	3.5	2	75	26	0	6
Latte, Caramel	1	420	18	12	210	53	0	10
Latte, Chai Tea	1	200	4.5	2.5	85	32	0	7
Lemonade	16 oz	100	0	0	10	25	0	0
Milk, Organic	1	120	4.5	3	115	12	0	8
Milk, Organic Chocolate	1	170	5	3	150	25	0	7
Orange Juice	sm	110	0	0	0	26	1	2
Smoothie, Black Cherry, Low-Fat	16 oz	290	1.5	1	90	63	2	6
Smoothie, Mango, Low-Fat	16 oz	230	1.5	1	90	51	2	6
Smoothie, Strawberry, Low-Fat w/ Ginseng	16 oz	260	1.5	1	90	59	2	6
Smoothie, Wild Berry, Low Fat	16 oz	290	1.5	1	90	67	1	6
BREAKFAST ITEMS								
Bagel, Asiago Cheese w/ Bacon	1	610	28	13	1350	55	2	34
Bagel, Asiago Cheese w/ Egg & Cheese	1	480	18	10	890	54	2	24
Bagel, Asiago Cheese w/ Sausage	1	640	32	15	1220	56	2	32
Bagel, French Toast w/ Sausage	1	670	31	14	1280	69	2	28

ITEM DESCRIPTION	Serving Size	Calories	Total Fat (g)	Saturated Fat (g)	Sodium (mg)	Carbohydrates (g)	Fiber (g)	Protein (g)
Bagel, Jalapeño & Cheddar w/ Bacon	1	590	25	11	1530	58	3	33
Bagel, Jalapeño & Cheddar w/ Egg & Cheese	1	470	16	8	1070	57	3	23
Bagel, Jalapeño & Cheddar w/ Sausage	1	630	29	12	1400	59	3	32
Bagel, Jalapeño & Cheddar w/ Smoked Ham	1	500	16	8	1280	58	3	28
Bagel, Sweet Onion & Poppyseed w/ Steak	1	660	27	10	970	74	5	34
Ciabatta w/ Bacon, Egg & Cheese	1	510	24	10	1160	44	2	29
Ciabatta w/ Egg & Cheese	1	390	15	7	710	43	2	19
Ciabatta w/ Sausage, Egg & Cheese	1	550	29	12	1040	44	2	27
Egg Soufflé, Four Cheese	1	480	29	16	700	36	2	16
Egg Soufflé, Ham & Swiss	1	490	30	16	740	35	2	20
Egg Soufflé, Spinach & Artichoke	1	540	34	19	910	38	2	19
Egg Soufflé, Spinach & Bacon	1	570	37	20	940	35	2	23
Granola Parfait, Strawberry	1	310	11	4	100	44	3	9
Power Sandwich	1	340	14	7	820	31	4	23
DESSERTS								
Bear Claw	1	550	28	12	360	67	3	10
Brownie, Double Fudge w/ Icing	1	480	17	9	290	76	2	5
Cake, Cinnamon Coffee Crumb	1 serv	470	25	9	310	54	1	6
Cinnamon Roll	1	620	24	14	480	89	3	13
Cobblestone	1	650	13	5	410	122	3	12
Cookie, Candy	1	420	19	10	280	59	1	4
Cookie, Chocolate Chipper	1	440	23	14	250	59	2	5
Cookie, Easter Egg	1	480	22	13	160	67	1	4
Cookie, Oatmeal Raisin	1	370	14	8	310	57	2	5
Cookie, Petite Chocolate Chipper	1	110	6	3.5	60	15	1	1
Cookie, Petite Spring	1	230	12	7	90	27	0	2
Cookie, Shortbread	1	350	21	12	160	36	1	3
Cookie, Toffee Nut	1	460	19	13	330	59	1	5
Croissant, French	1	310	18	11	260	30	1	7
Hot Cross Buns	1	220	5	3	280	38	1	5
Muffie, Chocolate Chip	1	320	14	4	200	46	2	4
Muffie, Cornbread	1	230	9	1.5	250	33	1	3
Muffie, Pumpkin	1	290	11	2	240	45	1	3

ITEM DESCRIPTION	Serving Size	Calories	Total Fat (g)	Saturated Fat (g)	Sodium (mg)	Carbohydrates (g)	Fiber (g)	Protein (g)
Muffin, Apple Crunch	1	450	12	3	340	80	2	7
Muffin, Carrot Walnut	1	500	21	4.5	580	72	3	8
Muffin, Pumpkin	1	580	22	4	470	89	2	7
Muffin, Wild Blueberry	1	440	17	3	330	66	2	6
Pastry Ring, Apple Cherry Cheese	1 pc	230	11	6	160	30	1	3
Pastry, Cheese	1	400	22	14	340	42	1	8
Pastry, Cherry	1	500	18	11	320	77	2	7
Pastry, Chocolate	1	410	24	14	260	46	2	8
Pastry, Fresh Apple	1	380	17	13	320	44	1	7
Pastry, Pecan Braid	1	470	26	12	270	52	2	8
Pecan Roll	1	730	39	12	310	87	5	11
Scone, Cinnamon Chip	1	600	31	19	370	73	2	9
Scone, Mini Orange	1	160	4	2.5	150	29	1	1
Scone, Mini Strawberries & Cream	1	140	6	4	260	19	0	2
Scone, Mini Wild Blueberry	1	160	6	4	290	21	1	2
Scone, Orange	1	470	11	7	460	87	3	4
Scone, Strawberries & Cream	1	420	19	12	770	57	1	6
Scone, Wild Blueberry	1	440	18	12	880	63	2	7
DRESSINGS AND SPREADS								
Asian Sesame Vinaigrette, Reduced-Sugar	half	45	4	0.5	190	3	0	0
Balsamic Vinaigrette, Reduced Fat	half	60	5	1	120	4	0	0
BBQ Ranch Dressing	half	70	6	1	180	4	0	0
Blue Cheese Vinaigrette	half	90	9	1.5	130	2	0	1
Caesar Dressing	half	80	8	1.5	95	1	0	0
Cream Cheese, Chive & Onion	2 oz	130	11	7	370	4	1	5
Cream Cheese, Plain	2 oz	180	18	11	210	2	0	3
Cream Cheese, Reduced Fat Hazelnut	2 oz	140	11	6	210	6	1	5
Cream Cheese, Reduced Fat Honey Walnut	2 oz	150	11	6	200	8	1	5
Cream Cheese, Reduced Fat Plain	2 oz	130	12	7	230	2	1	5
Cream Cheese, Reduced Fat Raspberry	2 oz	130	10	6	200	7	1	4
Cream Cheese, Reduced Fat Veggie	2 oz	120	10	6	210	3	1	5
Greek Dressing/Herb Vinaigrette	half	110	12	2	190	1	0	0
Light Buttermilk Ranch	half	40	2	0	170	4	0	0
Thai Chili Vinaigrette, Low Fat	half	30	1	0	220	5	0	0

ITEM DESCRIPTION	Serving Size	Calories	Total Fat (g)	Saturated Fat (g)	Sodium (mg)	Carbohydrates (g)	Fiber (g)	Protein (g)
White Balsamic Apple Vinaigrette	half	80	6	1	160	6	0	0
KIDS MENU								
Macaroni & Cheese	1	490	30	13	1020	37	1	17
Sandwich, Grilled Cheese	1	360	13	10	1020	46	4	17
Sandwich, Peanut Butter & Jelly	1	410	18	3.5	550	56	4	12
Sandwich, Roast Beef	1	320	10	6	820	35	3	23
Sandwich, Smoked Ham	1	300	9	6	1060	35	3	21
Sandwich, Smoked Turkey	1	290	8	5	1100	35	3	21
Yogurt, Organic (Blueberry or Strawberry)	1	60	.5	0	40	11	0	2
SALADS								
Caesar	half	200	14	4	310	13	1	6
Chicken Caesar	half	260	15	4.5	410	14	1	18
Chicken Cobb, Chopped	half	250	18	4.5	560	6	1	19
Chicken, Asian Sesame	half	200	10	2	410	16	2	15
Chicken, BBQ Chopped	half	250	11	1.5	380	25	3	16
Chicken, Thai Chopped	half	200	7	1	670	18	2	17
Classic Cafe	half	80	5	1	135	9	2	1
Fruit Cup	sm	60	0	0	15	17	1	1
Fuji Apple w/ Chicken	half	260	16	3.5	410	18	3	16
Greek	half	190	17	4	840	7	2	4
Steak, Chopped w/ Blue Cheese	half	430	32	10	800	18	2	18
SANDWICHES								
Bacon Turkey Bravo® on Tomato Basil	half	400	14	5	1400	42	2	26
Chicken Caesar on Three Cheese	half	360	16	5	640	35	2	22
Chicken Salad on Sesame Semolina	half	340	13	2	600	45	2	15
Chicken, Chipotle on Artisan French	half	420	19	6	1090	36	2	27
Ham & Swiss, Smoked on Stone-Milled Rye	half	290	8	4	930	32	2	22
Italian Combo on Ciabatta	half	490	21	8	1310	47	2	29
Panini, Cuban Chicken	half	430	18	5	880	43	2	23
Panini, Frontega Chicken® on Focaccia	half	430	19	4.5	960	39	2	24
Panini, Smokehouse Turkey® on Three Cheese	half	340	13	6	1170	32	2	26
Panini, Tomato & Mozzarella on Ciabatta	half	380	15	5	650	48	3	15
Panini, Turkey Artichoke on Focaccia	half	370	13	4	1100	43	2	21

ITEM DESCRIPTION	Serving Size	Calories	Total Fat (g)	Saturated Fat (g)	Sodium (mg)	Carbohydrates (g)	Fiber (g)	Protein (g)
Roast Beef, Asiago on Asiago Cheese	half	350	14	7	660	32	2	24
Steak & White Cheddar on French Baguette	half	480	18	7	900	56	2	21
Tuna Salad on Honey Wheat	half	240	8	2	490	32	3	10
Turkey Breast, Smoked on Country	half	210	1.5	0	820	33	2	16
Turkey, Sierra on Focaccia w/ Asiago Cheese	half	460	25	6	950	39	2	20
Veggie, Mediterranean on Tomato Basil	half	300	7	1.5	710	49	5	11
SIDES AND SNACKS								
Apple	1	80	0	0	0	21	4	0
Baguette, French	1	180	1	0	440	36	1	6
Baguette, Whole Grain	1	180	1.5	0	400	36	4	7
Potato Chips	1 bag	160	8	1	130	19	2	2
Potato Chips, Baked	1 bag	130	2	0	200	26	2	2
SOUPS								
Baked Potato, You Pick Two®	sm	250	15	9	850	24	2	7
Broccoli Cheddar, You Pick Two®	sm	190	10	6	1020	16	5	8
Chicken Noodle, Low-Fat, You Pick Two®	sm	100	2	1	990	16	0	4
Chili	sm	260	12	4.5	740	20	4	18
Chili w/ Cornbread	sm	390	18	5	890	39	4	19
Cream of Chicken & Wild Rice, You Pick Two®	sm	220	12	6	1030	20	2	7
French Onion, You Pick Two®	sm	210	9	4.5	1680	24	2	9
Macaroni & Cheese	sm	490	30	13	1020	37	1	17
New England Clam Chowder, You Pick Two®	sm	300	23	13	790	19	2	5
Tomato, You Pick Two®	sm	300	18	10	570	29	4	6
Vegetable w/ Pesto, Low-Fat, You Pick Two®	sm	110	2	0	830	19	4	4
Vegetarian Black Bean, Low-Fat, You Pick Two®	sm	110	2.5	1	980	18	3	6

Based on federal rounding and other applicable regulations. Nutritional information is calculated based on Panera's standardized recipes. Because our menu items are handcrafted and may be customized, variations in serving sizes, preparation techniques, ingredient substitutions, product testing, and sources of supply, as well as regional and seasonal differences may affect the nutrition values for each product. In addition, testing of new recipes of existing products may be conducted from time to time in certain markets. These new recipes may contain different/ additional ingredients, including allergens, as compared to the original version. Some bakery-cafes may serve menu items which are not listed on this Site. Panera cannot guarantee that the nutritional information provided on this Site or available in any bakery-cafe is completely accurate as it relates to the prepared menu items in every bakery-cafe. For the most up-to-date information, please call or visit your nearest bakery-cafe to speak with a manager.

PIZZA HUT

ITEM DESCRIPTION	Serving Size	Calories	Total Fat (g)	Saturated Fat (g)	Sodium (mg)	Carbohydrates (g)	Fiber (g)	Protein (g)
BEVERAGES								
Diet Pepsi®	16 oz	0	0	0	50	0	0	0
Mountain Dew®	16 oz	220	0	0	70	58	0	0
Pepsi®	16 oz	200	0	0	50	56	0	0
Sierra Mist®	16 oz	200	0	0	40	54	0	0
DESSERTS								
Cinnamon Sticks	2 pcs	170	6	1.5	200	26	1	4
Hershey's® Chocolate Dunkers™	2 pcs	200	9	4	210	26	1	5
Hershey's® Chocolate Sauce	1 pkg	120	2.5	1	75	24	1	1
Pie, Apple	2 pcs	330	160	17	190	40	2	2
White Icing	1 pkg	170	0	0	5	44	0	0
MAIN MENU								
Fit 'n Delicious Pizza w/ Chicken, Mushrooms & Jalapeño	1 pc /8	170	4.5	1.5	720	22	1	11
Fit 'n Delicious Pizza w/ Chicken, Red Onion & Green Pepper	1 pc /8	180	4.5	2	510	23	1	11
Fit 'n Delicious Pizza w/ Diced Red Tomato, Mushroom & Jalapeño	1 pc /8	150	4	1.5	610	23	2	6
Fit 'n Delicious Pizza w/ Green Pepper, Red Onion & Diced Red Tomato	1 pc /8	150	4	1.5	400	24	2	6
Fit 'n Delicious Pizza w/ Ham, Pineapple & Diced Red Tomato	1 pc /8	160	4.5	1.5	550	24	1	7
Fit 'n Delicious Pizza w/ Ham, Red Onion & Mushroom	1 pc /8	160	4.5	1.5	550	23	1	8
Hand-Tossed Pizza w/ Cheese, Medium	1 pc /8	220	8	4.5	560	26	1	10
Hand-Tossed Pizza w/ Ham & Pineapple, Medium	1 pc /8	200	7	3.5	560	27	1	9
Hand-Tossed Pizza w/ Italian Sausage & Red Onion, Medium	1 pc /8	240	11	4.5	590	27	2	10
Hand-Tossed Pizza w/ Pepperoni & Mushroom, Medium	1 pc /8	210	8	4	550	26	2	10
Hand-Tossed Pizza w/ Pepperoni, Medium	1 pc /8	230	10	4.5	620	25	1	10
Hand-Tossed Pizza, Dan's Original	1 pc /8	260	12	5	670	26	2	12

ITEM DESCRIPTION	Serving Size	Calories	Total Fat (g)	Saturated Fat (g)	Sodium (mg)	Carbohydrates (g)	Fiber (g)	Protein (g)
Hand-Tossed Pizza, Hawaiian Luau	1 pc /8	240	10	4.5	650	27	1	10
Hand-Tossed Pizza, Meat Lover's®, Medium	1 pc /8	300	16	7	870	25	1	14
Hand-Tossed Pizza, Spicy Sicilian	1 pc /8	250	11	5	740	26	2	10
Hand-Tossed Pizza, Supreme, Medium	1 pc /8	260	12	5	690	26	2	11
Hand-Tossed Pizza, Triple Meat Italiano	1 pc /8	260	12	5	740	25	1	12
Hand-Tossed Pizza, Veggie Lover's®, Medium	1 pc /8	200	7	3.5	540	27	2	9
Pan Pizza w/ Cheese, Medium	1 pc /8	240	11	4.5	530	27	1	11
Pan Pizza w/ Ham & Pineapple, Medium	1 pc /8	230	9	3.5	520	28	1	10
Pan Pizza w/ Italian Sausage & Red Onion, Medium	1 pc /8	270	13	4.5	560	28	1	11
Pan Pizza w/ Pepperoni & Mushroom, Medium	1 pc /8	240	10	4	520	27	1	10
Pan Pizza w/ Pepperoni, Medium	1 pc /8	250	12	4.5	590	26	1	11
Pan Pizza, Dan's Original, Medium	1 pc /8	280	14	5	630	27	1	12
Pan Pizza, Hawaiian Luau, Medium	1 pc /8	260	12	4.5	610	28	1	11
Pan Pizza, Meat Lover's®, Medium	1 pc /8	330	18	7	830	27	1	14
Pan Pizza, Spicy Sicilian, Medium	1 pc /8	270	13	5	700	27	2	11
Pan Pizza, Supreme, Medium	1 pc /8	290	14	5	650	27	2	12
Pan Pizza, Triple Meat Italiano, Medium	1 pc /8	290	15	5	700	27	1	13
Pan Pizza, Veggie Lover's®, Medium	1 pc /8	230	9	3.5	500	28	2	9
Pasta, Bacon Mac N Cheese	1	520	22	12	1170	54	4	24
Pasta, Chicken Alfredo	1	630	33	11	1180	56	4	27
Pasta, Lasagna	1	600	33	14	1600	43	5	31
Pasta, Meaty Marinara	1	520	24	10	1310	50	6	26
Personal Pan Pizza w/ Cheese	1	590	24	10	1290	69	3	26
Personal Pan Pizza w/ Ham & Pineapple	1	550	20	8	1260	71	3	23
Personal Pan Pizza w/ Italian Sausage & Red Onion	1	690	32	12	1440	71	4	28
Personal Pan Pizza w/ Pepperoni	1	610	26	10	1410	67	3	26
Personal Pan Pizza w/ Pepperoni & Mushroom	1	570	23	9	1250	68	4	24
Personal Pan Pizza, Dan's Original	1	720	36	13	1600	69	4	31
Personal Pan Pizza, Hawaiian Luau	1	620	25	10	1440	71	3	26

ITEM DESCRIPTION	Serving Size	Calories	Total Fat (g)	Saturated Fat (g)	Sodium (mg)	Carbohydrates (g)	Fiber (g)	Protein (g)
Personal Pan Pizza, Meat Lover's®	1	830	46	17	2110	68	3	36
Personal Pan Pizza, Spicy Sicilian	1	680	32	12	1730	69	4	29
Personal Pan Pizza, Supreme	1	720	36	14	1680	69	4	30
Personal Pan Pizza, Triple Meat Italiano	1	730	36	13	1770	68	3	32
Personal Pan Pizza, Veggie Lover's®	1	550	20	8	1190	70	4	22
Personal PANormous™ Pizza w/ Cheese	1	1100	45	19	2400	124	6	48
Personal PANormous™ Pizza w/ Ham & Pineapple	1	1020	37	14	2300	128	6	43
Personal PANormous™ Pizza w/ Italian Sausage & Red Onion	1	1210	56	21	2550	128	7	50
Personal PANormous™ Pizza w/ Pepperoni	1	1100	48	18	2540	121	6	47
Personal PANormous™ Pizza w/ Pepperoni & Mushroom	1	1050	42	16	2290	123	7	45
Personal PANormous™ Pizza, Dan's Original	1	1270	62	23	2810	124	7	55
Personal PANormous™ Pizza, Hawaiian Luau	1	1150	49	18	2670	129	6	49
Personal PANormous™ Pizza, Meat Lover's®	1	1470	80	30	3670	123	6	64
Personal PANormous™ Pizza, Spicy Sicilian	1	1220	57	22	3150	126	7	51
Personal PANormous™ Pizza, Supreme	1	1270	62	24	2920	125	7	54
Personal PANormous™ Pizza, Triple Meat Italiano	1	1280	62	23	3070	123	6	56
Personal PANormous™ Pizza, Veggie Lover's®	1	1010	38	14	2240	127	8	42
Pizza Mia Pizza w/ Cheese	1 pc /8	200	7	4	490	24	1	9
Pizza Mia Pizza w/ Pepperoni	1 pc /8	200	8	3.5	510	24	1	8
Pizza Rollers, Stuffed	1	230	10	4.5	590	24	1	9
P'Zone®, Classic	1	630	23	11	1460	77	3	28
P'Zone®, Meaty	1	710	31	14	1800	76	2	32
P'Zone®, Pepperoni	1	630	24	11	1570	76	2	29
Stuffed Crust w/ Cheese, Large	1 pc /8	350	14	8	910	39	2	16
Stuffed Crust w/ Ham & Pineapple, Large	1 pc /8	340	13	7	950	41	2	15

ITEM DESCRIPTION	Serving Size	Calories	Total Fat (g)	Saturated Fat (g)	Sodium (mg)	Carbohydrates (g)	Fiber (g)	Protein (g)
Stuffed Crust w/ Italian Sausage & Red Onion, Large	1 pc /8	390	18	8	980	40	2	17
Stuffed Crust w/ Pepperoni & Mushroom, Large	1 pc /8	350	15	7	940	39	2	16
Stuffed Crust w/ Pepperoni, Large	1 pc /8	380	17	8	1050	38	2	17
Stuffed Crust, Dan's Original, Large	1 pc /8	420	21	9	1090	39	2	19
Stuffed Crust, Hawaiian Luau, Large	1 pc /8	380	16	8	1070	41	2	17
Stuffed Crust, Meat Lover's®, Large	1 pc /8	480	26	12	1390	39	2	22
Stuffed Crust, Spicy Sicilian, Large	1 pc /8	400	19	9	1170	40	2	17
Stuffed Crust, Supreme, Large	1 pc /8	420	21	10	1140	40	2	18
Stuffed Crust, Triple Meat Italiano, Large	1 pc /8	420	21	10	1210	39	2	19
Stuffed Crust, Veggie Lover's®, Large	1 pc /8	330	13	7	900	40	3	14
Thin 'N Crispy® Pizza w/ Cheese, Medium	1 pc /8	190	8	4	550	22	1	9
Thin 'N Crispy® Pizza w/ Ham & Pineapple, Medium	1 pc /8	180	6	3	540	23	1	8
Thin 'N Crispy® Pizza w/ Italian Sausage & Red Onion, Medium	1 pc /8	220	10	4	580	23	1	9
Thin 'N Crispy® Pizza w/ Pepperoni & Mushroom, Medium	1 pc /8	190	8	3.5	540	22	1	9
Thin 'N Crispy® Pizza w/ Pepperoni, Medium	1 pc /8	200	9	4	610	21	1	9
Thin 'N Crispy® Pizza, Dan's Original	1 pc /8	240	12	5	650	22	1	11
Thin 'N Crispy® Pizza, Hawaiian Luau, Medium	1 pc /8	220	10	4	650	24	1	10
Thin 'N Crispy® Pizza, Meat Lover's®, Medium	1 pc /8	280	16	6	860	22	1	13
Thin 'N Crispy® Pizza, Spicy Sicilian	1 pc /8	220	10	4.5	750	22	1	9
Thin 'N Crispy® Pizza, Supreme, Medium	1 pc /8	240	12	5	670	23	1	10
Thin 'N Crispy® Pizza, Triple Meat Italiano	1 pc /8	240	12	5	720	22	1	11
Thin 'N Crispy® Pizza, Veggie Lover's® Medium	1 pc /8	180	6	3	530	23	1	8

ITEM DESCRIPTION

SIDES AND SNACKS

Item Description	Serving Size	Calories	Total Fat (g)	Saturated Fat (g)	Sodium (mg)	Carbohydrates (g)	Fiber (g)	Protein (g)
Breadsticks	1 pc	150	7	2	250	19	1	5
Breadsticks w/ Cheese	1 pc	180	7	3.5	370	20	1	7
Dipping Sauce, Blue Cheese	1 pkg	230	24	4.5	420	2	0	1
Dipping Sauce, Marinara	1 pkg	60	0	0	440	12	2	2
Dipping Sauce, Ranch	1 pkg	220	23	3.5	420	2	0	0
Fried Cheese Sticks	4 pcs	380	24	9	1020	29	2	13
Wedge Fries	1/2 order	320	18	3.5	530	35	3	4
Wings, Baked, Hot	2 pcs	100	6	2	430	1	0	10
Wings, Baked, Mild	2 pcs	110	7	2	430	1	0	10
Wings, Bone Out, All American	2 pcs	150	8	1.5	490	11	1	10
Wings, Bone Out, Buffalo Burnin Hot	2 pcs	190	8	1.5	1000	18	1	10
Wings, Bone Out, Buffalo Medium	2 pcs	190	9	1.5	990	18	1	10
Wings, Bone Out, Buffalo Mild	2 pcs	190	9	1.5	1020	18	1	10
Wings, Bone Out, Cajun	2 pcs	200	8	1.5	790	21	1	10
Wings, Bone Out, Garlic Parmesan	2 pcs	260	19	3.5	710	11	1	11
Wings, Bone Out, Honey BBQ	2 pcs	220	8	1.5	720	27	1	10
Wings, Bone Out, Spicy Asian	2 pcs	210	8	1.5	690	24	1	10
Wings, Bone Out, Spicy BBQ	2 pcs	200	8	1.5	940	21	1	10
Wings, Crispy Bone In, All American	2 pcs	200	14	2.5	500	8	1	9
Wings, Crispy Bone In, Buffalo Burnin Hot	2 pcs	230	15	3	1020	16	1	9
Wings, Crispy Bone In, Buffalo Medium	2 pcs	230	15	3	1010	16	2	9
Wings, Crispy Bone In, Buffalo Mild	2 pcs	230	15	3	1040	16	1	9
Wings, Crispy Bone In, Cajun	2 pcs	240	14	3	810	19	2	10
Wings, Crispy Bone In, Garlic Parmesan	2 pcs	300	25	5	730	9	1	10
Wings, Crispy Bone In, Honey BBQ	2 pcs	260	14	3	740	24	1	10
Wings, Crispy Bone In, Spicy Asian	2 pcs	250	14	2.5	710	21	1	10
Wings, Crispy Bone In, Spicy BBQ	2 pcs	240	14	2.5	950	19	1	9
Wings, Traditional, All American	2 pcs	80	5	1.5	290	0	0	7
Wings, Traditional, Buffalo Burnin Hot	2 pcs	110	6	1.5	810	8	1	8
Wings, Traditional, Buffalo Medium	2 pcs	110	6	1.5	800	8	1	8
Wings, Traditional, Buffalo Mild	2 pcs	110	6	1.5	830	8	1	8
Wings, Traditional, Cajun	2 pcs	120	5	1.5	600	11	1	8

ITEM DESCRIPTION	Serving Size	Calories	Total Fat (g)	Saturated Fat (g)	Sodium (mg)	Carbohydrates (g)	Fiber (g)	Protein (g)
Wings, Traditional, Garlic Parmesan	2 pcs	180	16	3.5	520	1	0	8
Wings, Traditional, Honey BBQ	2 pcs	140	5	1.5	530	16	0	8
Wings, Traditional, Spicy Asian	2 pcs	130	5	1.5	500	13	0	8
Wings, Traditional, Spicy BBQ	2 pcs	120	5	1.5	750	11	0	8

POPEYES

BEVERAGES

	Serving Size	Calories	Total Fat (g)	Saturated Fat (g)	Sodium (mg)	Carbohydrates (g)	Fiber (g)	Protein (g)
Coffee	16 oz	0	0	0	0	0	0	0
Coke	22 oz	230	0	0	22	59	0	0
Diet Coke	22 oz	0	0	0	38	0	0	0
Diet Pepsi	22 oz	0	0	0	0	50	0	0
Dr Pepper	22 oz	250	0	0	87.5	68	0	0
Fanta Orange	22 oz	300	0	0	25	80	0	0
Fanta Strawberry	22 oz	300	0	0	75	80	0	0
Hawaiian Punch	22 oz	175	0	0	265	43	0	0
Mountain Dew	22 oz	290	0	0	120	77	0	0
Orange Juice	10 oz	140	0	0	20	33	0	2
Pepsi	22 oz	200	0	0	150	70	0	0
Sprite	22 oz	210	0	0	77	56	0	0
Sweet Tea	22 oz	180	0	0	10	45	0	0
Unsweetened Tea	22 oz	0	0	0	10	0	0	0

BREAKFAST

	Serving Size	Calories	Total Fat (g)	Saturated Fat (g)	Sodium (mg)	Carbohydrates (g)	Fiber (g)	Protein (g)
Biscuit, Bacon	1	400	25	12	780	37	3	8
Biscuit, Chicken	1	490	26	14	1275	47	1	17
Biscuit, Egg	1	510	29	15	1155	41	1	13
Biscuit, Egg & Sausage	1	690	45	22	1520	43	1	20
Biscuit, Sausage & Gravy	1	510	33	14	1090	42	3	10

ITEM DESCRIPTION	Serving Size	Calories	Total Fat (g)	Saturated Fat (g)	Sodium (mg)	Carbohydrates (g)	Fiber (g)	Protein (g)
Grits	1	370	5	0.5	30	80	7	5
Hashbrowns	1	360	20	9	450	41	4	3
DESSERTS								
Cheesecake, Mardi Gras	1	310	19	10	290	32	1	4
Pie, Hot Cinnamon Apple	1	320	6	8	340	40	2	3
Pie, Hot Sweet Potato	1	350	19	8	370	41	2	4
Pie, Mississippi Mud	1	280	7	1.5	210	51	2	3
Pie, Sliced Pecan	1	410	21	6	220	52	2	4
MAIN MENU								
Breast, Mild	1	440	27	11	1330	16	2	35
Breast, Spicy	1	420	27	9	830	13	3	33
Catfish Fillet	2	460	29	12	1140	27	1	21
Chicken Biscuit	1	490	26	14	1275	47	1	17
Chicken Livers	10	1190	80	34	2070	65	6	54
Chicken & Sausage Jambalaya	1	220	11	3	760	20	1	10
Leg, Mild	1	160	9	4	460	5	1	14
Leg, Spicy	1	170	10	4	360	5	1	13
Nuggets	6 pcs	230	14	6	350	14	1	11
Sandwich, Catfish Po Boy	1	800	50	16	2015	65	3	27
Sandwich, Chicken Po Boy	1	660	34	9	1120	61	3	31
Sandwich, Shrimp Po Boy	1	690	42	13	2165	66	5	42
Shrimp, Butterfly	8 shrimp	290	17	8	820	21	3	12
Shrimp, Popcorn	1	330	9	9	1290	28	3	11
Tenders, Mild	3 pcs	340	14	6	1350	26	1	27
Tenders, Spicy	3 pcs	310	15	6	1240	16	2	28
Thigh, Mild	1	280	21	8	640	7	1	14
Thigh, Spicy	1	260	18	6	460	8	1	14
Wing, Mild	1	210	14	4	610	8	1	13
Wing, Spicy	1	210	14	6	410	8	1	13
Wrap, Loaded Chicken	1	310	13	6	890	33	3	14
SAUCES								
Cocktail	1	30	0	0	320	6	0	0
Confetti Sauce	1	65	0	0	90	16	0	0
Ranch	1	150	15	2.5	230	3	0	0

ITEM DESCRIPTION	Serving Size	Calories	Total Fat (g)	Saturated Fat (g)	Sodium (mg)	Carbohydrates (g)	Fiber (g)	Protein (g)
Spicy BBQ	1	45	0	0	320	10	0	0
Spicy Honey Mustard	1	100	8	1	170	7	0	0
Tartar Sauce	1	140	15	2.5	280	1	0	0
SIDES AND SNACKS								
Beans, Red & Rice	reg	230	14	4	580	23	5	7
Biscuit	1	260	15	7	450	26	2	4
Coleslaw	reg	220	15	2.5	300	19	2	1
Corn on the Cob	1	190	2	0.5	0	37	4	6
Fries, Cajun	1	260	14	5	570	30	2	3
Green Beans	reg	40	1.5	0	420	6	2	2
Jalapeños	1	6	0	0	368	1	1	0
Macaroni & Cheese	reg	200	7	3.5	490	26	1	8
Mashed Potatoes	reg	110	4	2	590	18	1	3
Onion Rings	12	560	38	17	920	50	5	6
Rice, Cajun	reg	170	5	2	530	25	1	7

The nutritional information provided in the "Nutrition Guide" and otherwise on the Popeyes® website or in its restaurants is comprised from data provided by an independent testing company commissioned by Popeyes (Silliker, Inc.) and our suppliers, and is current as of January of 2009. The data is based on standard product formulations and portion sizes, which can vary due to sampling differences, seasonal differences, ingredient substitutions, supplier variations, slight differences in product assembly on a restaurant by restaurant basis, and other factors.

All standard domestic Popeyes menu items are listed in the "Nutrition Guide." Some products may not be available at all restaurants. Products currently being tested & other limited time offerings and other regional menu alternatives may not be listed. Servings sizes may also vary slightly.

We encourage anyone with food sensitivities, allergies, or other special dietary needs or concerns to consult with your local physician or dietitian prior to eating at any Popeyes restaurant. Please periodically review the "Nutrition Guide" and our Popeyes website as information may be updated.

Updated January 16, 2009

RED LOBSTER

APPETIZERS

	Serving Size	Calories	Total Fat (g)	Saturated Fat (g)	Sodium (mg)	Carbohydrates (g)	Fiber (g)	Protein (g)
Calamari, Crispy w/ Vegetables	1 serv	1520	97	11	3050	115	n/a	n/a
Calamari, Crispy w/ Vegetables, in Combo platter	1 serv	760	49	6	1530	58	n/a	n/a
Chicken Breast Strips, in Combo platter	1 serv	410	24	2	1320	28	n/a	n/a
Chicken Wings, Buffalo*	1 serv	680	39	9	1750	0	n/a	n/a
Clam Strips, in Combo platter	1 serv	370	22	2	820	31	n/a	n/a
Clams, Steamed*	1 serv	430	15	3.5	1110	10	n/a	n/a
Crab Cakes, Pan-Seared	1 serv	280	14	2.5	1110	13	n/a	n/a
Crawfish, Fried*	1 serv	1190	69	7	2740	104	n/a	n/a
Lobster Nachos	1 serv	1090	64	19	1680	94	n/a	n/a
Lobster Pizza	1 serv	720	30	13	1390	69	n/a	n/a

ITEM DESCRIPTION	Serving Size	Calories	Total Fat (g)	Saturated Fat (g)	Sodium (mg)	Carbohydrates (g)	Fiber (g)	Protein (g)
Lobster, Artichoke & Seafood Dip	1 serv	1200	74	20	1950	101	n/a	n/a
Mozzarella Cheese Sticks	1 serv	680	39	14	1910	49	n/a	n/a
Mozzarella Cheese Sticks, in Combo platter	1 serv	340	20	7	950	24	n/a	n/a
Mushrooms Stuffed w/ Lobster, Crab & Seafood	1 serv	330	18	9	1110	18	n/a	n/a
Mushrooms, Stuffed, in Combo platter	1 serv	220	12	6	740	12	n/a	n/a
Oysters, Fried*	1 serv	590	31	3	1220	66	n/a	n/a
Scallops, Peach-Bourbon Barbecue	1 serv	430	27	5	1210	24	n/a	n/a
Seafood Sampler, New England	1 serv	750	42	10	2160	45	n/a	n/a
Shrimp Cocktail, Chilled Jumbo	1 serv	120	0.5	0	580	9	n/a	n/a
Shrimp, Grilled Bruschetta	1 serv	650	26	4.5	2380	58	n/a	n/a
Shrimp, Parrot Isle Jumbo Coconut	1 serv	530	36	9	1110	34	n/a	n/a
BEVERAGES								
Amaretto Sour	1	170	0	0	0	30	n/a	n/a
Appletini, Caramel	1	160	0	0	10	18	n/a	n/a
Bahama Mama	1	350	0	0	20	51	n/a	n/a
Bahama Mama, Non-alcoholic	1	230	0	0	25	57	n/a	n/a
Baileys® & Coffee	1	180	8	5	50	15	n/a	n/a
Baileys® Irish Cream	1	270	4.5	0	0	6	n/a	n/a
Biscayne Bay Breeze	1	240	0	0	10	46	n/a	n/a
Bloody Mary	1	140	0	0	1170	16	n/a	n/a
Blue Moon®	16 oz	220	0	0	20	20	n/a	n/a
Bud Light®	16 oz	160	0	0	20	19	n/a	n/a
Coffee	1	0	0	0	5	0	n/a	n/a
Coffee Nudge	1	130	2	1.5	15	13	n/a	n/a
Cognac	1	70	0	0	0	0	n/a	n/a
Coke®	1	100	0	0	35	27	n/a	n/a
Colada, Alotta	1	700	16	14	55	95	n/a	n/a
Colada, Piña	1	320	6	5	35	55	n/a	n/a
Colada, Piña, Non-alcoholic	1	280	7	6	20	52	n/a	n/a
Colada, Red Passion	1	310	4.5	4	35	55	n/a	n/a
Colada, Sunset Passion	1	360	8	7	15	63	n/a	n/a

ITEM DESCRIPTION	Serving Size	Calories	Total Fat (g)	Saturated Fat (g)	Sodium (mg)	Carbohydrates (g)	Fiber (g)	Protein (g)
Colada, Sunset Passion, Non-alcoholic	1	330	8	7	25	62	n/a	n/a
Cosmopolitan	1	220	0	0	0	15	n/a	n/a
Daiquiri, Berry Mango	1	350	0	0	30	62	n/a	n/a
Daiquiri, Berry Mango, Non-alcoholic	1	210	0	0	20	52	n/a	n/a
Daiquiri, Big Berry	1	350	0	0	20	65	n/a	n/a
Daiquiri, Strawberry	1	250	0	0	10	46	n/a	n/a
Daiquiri, Strawberry, Non-alcoholic	1	230	0	0	5	56	n/a	n/a
Diet Coke®	1	0	0	0	30	0	n/a	n/a
Disaronno Amaretto®	1	80	0	0	0	12	n/a	n/a
Distilled Spirits, 80 Proof	1	100	0	0	0	0	n/a	n/a
Dr Pepper®	1	150	0	0	35	27	n/a	n/a
Fat Tire®	16 oz	210	0	0	20	20	n/a	n/a
Frangelico®	1	70	0	0	0	12	n/a	n/a
Grand Marnier®	1	80	0	0	0	6	n/a	n/a
Iced Tea, Boston	1	50	0	0	10	12	n/a	n/a
Irish Coffee	1	90	2	1	25	4	n/a	n/a
Juice	1	140	0	0	25	30	n/a	n/a
Kahlua®	1	90	0	0	0	15	n/a	n/a
Lemonade, Minute Maid® Light	1	0	0	0	55	0	n/a	n/a
Lemonade, Minute Maid® Raspberry	1	180	0	0	20	30	n/a	n/a
Lobsterita®, Raspberry	1	690	0	0	50	131	n/a	n/a
Lobsterita®, Strawberry	1	700	0	0	55	135	n/a	n/a
Lobsterita®, Traditional	1	890	0	0	860	183	n/a	n/a
Long Island Iced Tea, Top-Shelf	1	190	0	0	0	21	n/a	n/a
Mai Tai, Mango	1	190	0	0	5	34	n/a	n/a
Malibu Hurricane	1	200	0	0	15	35	n/a	n/a
Manhattan	1	150	0	0	0	5	n/a	n/a
Margarita, Classic Frozen	1	470	0	0	590	96	n/a	n/a
Margarita, Classic Frozen, Non-alcoholic	1	280	0	0	510	69	n/a	n/a
Margarita, Classic On the Rocks	1	250	0	0	770	22	n/a	n/a
Margarita, Classic On the Rocks, Non-alcoholic	1	150	0	0	750	22	n/a	n/a
Margarita, Frozen Raspberry	1	320	0	0	0	61	n/a	n/a
Margarita, Frozen Strawberry	1	350	0	0	20	68	n/a	n/a

ITEM DESCRIPTION	Serving Size	Calories	Total Fat (g)	Saturated Fat (g)	Sodium (mg)	Carbohydrates (g)	Fiber (g)	Protein (g)
Margarita, Raspberry, Non-alcoholic	1	330	0	0	0	81	n/a	n/a
Margarita, Strawberry, Non-alcoholic	1	340	0	0	10	85	n/a	n/a
Margarita, Top-Shelf Frozen	1	520	0	0	640	97	n/a	n/a
Margarita, Top-Shelf On the Rocks	1	300	0	0	810	25	n/a	n/a
Martini, Classic w/ Gin	1	140	1.5	0	330	0	n/a	n/a
Martini, Classic w/ Vodka	1	150	0.5	0	170	0	n/a	n/a
Milk	1	130	5	3	125	13	n/a	n/a
Mudslide	1	520	21	13	160	52	n/a	n/a
Red Rockin' Shirley T	1	170	0	0	0	43	n/a	n/a
Rob Roy	1	160	0	0	10	3	n/a	n/a
Sam Adams®	16 oz	210	0	0	15	24	n/a	n/a
Sangria, Triple Berry	1	200	0	0	30	35	n/a	n/a
Scotches, Single Malt	1	70	0	0	0	0	n/a	n/a
Screwdriver	1	100	0	0	0	8	n/a	n/a
Shiner Bock®	16 oz	190	0	0	15	16	n/a	n/a
Slushy, Cherry Wave	1	290	0	0	10	73	n/a	n/a
Smoothie, Banana Bay Chocolate	1	460	14	9	10	78	n/a	n/a
Smoothie, Berry Strawberry Banana	1	340	9	6	85	63	n/a	n/a
Smoothie, Sunset Strawberry	1	250	6	4	45	47	n/a	n/a
Sprite®	1	100	0	0	45	26	n/a	n/a
Tea, Iced or Hot, Unsweetened	1	0	0	0	0	0	n/a	n/a
Tequila Sunrise	1	170	0	0	10	24	n/a	n/a
Tropical Freeze, Orange	1	250	6	5	20	49	n/a	n/a
Tropical Freeze, Pineapple	1	250	5	4.5	180	50	n/a	n/a
Wine, Sparkling, Bottle	1	420	0	0	60	6	n/a	n/a
Wine, Sparkling, Glass	1	100	0	0	15	2	n/a	n/a
Wine, White, Blush or Red, Bottle	1	490	0	0	70	27	n/a	n/a
Wine, White, Blush or Red, Glass	1	120	0	0	20	7	n/a	n/a
Yuengling®	16 oz	190	0	0	15	16	n/a	n/a
DESSERTS								
Apple Crumble, Warm a La Mode	1	770	31	13	200	117	n/a	n/a
Cheesecake, New York-Style w/ Strawberries	1	520	36	21	270	39	n/a	n/a
Chocolate Wave	1	1490	81	25	950	172	n/a	n/a

ITEM DESCRIPTION	Serving Size	Calories	Total Fat (g)	Saturated Fat (g)	Sodium (mg)	Carbohydrates (g)	Fiber (g)	Protein (g)
Cookie, Warm Chocolate Chip Lava	1	1070	51	23	470	142	n/a	n/a
Pie, Key Lime	1	580	22	12	450	88	n/a	n/a
DRESSINGS AND SPREADS								
Dipping Sauce, Butter, Melted	1 serv	350	38	23	30	2	n/a	n/a
Dipping Sauce, Cocktail	1 serv	40	0	0	480	9	n/a	n/a
Dipping Sauce, Honey Mustard	1 serv	280	26	4	360	12	n/a	n/a
Dipping Sauce, Ketchup	1 serv	50	0	0	460	11	n/a	n/a
Dipping Sauce, Marinara	1 serv	25	1	0	170	4	n/a	n/a
Dipping Sauce, Pico de Gallo	1 serv	10	0	0	160	2	n/a	n/a
Dipping Sauce, Piña Colada Sauce	1 serv	80	4	3	20	12	n/a	n/a
Dipping Sauce, Remoulade	1 serv	230	22	3.5	220	6	n/a	n/a
Dipping Sauce, Tartar	1 serv	190	19	3	170	6	n/a	n/a
Dressing, Balsamic Vinaigrette	1 serv	80	6	1	190	4	n/a	n/a
Dressing, Blue Cheese	1 serv	240	26	4.5	260	2	n/a	n/a
Dressing, Caesar	1 serv	280	30	5	560	1	n/a	n/a
Dressing, French	1 serv	160	14	2	390	9	n/a	n/a
Dressing, Honey Mustard	1 serv	190	17	2.5	250	8	n/a	n/a
Dressing, Ranch	1 serv	160	16	2.5	380	3	n/a	n/a
Dressing, Thousand Island	1 serv	200	20	3	180	6	n/a	n/a
FRESH FISH—WOOD-GRILLED, BROILED, OR BLACKENED								
Arctic Char	half	340	15	3	460	13	n/a	n/a
Barramundi	half	230	5	1.5	270	8	n/a	n/a
Cobia	half	400	26	8	250	8	n/a	n/a
Cod	half	170	2	0	500	8	n/a	n/a
Corvina	half	180	1.5	0	300	7	n/a	n/a
Flounder	half	200	1.5	0	350	8	n/a	n/a
Grouper	half	210	1.5	0	280	6	n/a	n/a
Haddock	half	180	1.5	0	520	6	n/a	n/a
Halibut	half	180	2	0	610	6	n/a	n/a
Lake Whitefish	half	210	2.5	0.5	400	6	n/a	n/a
Mahi-Mahi	half	200	1.5	0	270	6	n/a	n/a
Monchong	half	190	1.5	0	290	7	n/a	n/a
Opah	half	280	12	3.5	280	8	n/a	n/a

ITEM DESCRIPTION	Serving Size	Calories	Total Fat (g)	Saturated Fat (g)	Sodium (mg)	Carbohydrates (g)	Fiber (g)	Protein (g)
Perch	half	170	2	0	550	6	n/a	n/a
Pompano	half	240	8	3.5	310	6	n/a	n/a
Rainbow Trout	half	220	10	2.5	380	6	n/a	n/a
Red Rockfish	half	170	2.5	0	580	6	n/a	n/a
Salmon	half	270	9	2	310	6	n/a	n/a
Seabass	half	230	6	1.5	450	6	n/a	n/a
Snapper	half	210	1.5	0	330	8	n/a	n/a
Sole	half	140	2	0	860	6	n/a	n/a
Tilapia	half	210	3	1	230	9	n/a	n/a
Tuna	half	200	1	0	420	7	n/a	n/a
Wahoo	half	220	2.5	0.5	340	8	n/a	n/a
Walleye	half	170	2	0	400	7	n/a	n/a
KIDS MENU								
Broccoli	1 serv	45	0.5	0	200	6	n/a	n/a
Chicken Fingers	1 serv	410	24	2	1320	28	n/a	n/a
Chicken, Grilled	1 serv	210	4	1	710	14	n/a	n/a
Crab Legs, Snow	1 serv	90	1	0	790	0	n/a	n/a
Fish, Broiled	1 serv	200	1.5	0	350	8	n/a	n/a
Fruit	1 serv	40	0	0	0	10	n/a	n/a
Macaroni & Cheese	1	280	7	2	590	42	n/a	n/a
Salad, Caesar	1	270	21	4.5	560	13	n/a	n/a
Salad, Garden	1	90	3	0	105	13	n/a	n/a
Shrimp, Garlic-Grilled	1 serv	60	1	0	580	<1	n/a	n/a
Shrimp, Popcorn	1 serv	140	7	0.5	530	13	n/a	n/a
Sundae, Surf's Up	1	170	9	6	45	20	n/a	n/a
MAIN MENU								
Admiral's Feast	1 serv	1280	73	6	4300	92	n/a	n/a
Cajun Chicken Linguini Alfredo	half	630	27	10	1550	45	n/a	n/a
Catfish, Blackened Farm-Raised	1 serv	190	9	1.5	150	0	n/a	n/a
Catfish, Fried Farm-Raised	1 serv	220	12	1.5	280	3	n/a	n/a
Chicken Breast Strips	1 serv	690	40	3.5	2200	47	n/a	n/a
Chicken Breast Strips, Create Your Own Lunch	1 serv	410	24	2	1320	28	n/a	n/a
Chicken, Maple-Glazed	1 serv	570	9	2.5	1950	62	n/a	n/a

ITEM DESCRIPTION	Serving Size	Calories	Total Fat (g)	Saturated Fat (g)	Sodium (mg)	Carbohydrates (g)	Fiber (g)	Protein (g)
Chicken Sandwich, Grilled	1	810	32	4.5	2080	89	n/a	n/a
Clam Strips, Lightly Breaded, Create Your Own Lunch	1 serv	370	22	2	820	31	n/a	n/a
Coastal Soup & Salad w/ New England Clam Chowder	1 serv	710	30	12	1670	79	n/a	n/a
Coastal Soup & Salad w/ Potato Bacon Soup	1 serv	700	29	11	1780	84	n/a	n/a
Coastal Soup & Salad w/ Seafood Gumbo	1 serv	680	22	4.5	1950	87	n/a	n/a
Crab Legs, North Pacific King	1 serv	390	3.5	1	3520	2	n/a	n/a
Crab Legs, Snow	1 serv	180	2	0	1580	0	n/a	n/a
Crab Legs, Steamed Snow, Create Your Own Feast	1 serv	90	1	0	790	0	n/a	n/a
Crab Linguini Alfredo	half	560	25	12	1310	47	n/a	n/a
Crawfish, Fried*, Create Your Own Feast	1 serv	750	47	4.5	1480	49	n/a	n/a
Fish & Chips	1 serv	730	33	3	1980	64	n/a	n/a
Fish Sandwich, Crunch-Fried	1	730	37	9	1540	67	n/a	n/a
Fish, Broiled	1 serv	320	2	0	470	10	n/a	n/a
Fish, Crunch-Fried, Create Your Own	1 serv	410	24	2	1200	27	n/a	n/a
Fish, Fried	1 serv	440	16	1.5	560	5	n/a	n/a
Fish, Seafood-Stuffed	1 serv	320	11	3.5	1520	13	n/a	n/a
Fish, Seafood-Stuffed, Create Your Own Feast	1 serv	160	5	1.5	760	6	n/a	n/a
Lobster & Shrimp Pasta, Chef's Signature	half	510	25	11	1090	43	n/a	n/a
Lobster-and-Shrimp Trio, Bar Harbor	1 serv	820	39	16	3370	50	n/a	n/a
Lobster, Grilled Maine w/ Shrimp	1 serv	490	18	9	2850	39	n/a	n/a
Lobster, Live Maine	1 serv	230	1.5	0	840	0	n/a	n/a
Lobster, Shrimp & Scallops, Grilled	1 serv	500	11	2.5	3220	42	n/a	n/a
Lobster, Stuffed Maine	1 serv	330	12	3.5	1090	2	n/a	n/a
Lobster Lover's Dream	1 serv	680	30	11	2240	42	n/a	n/a
Lobster Rolls	1 serv	600	34	4	1530	47	n/a	n/a
Oysters, Fried, Create Your Own Feast	1 serv	590	32	3.5	1100	58	n/a	n/a
Rock Lobster, Crab & Shrimp	1 serv	310	10	2	2290	0	n/a	n/a
Rock Lobster Tail	1 serv	90	1	0	490	0	n/a	n/a

ITEM DESCRIPTION	Serving Size	Calories	Total Fat (g)	Saturated Fat (g)	Sodium (mg)	Carbohydrates (g)	Fiber (g)	Protein (g)
Rockzilla*	1 serv	130	1.5	0	690	0	n/a	n/a
Sailor's Platter	1 serv	330	10	1.5	1220	8	n/a	n/a
Salmon, Wood-Grilled Fresh, Create Your Own Feast	1 serv	210	9	2	240	0	n/a	n/a
Scallops, Bay, Broiled, Create Your Own Lunch	1 serv	70	1	0	490	2	n/a	n/a
Scallops, Bay, Fried, Create Your Own Lunch	1 serv	140	7	0.5	760	9	n/a	n/a
Scallops, Shrimp & Chicken, Wood-Grilled	1 serv	600	13	3	3190	42	n/a	n/a
Seafood Platter, Broiled	1 serv	300	10	3	1880	9	n/a	n/a
Shrimp & Chips, Beer-Battered	1 serv	540	35	3	1170	40	n/a	n/a
Shrimp & Chicken w/ Garlic Shrimp Scampi	1 serv	400	11	2.5	1970	34	n/a	n/a
Shrimp & Chicken w/ Hand-Breaded Shrimp	1 serv	550	17	2.5	2190	45	n/a	n/a
Shrimp & Chicken w/ Shrimp Skewer, Grilled	1 serv	380	8	2	1490	34	n/a	n/a
Shrimp & Salmon, Maple-Glazed	1 serv	670	17	3.5	2690	57	n/a	n/a
Shrimp & Scallops, Peach-Bourbon Barbecue	1 serv	540	27	4.5	1440	36	n/a	n/a
Shrimp Flatbread & Grilled Shrimp Salad	1	720	33	10	1900	66	n/a	n/a
Shrimp Jambalaya	1 serv	590	34	10	1860	47	n/a	n/a
Shrimp Linguini Alfredo	half	550	29	10	1580	41	n/a	n/a
Shrimp Linguini Alfredo, Create Your Own Feast	1 serv	550	29	10	1580	41	n/a	n/a
Shrimp Lover's Monday & Tuesday Coconut Shrimp Bites	1 serv	290	18	3	830	19	n/a	n/a
Shrimp Lover's Monday & Tuesday Fried Shrimp	1 serv	210	11	1	860	11	n/a	n/a
Shrimp Lover's Monday & Tuesday Popcorn Shrimp	1 serv	180	9	1	670	16	n/a	n/a
Shrimp Lover's Monday & Tuesday Scampi	1 serv	130	8	1.5	990	0	n/a	n/a
Shrimp Scampi, Garlic, Create Your Own Feast	1 serv	180	11	2	1440	0	n/a	n/a

ITEM DESCRIPTION	Serving Size	Calories	Total Fat (g)	Saturated Fat (g)	Sodium (mg)	Carbohydrates (g)	Fiber (g)	Protein (g)
Shrimp Scampi, Garlic, Create Your Own Lunch	1 serv	70	4	1	640	0	n/a	n/a
Shrimp Skewers, Wood-Grilled	1 serv	360	7	1.5	1290	47	n/a	n/a
Shrimp, Coconut Bites	1 serv	290	18	3	830	19	n/a	n/a
Shrimp, Crunchy Popcorn	1 serv	560	27	2.5	2100	51	n/a	n/a
Shrimp, Fried	1 serv	210	11	1	860	11	n/a	n/a
Shrimp, Garlic-Grilled Jumbo	1 serv	370	9	2	2160	40	n/a	n/a
Shrimp, Garlic-Grilled Jumbo, Create Your Own Feast	1 serv	60	1	0	580	<1	n/a	n/a
Shrimp, Hand-Breaded	1 serv	260	13	1	1060	13	n/a	n/a
Shrimp, Hand-Breaded, Create Your Own Lunch	1 serv	150	8	.5	620	8	n/a	n/a
Shrimp, Maple-Glazed	1 serv	110	1	0	780	11	n/a	n/a
Shrimp, Parrot Isle Jumbo Coconut	1 serv	880	60	15	1860	56	n/a	n/a
Shrimp, Parrot Isle Jumbo Coconut, Create Your Own Feast	1 serv	710	48	12	1490	45	n/a	n/a
Shrimp, Pecan-Crusted Jumbo	1 serv	735	25	4	3780	60	n/a	n/a
Shrimp, Popcorn	1 serv	180	9	1	670	16	n/a	n/a
Shrimp, Scampi	1 serv	130	8	1.5	990	0	n/a	n/a
Shrimp, Seaside Trio	1 serv	1010	55	13	3940	65	n/a	n/a
Shrimp, Walt's Favorite	1 serv	550	30	2.5	2270	39	n/a	n/a
Shrimp, Walt's Favorite, Create Your Own Feast	1 serv	370	20	2	1500	25	n/a	n/a
Sirloin & Shrimp, Wood-Grilled Peppercorn	1 serv	590	22	10	2230	30	n/a	n/a
Sirloin Surf & Turf, Wood-Grilled	1 serv	630	20	5	2050	34	n/a	n/a
Sirloin, Wood-Grilled Peppercorn, Create Your Own Feast	1 serv	280	10	4	850	0	n/a	n/a
Steak, Center-Cut New York Strip	1 serv	590	33	14	1420	0	n/a	n/a
Steak, Lobster & Shrimp Oscar	1 serv	1170	77	33	2770	20	n/a	n/a
Steak, New York Strip & Rock Lobster Tail	1 serv	690	35	14	1930	0	n/a	n/a
Tilapia, Parmesan-Crusted	half	430	20	8	990	19	n/a	n/a
Tilapia, Rock Island Stuffed	1 serv	410	16	6	1360	22	n/a	n/a
Ultimate Feast®	1 serv	600	28	3.5	3660	25	n/a	n/a

ITEM DESCRIPTION	Serving Size	Calories	Total Fat (g)	Saturated Fat (g)	Sodium (mg)	Carbohydrates (g)	Fiber (g)	Protein (g)
Walleye, Beer Battered*	1 serv	700	42	4	1200	24	n/a	n/a
Walleye, Blackened*	1 serv	300	7	1	410	9	n/a	n/a
Walleye, Broiled*	1 serv	260	3.5	1	540	0	n/a	n/a
Walleye, Fried*	1 serv	600	29	2.5	990	35	n/a	n/a
SIDES AND SNACKS								
Asparagus	1 serv	60	3	1.5	270	5	n/a	n/a
Broccoli	1 serv	45	0.5	0	200	6	n/a	n/a
Butter for Potato	1 serv	90	10	6	80	1	n/a	n/a
Cheddar Bay Biscuit™	1	150	8	2.5	350	16	n/a	n/a
Clam Chowder, Manhattan*	1 cup	80	1	0	690	12	n/a	n/a
Clam Chowder, New England	1 cup	230	17	10	680	13	n/a	n/a
Coleslaw	1 serv	200	15	2.5	250	13	n/a	n/a
Crab Legs, North Pacific King	1/2 lb	130	1	0	1190	<1	n/a	n/a
Crab Legs, Snow	1/2 lb	90	1	0	790	0	n/a	n/a
French Fries	1 serv	330	17	1.5	740	40	n/a	n/a
Lemon Wedge	1	5	0	0	0	1	n/a	n/a
Lobster Tail, Maine	1 serv	60	0.5	0	490	0	n/a	n/a
Potato, Baked	1 serv	220	1	0	730	47	n/a	n/a
Potato, Baked w/ Creamy Lobster	1 serv	380	14	4.5	1100	50	n/a	n/a
Potato Chips, Freshly Cooked	1 serv	300	19	1.5	580	28	n/a	n/a
Potato, Mashed w/ Creamy Lobster	1 serv	370	22	10	1000	30	n/a	n/a
Potatoes, Mashed Home-Style	1 serv	210	10	6	620	27	n/a	n/a
Rice Pilaf, Wild	1 serv	180	3	0.5	650	34	n/a	n/a
Salad, Caesar	1 serv	270	21	4.5	560	13	n/a	n/a
Salad, Garden	1 serv	90	3	0	105	13	n/a	n/a
Salad, Hand-Tossed Caesar w/ Chicken	1	670	52	10	1750	14	n/a	n/a
Salad, Hand-Tossed Caesar w/ Shrimp	1	620	51	10	1370	14	n/a	n/a
Seafood Gumbo*	1 cup	230	8	2.5	1160	25	n/a	n/a
Shrimp, Maple-Glazed Skewer	1	110	1	0	780	11	n/a	n/a
Shrimp, Parrot Isle Jumbo Coconut	5 pcs	450	30	8	950	29	n/a	n/a
Shrimp, Petite for Salad	1 serv	15	0	0	125	0	n/a	n/a
Shrimp, Walt's Favorite	6 pcs	280	15	1.5	1140	19	n/a	n/a

ITEM DESCRIPTION	Serving Size	Calories	Total Fat (g)	Saturated Fat (g)	Sodium (mg)	Carbohydrates (g)	Fiber (g)	Protein (g)
Soup, Creamy Potato Bacon	1 cup	220	15	9	790	19	n/a	n/a
Soup, Lobster Bisque	1 cup	210	14	8	830	12	n/a	n/a
Sour Cream for Potato	1 serv	30	2.5	1.5	10	1	n/a	n/a

* = Regional Items availability varies by restaurant. Due to the handcrafted nature of our menu items and the inherent size variations of seafood, nutritional content may vary. Guests who have special food sensitivities or dietary needs should not rely solely on this information. Nutritional information valid only for U.S. restaurants. Nutritional content does not include condiments, dipping sauces, or optional accompaniments.

RUBY TUESDAY

APPETIZERS

Asian Dumplings	1/4 dish	114	20	n/a	304	49	1	5
Chicken Tenders, Traditional	1/4 dish	94	17	n/a	222	11	0	11
Crab Cake, Jumbo Lump	1/4 dish	91	6	n/a	219	5	1	4
Dip, Fresh Guacamole	1/4 dish	358	24	n/a	429	32	10	5
Dip, Spinach Artichoke	1/4 dish	310	19	n/a	470	27	3	8
Mozzarella, Fried	1/4 dish	145	6	n/a	428	12	1	9
Quesadilla, California Club	1/4 dish	362	23	n/a	684	12	2	25
Quesadilla, Fresh Avocado	1/4 dish	266	19	n/a	346	13	2	14
Quesadilla, Grilled Chicken	1/4 dish	294	18	n/a	568	11	0	22
Queso & Chips	1/4 dish	317	20	n/a	535	28	3	11
Sampler, Four Way	1/4 dish	295	14	n/a	808	19	2	22
Shrimp, Buffalo	1/4 dish	126	23	n/a	580	48	1	7
Shrimp Fondue	1/4 dish	303	19	n/a	603	24	2	9
Shrimp Sampler	1/4 dish	225	12	n/a	784	19	1	10
Shrimp, Thai Phoon	1/4 dish	191	13	n/a	502	11	1	7
Spring Rolls, Southwestern	1/4 dish	158	8	n/a	305	18	1	4
Wings, Fire	1/4 dish	178	11	n/a	603	4	1	16

BEVERAGES

Berry Fusion	1	148	0	n/a	89	5	0	0
Fruit Punch, Honest Kids	1	40	0	n/a	5	10	0	0
Fruit Tea, Blackberry	1	142	2	n/a	60	10	1	1
Fruit Tea, Mango	1	94	3	n/a	128	9	0	2
Fruit Tea, Peach	1	137	2	n/a	66	9	0	1
Fruit Tea, Raspberry	1	142	2	n/a	60	10	1	1
Fruit Tea, Wild Berry	1	142	2	n/a	32	9	0	1
Lemonade, Blackberry	1	142	2	n/a	60	10	1	1

ITEM DESCRIPTION	Serving Size	Calories	Total Fat (g)	Saturated Fat (g)	Sodium (mg)	Carbohydrates (g)	Fiber (g)	Protein (g)
Lemonade, Pomegranate	1	195	0	n/a	1	12	0	0
Lemonade, Raspberry	1	199	0	n/a	3	8	0	0
Lemonade, Strawberry	1	206	0	n/a	3	16	0	0
Lemonade, Wild Berry	1	203	0	n/a	1	8	0	0
Peach Splash	1	152	0	n/a	38	9	0	0
POM Tea	1	94	2	n/a	32	13	0	1
RT Palmer	1	105	2	n/a	36	15	0	1
Tropical Sunrise	1	193	2	n/a	238	22	3	2
Watermelon Fizz	1	111	15	n/a	519	342	0	3
BRUNCH ITEMS								
Biscuit, Garlic Cheese	1 serv	102	5	n/a	230	13	0	2
Crêpe, Bella Chicken	1 serv	1052	56	n/a	2528	60	7	73
Crêpes, Cranapple	1 serv	1151	36	n/a	1282	192	12	11
Eggscellent Combo, Kids'	1	221	16	n/a	429	3	1	17
French Toast, Kids'	1 serv	285	13	n/a	420	29	5	12
French Toast	1 serv	570	26	n/a	840	58	10	24
Mini Benedicts, Crispy Southern Chicken	1	639	33	n/a	1526	46	4	36
Mini Benedicts, Steak	1	483	26	n/a	1261	31	2	32
Omelet, Bella Chicken	1	1162	75	n/a	2668	25	5	96
Omelet, Crabacado	1	808	61	n/a	1392	12	5	55
Omelet, Spinach & Mushroom	1	979	65	n/a	2201	24	4	57
Omelet, Western	1	1051	75	n/a	2309	11	1	62
Patty Cakes, Kids'	1	511	27	n/a	883	54	2	12
Steak & Eggs	1 serv	633	36	n/a	2015	7	3	69
Sunrise Quesadilla, Bacon Avocado	1	1595	114	n/a	2983	52	8	87
Sunrise Quesadilla, California Club	1	1795	117	n/a	3395	52	9	125
Yogurt Parfait, Berry Good	1	162	3	n/a	127	28	1	5
DESSERTS								
Blondie for One	1	630	27	n/a	222	88	3	11
Blondie for Two	1	1058	44	n/a	377	152	4	17
Cake, Double Chocolate	1 pc	902	40	n/a	617	125	1	13
Cake, Italian Cream	1 pc	990	56	n/a	550	110	2	12
Cheesecake, New York	1 pc	736	60	n/a	740	84	2	14
Cookie, Chocolate Chip	1	180	9	n/a	190	24	1	2

ITEM DESCRIPTION	Serving Size	Calories	Total Fat (g)	Saturated Fat (g)	Sodium (mg)	Carbohydrates (g)	Fiber (g)	Protein (g)
Cookie, White Chocolate Macadamia Nut	1	200	12	n/a	190	23	1	4
Cupcake, Carrot Cake	1	325	16	n/a	170	45	1	2
Cupcake, Red Velvet	1	285	11	n/a	305	45	1	2
Tiramisu	1	545	29	n/a	60	66	0	5
Yogurt Parfait, Berry Good	1	162	3	n/a	127	28	1	5
DRESSING AND SPREADS								
Dressing, Balsamic Vinaigrette	1 serv	40	2	n/a	530	5	0	0
Dressing, Blue Cheese	1 serv	180	19	n/a	250	1	0	2
Dressing, French	1 serv	120	11	n/a	260	6	0	0
Dressing, Honey Mustard	1 serv	90	8	n/a	150	5	0	0
Dressing, Italian	1 serv	60	6	n/a	330	2	0	0
Dressing, Ranch	1 serv	100	11	n/a	300	1	0	0
Dressing, Ranch Lite	1 serv	50	5	n/a	300	1	0	0
Dressing, Ranch, Sriracha	1 serv	75	8	n/a	273	1	0	0
Dressing, Signature Parmesan	1 serv	150	16	n/a	230	1	0	1
Dressing, Thousand Island	1 serv	70	7	n/a	220	3	0	0
Salsa	1 serv	8	0	n/a	170	2	0	0
Sauce, Asian BBQ	1 serv	59	32	n/a	243	7	0	0
Sauce, BBQ	1 serv	50	0	n/a	330	13	0	0
Sauce, Boston BBQ	1 serv	42	0	n/a	289	10	0	0
Sauce, Caramel	1 serv	100	0	n/a	110	25	0	1
Sauce, Chocolate	1 serv	120	3	n/a	60	22	1	1
Sauce, Lemon Butter	1 serv	88	9	n/a	160	1	0	1
Sauce, Marinara	1 serv	17	1	n/a	43	2	1	0
Sauce, Parmesan Cream	1 serv	64	6	n/a	181	2	0	2
Sauce, Sweet Chile	1 serv	170	17	n/a	150	2	0	0
Sour Cream	1 serv	35	2	n/a	16	3	0	1
KIDS MENU								
Apples	side	59	0	n/a	1	16	3	0
Broccoli, Steamed	side	91	6	n/a	227	8	3	3
Chicken Breast	1 serv	300	12	n/a	1000	20	5	31
Chicken Tenders	1 serv	492	29	n/a	1170	30	4	32
Grapes	side	27	0	n/a	0	7	0	0
Green Beans, Grilled	side	45	2	n/a	385	5	2	2

ITEM DESCRIPTION	Serving Size	Calories	Total Fat (g)	Saturated Fat (g)	Sodium (mg)	Carbohydrates (g)	Fiber (g)	Protein (g)
Grilled Cheese	1 serv	676	32	n/a	1667	77	6	26
Macaroni & Cheese	1 serv	680	37	n/a	1565	61	3	27
Minis, Beef	1 serv	775	41	n/a	1732	68	7	36
Minis, Turkey	1 serv	715	37	n/a	2162	68	7	34
Pasta Marinara	1 serv	469	7	n/a	978	86	8	16
Potatoes, White Cheddar Mashed	side	85	5	n/a	260	11	1	2
Shrimp, Fried	1 serv	387	19	n/a	1342	39	5	19
Steak, Chop	1 serv	440	30	n/a	1032	20	5	26
Sugar Snap Peas	side	113	6	n/a	202	8	3	3
Sundae	1 serv	574	29	n/a	193	71	1	11
Zucchini, Grilled	side	41	2	n/a	561	4	1	1
MAIN MENU								
Burger, Alpine Swiss	1	1048	62	n/a	1976	70	5	53
Burger, Avocado Turkey	1	886	54	n/a	2712	53	6	49
Burger, Boston Blue	1	1199	71	n/a	2706	87	6	54
Burger, Boston Blue Triple Prime	1	1382	98	n/a	2620	71	5	57
Burger, Buffalo Chicken	1	788	41	n/a	2009	64	3	43
Burger, Jumbo Lump Crab	1	707	40	n/a	1373	61	6	28
Burger, Ruby's Classic	1	929	55	n/a	1759	65	5	44
Burger, Smokehouse	1	1217	72	n/a	2593	89	6	54
Burger, Smokehouse Triple Prime	1	1400	99	n/a	2507	73	5	57
Burger, Triple Prime	1	1112	82	n/a	1673	49	4	47
Burger, Triple Prime Bacon Cheddar	1	1332	101	n/a	2163	49	4	60
Burger, Triple Prime Cheddar	1	1272	96	n/a	1953	49	4	57
Burger, Turkey	1	699	39	n/a	2459	50	3	40
Cheeseburger, Bacon	1	1059	66	n/a	2209	66	5	51
Cheeseburger, Classic	1	999	61	n/a	1999	66	5	48
Chicken & Broccoli Pasta	1 serv	1564	96	n/a	2811	94	7	81
Chicken & Mushroom Alfredo	1 serv	1220	59	n/a	3007	89	8	83
Chicken Bella	1 serv	397	15	n/a	1526	10	1	57
Chicken Florentine	1 serv	391	14	n/a	1692	9	2	57
Chicken Fresco	1 serv	412	19	n/a	1539	10	1	53
Chicken Fresco, Petite	1 serv	416	23	n/a	1431	26	5	33
Chicken, Barbecue Grilled	1 serv	290	4	n/a	1314	12	0	52

ITEM DESCRIPTION	Serving Size	Calories	Total Fat (g)	Saturated Fat (g)	Sodium (mg)	Carbohydrates (g)	Fiber (g)	Protein (g)
Chicken, Grilled	1 serv	240	4	n/a	75	0	0	51
Chicken Pasta w/ Parmesan	1 serv	1418	77	n/a	3187	111	7	72
Chicken Sandwich, Grilled	1	869	41	n/a	1841	51	5	74
Chili, White Bean Chicken	1 serv	229	8	n/a	1441	29	8	16
Crab Cake Dinner	1 serv	271	17	n/a	800	13	3	17
Creole Catch	1 serv	196	8	n/a	383	1	1	30
Filet	1	401	21	n/a	1215	2	0	51
Lobster Carbonara	1 serv	1426	94	n/a	3613	82	7	60
Lobster Tails	2 tails	511	34	n/a	1433	5	2	46
Mahi Mahi, Pesto	1 serv	494	21	n/a	609	1	0	77
Mediterranean Shrimp Pasta	1 serv	1086	63	n/a	3933	80	9	40
New Orleans Seafood	1 serv	316	18	n/a	945	3	1	37
Rib Eye	1 serv	821	63	n/a	1495	2	0	61
Ribs, Asian Sesame Glazed	half	548	30	n/a	728	23	1	47
Ribs, Classic Barbecue	half	485	24	n/a	590	26	0	45
Ribs, Memphis Dry Rub	half	460	29	n/a	150	6	0	44
Salad, Carolina Chicken	1	707	38	n/a	1536	39	8	54
Salad, Garden	1	396	17	n/a	985	50	10	14
Salad, Grilled Chicken	1	701	26	n/a	2241	46	9	69
Salad, Grilled Salmon	1	621	27	n/a	1546	45	10	51
Salad, Petite Carolina Chicken	1	436	23	n/a	985	30	6	29
Salad, Petite Grilled Chicken	1	362	13	n/a	1142	26	5	35
Salmon Florentine	1 serv	392	21	n/a	1271	8	3	43
Salmon, Asian Glazed	1 serv	353	16	n/a	1028	18	4	40
Salmon, Grilled	1 serv	249	11	n/a	604	1	1	37
Salmon, Petite Grilled	1 serv	398	25	n/a	951	26	7	26
Sandwich, Chicken BLT	1	798	40	n/a	1759	64	3	46
Seafood Trio	1 serv	435	20	n/a	1444	13	5	55
Shellfish Trio	1 serv	575	40	n/a	1664	12	4	40
Shrimp, Jumbo Skewered	1 serv	388	31	n/a	1577	6	3	26
Shrimp, Louisiana Fried	1 serv	423	17	n/a	1709	40	2	27
Shrimp Pasta, Parmesan	1 serv	1050	57	n/a	3270	88	5	43
Shrimp Pasta, Petite Parmesan	1 serv	692	38	n/a	2036	58	3	27
Shrimp Scampi, Petite Jumbo	1 serv	361	22	n/a	1460	24	7	23

ITEM DESCRIPTION	Serving Size	Calories	Total Fat (g)	Saturated Fat (g)	Sodium (mg)	Carbohydrates (g)	Fiber (g)	Protein (g)
Sirloin, Chef's Cut	12 oz	741	50	n/a	1555	2	0	69
Sirloin, Grilled Petite	1 serv	200	6	n/a	240	0	0	36
Sirloin, Grilled Top	1 serv	290	12	n/a	420	0	0	44
Sirloin, Petite	1 serv	301	16	n/a	1285	2	0	36
Sirloin, Petite Sliced	1 serv	371	22	n/a	1220	20	5	28
Sirloin, Top	1 serv	391	22	n/a	1465	2	0	44
Spaghetti Squash Marinara	1 serv	355	18	n/a	862	40	5	7
Spaghetti Squash Marinara Petite	1 serv	214	11	n/a	666	21	3	5
Steak (7 oz) & Lobster Tail	1 serv	691	47	n/a	2110	2	1	59
Tilapia, Basil Pesto	1 serv	535	39	n/a	1820	10	5	34
Tilapia, Blackened w/ Mango Salsa	1 serv	230	8	n/a	436	11	4	31
Tilapia, Herb Crusted	1 serv	402	24	n/a	944	11	2	39
Tilapia, Tuscan Crab	1 serv	439	23	n/a	1752	14	4	43
Trout Almondine	1 serv	586	39	n/a	398	7	3	54
Trout Almondine, Petite	1 serv	523	35	n/a	768	28	8	34
Wrap, Grilled Chicken	1	459	17	n/a	1369	47	4	29
Wrap, Turkey Burger	1	590	27	n/a	2656	47	2	39
Zucchini Cakes, Petite	1 serv	409	20	n/a	1473	39	7	11
SIDES AND SNACKS								
Asparagus, Grilled	1 serv	78	5	n/a	458	5	3	3
Biscuit, Garlic Cheese	1	102	5	n/a	230	13	0	2
Broccoli, Fresh Steamed	1 serv	91	6	n/a	227	8	3	3
Cauliflower, Creamy Mashed	1 serv	136	8	n/a	714	14	3	3
French Fries	1 serv	396	18	n/a	1389	55	5	5
Garden Salad	side	186	8	n/a	470	22	4	7
Green Beans, Fresh Grilled	1 serv	45	2	n/a	385	5	2	2
Lobster Mac 'n' Cheese	1 serv	637	37	n/a	1426	33	2	44
Lobster Tail Add-On	1 serv	113	3	n/a	608	0	0	23
Mac 'n' Cheese	1 serv	570	37	n/a	1067	33	2	30
Minis, Buffalo Chicken	4 pcs	619	23	n/a	1703	69	5	31
Minis, Ruby	4 pcs	635	35	n/a	1418	51	2	30
Minis, Turkey	4 pcs	551	28	n/a	1703	53	3	27
Minis, Zucchini Cake	1 serv	580	22	n/a	1714	83	5	14
Onion Rings	1 serv	342	21	n/a	538	37	2	5

ITEM DESCRIPTION	Serving Size	Calories	Total Fat (g)	Saturated Fat (g)	Sodium (mg)	Carbohydrates (g)	Fiber (g)	Protein (g)
Portabella Mushrooms, Sautéed Baby	1 serv	98	4	n/a	353	10	0	6
Potato, Baked w/ Butter & Sour Cream	1 serv	441	17	n/a	228	59	10	10
Potato, Loaded Baked	1 serv	591	29	n/a	545	59	10	20
Potato, Plain Baked	1 serv	282	2	n/a	113	57	10	10
Potatoes, White Cheddar Mashed	1 serv	169	10	n/a	520	22	2	5
Rice Pilaf, Brown	1 serv	230	9	n/a	981	27	3	6
Shrimp, Fried Add-On	sm	381	26	n/a	1005	22	1	13
Shrimp, Jumbo Skewered Add-On	1 skewer	87	6	n/a	486	0	0	18
Soup, Broccoli & Cheese	1 serv	378	32	n/a	1438	13	1	9
Soup, Clam Chowder	1 serv	318	20	n/a	635	18	2	18
Soup, Tortilla	1 serv	286	13	n/a	1592	30	2	13
Spaghetti Squash, Roasted	1 serv	54	3	n/a	69	6	2	1
Sugar Snap Peas	1 serv	113	6	n/a	202	8	3	3
Sweet Potato Fries	1 serv	330	12	n/a	660	54	9	6
Tomatoes, Sliced w/ Balsamic Vinaigrette	1 serv	52	1	n/a	288	15	0	2
Zucchini, Fresh Grilled	1 serv	41	2	n/a	561	4	1	1

SONIC DRIVE-IN

BEVERAGES

ITEM DESCRIPTION	Serving Size	Calories	Total Fat (g)	Saturated Fat (g)	Sodium (mg)	Carbohydrates (g)	Fiber (g)	Protein (g)
Apple Juice, Minute Maid®	sm (14 oz)	160	0	0	20	40	0	0
Apple Juice, Minute Maid® (box)	1	100	0	0	15	23	0	0
Coca-Cola®	sm (14 oz)	140	0	0	10	39	0	0
Coffee	reg (14 oz)	10	0	0	35	2	1	1
Coke Zero®	sm (14 oz)	0	0	0	40	0	0	0
Cranberry Juice, Minute Maid®	reg (14 oz)	170	0	0	20	46	0	0
Diet Coke®	sm (14 oz)	0	0	0	15	0	0	0
Diet Dr Pepper®	sm (14 oz)	0	0	0	70	0	0	0
Dr Pepper®	sm (14 oz)	130	0	0	45	37	0	0
Espresso Shot, Sonic Boom®	1	5	0	0	5	1	0	0
Fanta®, Orange	sm (14 oz)	150	0	0	10	42	0	0
Fruit Punch, Hi-C®	sm (14 oz)	150	0	0	15	40	0	0
Iced Latté, Caramel	14 oz	280	9	6	180	47	0	3
Iced Latté, Caramel/Hazelnut	14 oz	270	8	5	135	46	0	3
Iced Latté, Chocolate	14 oz	270	7	5	115	47	0	3

ITEM DESCRIPTION	Serving Size	Calories	Total Fat (g)	Saturated Fat (g)	Sodium (mg)	Carbohydrates (g)	Fiber (g)	Protein (g)
Iced Latté, Chocolate/Caramel	14 oz	280	8	5	150	47	0	3
Iced Latté, Chocolate/Hazelnut	14 oz	260	7	5	105	46	0	3
Iced Latté, Hazelnut	14 oz	260	7	5	90	44	0	3
Iced Tea	sm (14 oz)	5	0	0	10	1	0	0
Iced Tea, Peach	sm (14 oz)	5	0	0	15	1	0	0
Iced Tea, Raspberry	sm (14 oz)	5	0	0	15	1	0	0
Iced Tea, Sweet	sm (14 oz)	150	0	0	10	39	0	0
Java Chiller, Caramel	14 oz	520	25	18	350	66	0	7
Java Chiller, Caramel/Hazelnut	14 oz	500	24	17	310	65	0	7
Java Chiller, Chocolate	14 oz	510	24	17	290	66	0	7
Java Chiller, Chocolate/Caramel	14 oz	510	24	17	320	66	0	7
Java Chiller, Chocolate/Hazelnut	14 oz	500	24	17	280	65	0	7
Java Chiller, Hazelnut	14 oz	490	24	17	260	64	0	7
Lemonade, Minute Maid®	sm (14 oz)	140	0	0	60	37	0	0
Lemonade, Minute Maid® Light	sm (14 oz)	5	0	0	5	1	0	0
Limeade	sm (14 oz)	140	0	0	30	38	0	0
Limeade, Cherry	sm (14 oz)	170	0	0	35	45	0	0
Limeade Chiller	med (14 oz)	620	27	19	300	92	0	8
Limeade Chiller, Cherry	med (14 oz)	650	27	19	300	100	0	8
Limeade Chiller, Strawberry	med (14 oz)	680	27	19	310	108	1	8
Limeade, Cranberry, Minute Maid®	sm (14 oz)	150	0	0	35	41	0	0
Limeade, Lo-Cal Diet	sm (14 oz)	5	0	0	10	1	0	0
Limeade, Lo-Cal Diet Cherry	sm (14 oz)	10	0	0	10	2	0	0
Limeade, Strawberry	sm (14 oz)	150	0	0	35	41	0	0
Mello Yello®	sm (14 oz)	150	0	0	10	42	0	0
Milk, 1%	1	110	2.5	1.5	130	13	0	8
Milk, 1% Chocolate	1	160	2.5	1.5	210	27	0	8
Ocean Water®	sm (14 oz)	150	0	0	35	41	0	0
Orange Juice, Minute Maid®	sm (14 oz)	150	0	0	20	36	0	2
Powerade® Mountain Blast®	sm (14 oz)	90	0	0	75	24	0	0
Powerade® Mountain Blast® Slush	sm (14 oz)	200	0	0	50	53	0	0
Root Beer, Barq's®	sm (14 oz)	160	0	0	35	43	0	0
Slush, Blue Coconut	sm (14 oz)	190	0	0	30	51	0	0
Slush, Bubble Gum	sm (14 oz)	190	0	0	35	51	0	0

ITEM DESCRIPTION	Serving Size	Calories	Total Fat (g)	Saturated Fat (g)	Sodium (mg)	Carbohydrates (g)	Fiber (g)	Protein (g)
Slush, Cherry	sm (14 oz)	190	0	0	30	52	0	0
Slush, Cranberry Juice, Minute Maid®	sm (14 oz)	190	0	0	30	51	0	0
Slush, Grape	sm (14 oz)	190	0	0	35	51	0	0
Slush, Green Apple	sm (14 oz)	200	0	0	30	54	0	0
Slush, Lemon	sm (14 oz)	190	0	0	30	52	0	0
Slush, Lemon-Berry	sm (14 oz)	190	0	0	30	51	0	0
Slush, Lime	sm (14 oz)	190	0	0	30	52	0	0
Slush, Orange	sm (14 oz)	190	0	0	30	51	0	0
Slush, Strawberry	sm (14 oz)	190	0	0	30	50	0	0
Slush, Watermelon	sm (14 oz)	190	0	0	30	52	0	0
Smoothie, Strawberry	reg (14 oz)	420	0	0	115	106	4	3
Smoothie, Strawberry-Banana	reg (14 oz)	380	0	0	100	96	4	3
Smoothie, Tropical	reg (14 oz)	440	0	0	105	109	2	2
Sprite®	sm (14 oz)	140	0	0	30	37	0	0
Sprite® Zero	sm (14 oz)	5	0	0	10	0	0	0
Strawberry Soda, Minute Maid®	sm (14 oz)	160	0	0	0	45	0	0
Tea, Cranberry	sm (14 oz)	20	0	0	10	6	0	0
Tea, Diet Green	sm (14 oz)	5	0	0	10	0	0	0
Tea, Green	sm (14 oz)	110	0	0	10	32	0	0
BREAKFAST ITEMS								
Breakfast Burrito	jr	340	21	7	930	24	0	12
Breakfast Burrito w/ Bacon, Egg & Cheese	1	470	28	10	1470	37	1	19
Breakfast Burrito w/ Ham, Egg & Cheese	1	460	23	8	1810	37	2	25
Breakfast Burrito w/ Sausage, Egg & Cheese	1	500	31	11	1380	37	1	18
Breakfast Burrito w/ Steak & Egg	1	590	33	11	1450	45	3	28
Breakfast Burrito, Super Sonic®	1	590	36	12	1830	47	3	18
Breakfast Toaster® w/ Bacon, Egg & Cheese	1	530	33	10	1460	39	2	21
Breakfast Toaster® w/ Ham, Egg & Cheese	1	490	27	7	1720	39	2	24
Breakfast Toaster® w/ Sausage, Egg & Cheese	1	620	42	13	1400	39	2	21
CroisSonic® Breakfast Sandwich w/ Bacon	1	510	36	14	1410	28	0	19
CroisSonic® Breakfast Sandwich w/ Ham	1	430	27	12	1520	24	1	21

ITEM DESCRIPTION	Serving Size	Calories	Total Fat (g)	Saturated Fat (g)	Sodium (mg)	Carbohydrates (g)	Fiber (g)	Protein (g)
CroisSonic® Breakfast Sandwich w/ Sausage	1	600	46	17	1350	28	0	19
French Toast Sticks	4 pcs	500	31	5	490	49	2	7
Sausage Biscuit Dippers w/ Gravy	3 pcs	690	44	18	1770	57	0	16
DESSERTS								
Banana Split	reg	490	18	13	210	76	2	6
Banana Split	jr	200	6	4.5	80	35	1	2
CreamSlush® Treat, Blue Coconut	reg (14 oz)	350	14	10	170	53	0	4
CreamSlush® Treat, Cherry	reg (14 oz)	350	14	10	170	54	0	4
CreamSlush® Treat, Grape	reg (14 oz)	350	14	10	170	53	0	4
CreamSlush® Treat, Lemon	reg (14 oz)	350	14	10	170	54	0	4
CreamSlush® Treat, Lemon-Berry	reg (14 oz)	370	14	10	180	59	1	4
CreamSlush® Treat, Lime	reg (14 oz)	350	14	10	170	54	0	4
CreamSlush® Treat, Orange	reg (14 oz)	350	14	10	170	54	0	4
CreamSlush® Treat, Strawberry	reg (14 oz)	370	14	10	180	58	1	4
CreamSlush® Treat, Watermelon	reg (14 oz)	350	14	10	170	54	0	4
Float, Coca-Cola®	reg (14 oz)	330	14	10	160	49	0	4
Float, Coke Zero®	reg (14 oz)	260	14	10	180	29	0	4
Float, Diet Coke®	reg (14 oz)	260	14	10	160	29	0	4
Float, Diet Dr Pepper®	reg (14 oz)	260	14	10	190	28	0	4
Float, Dr Pepper®	reg (14 oz)	320	14	10	180	48	0	4
Float, Fanta® Orange	reg (14 oz)	340	14	10	160	51	0	4
Float, Root Beer, Barq's®	reg (14 oz)	340	14	10	170	51	0	4
Float, Sprite®	reg (14 oz)	330	14	10	170	48	0	4
Float, Sprite Zero™	reg (14 oz)	260	14	10	160	28	0	4
Ice Cream, Vanilla Cone	1	250	13	9	150	31	0	4
Ice Cream, Vanilla Dish	1	240	13	9	140	26	0	4
Malt, Banana	reg (14 oz)	510	26	18	290	62	1	8
Malt, Caramel	reg (14 oz)	600	28	19	410	78	0	8
Malt, Chocolate	reg (14 oz)	580	26	18	330	78	0	8
Malt, Hot Fudge	reg (14 oz)	610	31	23	350	72	1	8
Malt, Peanut Butter	reg (14 oz)	690	45	22	420	63	0	12
Malt, Peanut Butter Fudge	reg (14 oz)	650	38	22	380	67	1	10
Malt, Pineapple	reg (14 oz)	520	26	18	300	64	0	8

ITEM DESCRIPTION	Serving Size	Calories	Total Fat (g)	Saturated Fat (g)	Sodium (mg)	Carbohydrates (g)	Fiber (g)	Protein (g)
Malt, Strawberry	reg (14 oz)	510	26	18	300	63	1	8
Malt, Vanilla	reg (14 oz)	480	26	18	290	53	0	8
Shake, Banana	reg (14 oz)	500	26	18	280	60	1	8
Shake, Banana Cream Pie	reg (14 oz)	640	29	20	330	87	1	9
Shake, Caramel	reg (14 oz)	580	27	19	400	76	0	8
Shake, Chocolate	reg (14 oz)	570	26	18	320	77	0	8
Shake, Chocolate Cream Pie	reg (14 oz)	710	29	20	370	103	0	8
Shake, Coconut Cream Pie	reg (14 oz)	600	29	20	330	78	0	8
Shake, Hot Fudge	reg (14 oz)	590	31	22	340	70	1	8
Shake, Peanut Butter	reg (14 oz)	660	44	21	400	60	0	12
Shake, Peanut Butter Fudge	reg (14 oz)	630	38	22	370	65	1	10
Shake, Pineapple	reg (14 oz)	510	26	18	290	62	0	8
Shake, Strawberry	reg (14 oz)	500	26	18	290	61	1	8
Shake, Strawberry Cream Pie	reg (14 oz)	640	29	20	340	88	1	8
Shake, Vanilla	reg (14 oz)	460	26	18	280	51	0	8
Sonic Blast®, Butterfinger®	reg (14 oz)	730	38	26	410	87	0	11
Sonic Blast®, M&M's®	reg (14 oz)	750	40	28	380	86	1	11
Sonic Blast®, Oreo®	reg (14 oz)	680	37	25	460	78	1	11
Sonic Blast®, Red Velvet Cheesecake	reg (14 oz)	850	44	30	520	104	1	12
Sonic Blast®, Reese's Peanut Butter Cups®	reg (14 oz)	710	35	25	430	88	1	13
Sonic Blast®, Snickers®	reg (14 oz)	680	37	25	400	76	0	11
Sundae, Banana Fudge	1	540	26	19	280	71	2	6
Sundae, Butterfinger®	jr	210	10	6	105	26	0	3
Sundae, Caramel	1	510	23	17	340	69	0	6
Sundae, Chocolate	1	500	22	16	260	69	0	6
Sundae, Hot Fudge	1	520	27	20	280	63	1	6
Sundae, M&M®	jr	210	11	7	90	26	0	3
Sundae, Oreo®	jr	180	9	6	130	22	0	2
Sundae, Pineapple	1	440	22	16	230	55	0	6
Sundae, Reese's Peanut Butter Cups®	jr	200	8	6	115	27	0	4
Sundae, Snickers®	jr	210	11	7	115	25	0	3
Sundae, Strawberry	1	410	20	14	230	52	1	6

ITEM DESCRIPTION

ITEM DESCRIPTION	Serving Size	Calories	Total Fat (g)	Saturated Fat (g)	Sodium (mg)	Carbohydrates (g)	Fiber (g)	Protein (g)
DRESSINGS AND SPREADS								
Dressing, Honey Mustard	1 pkg	180	16	2.5	260	8	0	0
Dressing, Italian, Fat Free	1 pkg	25	0	0	390	5	0	0
Dressing, Ranch	1 pkg	210	22	3.5	370	2	0	1
Dressing, Ranch Light	1 pkg	70	4	.5	310	8	0	1
Dressing, Thousand Island	1 pkg	220	21	3.5	350	7	0	0
Ketchup	1	10	0	0	110	2	0	0
Mayonnaise	1	80	9	1.5	60	0	0	0
Mustard	1	5	0	0	55	0	0	0
Sauce, Barbecue	1	45	0	0	390	11	0	0
Sauce, French Fry	1	25	0	0	130	7	1	0
Sauce, Honey Mustard	1	90	7	1	190	7	0	0
Sauce, Marinara	1	15	0	0	270	3	1	0
Sauce, Picante	1	5	0	0	140	1	0	0
Sauce, Ranch	1	150	16	2.5	230	1	0	0
Syrup	1 pkg	90	0	0	0	22	0	0
KIDS MENU								
Apple Slices	1 serv	35	0	0	0	9	2	0
Apple Slices w/ Fat-Free Caramel Dipping Sauce	1 serv	110	0	0	60	28	2	0
Banana	1	110	0	0	0	27	3	1
Burger	jr	310	15	5	610	30	3	15
Burger, Deluxe	jr	350	20	6	440	28	3	15
Cheeseburger, Bacon	jr	410	23	9	1070	30	3	20
Cheeseburger, Double	jr	570	36	16	1330	31	3	31
Chicken Strips	2 pcs	200	11	2	470	10	1	14
Corn Dog	1	210	11	3.5	530	23	2	6
Grilled Cheese	1	380	20	7	1050	37	2	13
MAIN MENU								
Burger, Jalapeño	1	700	38	14	900	53	5	36
Burger w/ Ketchup	1	710	38	14	840	57	5	36
Burger w/ Mayonnaise	1	800	49	15	740	55	5	36
Burger w/ Mustard	1	700	38	14	770	54	5	36
Burger, Thousand Island	1	760	44	15	830	56	5	36

ITEM DESCRIPTION	Serving Size	Calories	Total Fat (g)	Saturated Fat (g)	Sodium (mg)	Carbohydrates (g)	Fiber (g)	Protein (g)
Ched 'R' Bites®	12 pcs	280	15	6	740	22	1	13
Ched 'R' Peppers®	4 pcs	330	17	6	1110	36	2	8
Cheeseburger w/ Bacon & Mayonnaise	1	930	60	20	1330	56	5	44
Cheeseburger w/ Ketchup	1	770	43	7	1170	58	5	40
Cheeseburger w/ Mayonnaise	1	860	54	18	1070	55	5	39
Cheeseburger w/ Mustard	1	770	43	17	1100	54	5	39
Cheeseburger, California	1	830	50	18	1100	56	5	39
Cheeseburger, Chili	1	800	47	18	1020	55	5	42
Cheeseburger, Green Chili	1	770	43	17	1100	55	5	39
Cheeseburger, Hickory	1	780	43	17	1200	60	5	39
Cheeseburger, Jalapeño	1	760	43	17	960	52	5	39
Cheeseburger, Super Sonic® Jalapeño	1	1180	76	32	1660	54	5	67
Cheeseburger, Super Sonic® w/ Ketchup	1	1190	76	32	1600	58	5	68
Cheeseburger, Super Sonic® w/ Mayonnaise	1	1270	87	34	1500	56	5	68
Cheeseburger, Super Sonic® w/ Mustard	1	1180	76	32	1530	55	5	68
Chicken Strip Dinner	4 pcs	970	45	8	1970	106	8	37
Chicken, Crispy Bacon Ranch	1	610	35	9	1750	47	4	30
Chicken, Crispy Sandwich	1	550	32	4.5	1070	46	4	22
Chicken, Grilled Bacon Ranch	1	470	22	7	1630	34	3	36
Chicken, Grilled Sandwich	1	400	19	2.5	960	32	3	28
Chicken®, Jumbo Popcorn	sm	380	22	4	1250	27	3	18
Chicken®, Jumbo Popcorn	lg	560	32	6	1890	41	5	27
Coney, Footlong	1	830	53	22	1980	55	4	32
Corn Dog	1	210	11	3.5	530	23	2	6
French Fries	sm	200	8	1.5	270	30	2	2
French Fries	lg	450	18	3.5	600	67	5	5
French Fries w/ Cheese	lg	740	36	11	1480	92	7	14
French Fries w/ Chili & Cheese	lg	850	43	14	1680	98	8	19
Fritos® Chili Pie	lg	970	64	18	1780	71	6	25
Hot Dog, All-American	1	390	18	7	1230	43	2	13
Hot Dog, Chicago Dog	1	430	20	7	2310	49	1	14
Hot Dog, Chili Cheese Coney	1	420	25	11	1180	33	2	19
Hot Dog, New York Dog	1	350	19	7	1290	33	3	14

ITEM DESCRIPTION	Serving Size	Calories	Total Fat (g)	Saturated Fat (g)	Sodium (mg)	Carbohydrates (g)	Fiber (g)	Protein (g)
Mozzarella Sticks	1 serv	440	22	9	1050	40	2	19
Onion Rings	med	440	21	3.5	430	55	3	6
Onion Rings	lg	640	31	5	630	80	4	9
Pickle-O's®	1 serv	310	16	3	1020	36	2	5
Salad, Crispy Chicken	1	340	19	5	970	24	5	20
Salad, Grilled Chicken	1	250	10	6	1070	12	3	29
Sandwich, Bacon Cheeseburger Toaster®	1	820	51	19	1500	51	3	39
Sandwich, BLT Toaster®	1	490	31	7	960	39	2	14
Sandwich, Chicken Club Toaster®	1	740	46	11	1760	54	4	30
Sandwich, Chicken Strip	1	420	22	3.5	710	39	3	18
Sandwich, Country Fried Steak Toaster®	1	670	37	10	1370	71	4	14
Sandwich, Fish	1	650	31	5	1160	71	7	22
Tater Tots	sm	130	8	1.5	270	13	1	1
Tater Tots	lg	330	21	4	720	33	4	2
Tater Tots w/ Cheese	lg	540	37	11	1550	42	4	10
Tater Tots w/ Chili & Cheese	lg	680	46	15	1820	49	6	17
Wrap, Crispy Chicken	1	490	23	5	1280	49	3	21
Wrap, Fritos® Chili Cheese	1	700	39	13	1600	65	4	21
Wrap, Fritos® Chili Cheese	jr	340	18	6	710	33	1	11
Wrap, Grilled Chicken	1	390	14	3.5	1420	39	2	28
TOPPINGS AND EXTRAS								
Bacon	1 serv	70	5	2	260	0	0	4
Caramel Topping	sm	60	1	.5	60	13	0	0
Cheese	1 serv	70	6	3	330	1	0	4
Chili	1 serv	50	3.5	1.5	160	2	1	3
Chocolate Topping	sm	50	0	0	20	13	0	0
Cole Slaw	1 serv	45	3	0.5	45	4	1	0
Green Chiles	1 serv	5	0	0	5	1	0	0
Jalapeño	1 serv	5	0	0	280	1	1	0
Nuts, Sundae Topping	1 serv	20	1.5	0	0	1	0	1
Onions, Grilled	1 serv	25	2	0	200	2	1	0
Pineapple Topping	sm	25	0	0	0	6	0	0
Strawberry Topping	sm	35	0	0	0	8	0	0

* Coffee products not currently available in all markets.
Consumer Information Center • 300 Johnny Bench Drive, Suite 400 • Oklahoma City, OK 73104 • 1-866-657-6642 (Toll-free)

SUBWAY

ITEM DESCRIPTION	Serving Size	Calories	Total Fat (g)	Saturated Fat (g)	Sodium (mg)	Carbohydrates (g)	Fiber (g)	Protein (g)
BEVERAGES								
Juice Box	1	100	0	0	15	24	0	0
Milk, Chocolate Flavored Reduced Fat***	1	300	8	5	300	43	<1	15
Milk, Low Fat***	1	160	3.5	2.5	180	19	0	12
Milk, Strawberry Flavored Reduced Fat***	1	300	7	4.5	220	44	0	15
BREAKFAST ITEMS								
Bacon, Egg & Cheese	6 in	410	16	6	1080	45	5	23
Bacon, Egg White & Cheese	6 in	370	11	4.5	1120	45	4	23
Breakfast BMT®	6 in	500	22	8	1640	47	5	29
Breakfast BMT® w/ Egg White	6 in	460	17	7	1680	48	5	29
Egg & Cheese	6 in	360	12	4.5	890	44	5	19
Egg Mega**	6 in	650	39	15	1600	45	5	30
Egg Muffin Breakfast BMT®	1	240	10	4	830	25	6	16
Egg Muffin Breakfast BMT® w/ Egg White	1	220	8	3	860	25	5	16
Egg Muffin Sunrise Subway® Melt	1	230	8	3	810	26	6	18
Egg Muffin Sunrise Subway® Melt w/ Egg White	1	210	6	2.5	830	26	5	18
Egg Muffin w/ Bacon, Egg & Cheese	1	200	7	3	550	24	6	13
Egg Muffin w/ Bacon, Egg White & Cheese	1	180	5	2	580	24	5	13
Egg Muffin w/ Egg & Cheese	1	170	6	2	460	24	6	12
Egg Muffin w/ Egg White & Cheese	1	150	1.5	1	480	24	5	12
Egg Muffin w/ Ham, Egg & Cheese	1	190	6	2	590	24	6	14
Egg Muffin w/ Ham, Egg White & Cheese	1	170	4	1.5	610	24	5	14
Egg Muffin w/ Sausage, Egg & Cheese	1	290	17	7	720	24	6	15
Egg Muffin w/ Sausage, Egg White & Cheese	1	270	15	6	740	24	5	15
Egg Muffin w/ Steak, Egg & Cheese	1	200	6	2.5	610	25	6	15
Egg Muffin w/ Steak, Egg White & Cheese	1	180	4	1.5	620	25	5	15
Egg Muffin, Egg Mega**	1	320	19	7	810	24	6	17
Egg Muffin, Egg White Mega**	1	300	17	7	840	24	5	17
Egg White & Cheese	6 in	320	8	3	940	44	4	19
Egg White Mega**	6 in	610	35	14	1640	45	4	30

ITEM DESCRIPTION	Serving Size	Calories	Total Fat (g)	Saturated Fat (g)	Sodium (mg)	Carbohydrates (g)	Fiber (g)	Protein (g)
Flatbread Breakfast BMT®	6 in	510	24	8	1780	45	3	28
Flatbread Breakfast BMT® w/ Egg White	6 in	470	20	7	1830	45	2	28
Flatbread w/ Bacon, Egg & Cheese	6 in	420	18	7	1220	42	3	22
Flatbread w/ Bacon, Egg White & Cheese	6 in	380	13	5	1270	43	2	22
Flatbread w/ Egg & Cheese	6 in	370	14	5	1030	42	3	19
Flatbread w/ Egg White & Cheese	6 in	330	10	3.5	1080	42	2	19
Flatbread w/ Ham, Egg & Cheese	6 in	400	15	5	1290	43	3	27
Flatbread w/ Ham, Egg White & Cheese	6 in	360	11	3.5	1340	43	2	23
Flatbread w/ Sausage, Egg & Cheese	6 in	610	38	14	1550	43	3	26
Flatbread w/ Sausage, Egg White & Cheese	1	570	34	13	1600	43	2	26
Flatbread w/ Steak, Egg & Cheese	1	440	17	6	1363	44	3	28
Flatbread w/ Steak, Egg White & Cheese	1	400	12	4.5	1450	45	2	28
Flatbread Sunrise Subway Melt®	1	480	20	7	1730	46	3	32
Flatbread Sunrise Subway Melt® w/ Egg White	1	440	15	6	1780	46	2	31
Flatbread, Egg Mega**	1	660	42	16	1740	43	3	29
Flatbread, Egg White Mega**	1	620	37	14	1790	43	2	29
Ham, Egg & Cheese	6 in	390	13	5	1150	45	5	24
Ham, Egg White & Cheese	6 in	360	11	3.5	1340	43	2	23
Hashbrowns	4 pcs	150	9	1	440	17	2	1
Mornin' Flatbread Breakfast BMT®	1	250	12	4	890	22	1	14
Mornin' Flatbread Breakfast BMT® w/ Egg White	1	230	10	3.5	910	22	1	14
Mornin' Flatbread Sunrise Subway® Melt	1	240	10	3.5	870	23	1	16
Mornin' Flatbread Sunrise Subway® Melt w/ Egg White	1	220	8	3	890	23	1	16
Mornin' Flatbread w/ Bacon, Egg & Cheese	1	210	9	3.5	620	21	1	11
Mornin' Flatbread w/ Bacon, Egg White & Cheese	1	190	7	2.5	630	21	1	11
Mornin' Flatbread w/ Egg & Cheese	1	190	7	2.5	520	21	1	9
Mornin' Flatbread w/ Egg White & Cheese	1	170	5	1.5	540	21	1	9
Mornin' Flatbread w/ Ham, Egg & Cheese	1	200	8	2.5	650	22	1	12
Mornin' Flatbread w/ Ham, Egg White & Cheese	1	180	5	2	670	22	1	12

ITEM DESCRIPTION	Serving Size	Calories	Total Fat (g)	Saturated Fat (g)	Sodium (mg)	Carbohydrates (g)	Fiber (g)	Protein (g)
Mornin' Flatbread w/ Sausage, Egg & Cheese	1	310	19	7	770	21	1	13
Mornin' Flatbread w/ Sausage, Egg White & Cheese	1	290	17	6	800	21	1	13
Mornin' Flatbread w/ Steak, Egg & Cheese	1	210	8	3	650	22	1	13
Mornin' Flatbread w/ Steak, Egg White & Cheese	1	190	6	2	670	22	1	13
Mornin' Flatbread, Egg Mega	1	310	19	7	770	21	1	13
Mornin' Flatbread, Egg White Mega	1	310	19	7	830	22	1	15
Sausage, Egg & Cheese	6 in	610	36	14	1410	45	5	26
Sausage, Egg White & Cheese	6 in	570	31	12	1460	45	4	26
Steak, Egg & Cheese	6 in	430	15	5	1260	47	5	28
Steak, Egg White & Cheese	6 in	390	10	4	1300	47	4	28
Sunrise Subway® Melt	6 in	470	17	7	1600	48	5	32
Sunrise Subway® Melt w/ Egg White	6 in	430	13	5	1640	48	4	32
DESSERTS								
Cheesecake, Raspberry	1 serv	210	9	4.5	180	29	0	2
Cookie, Chocolate Chip	1	210	10	6	150	30	1	2
Cookie, Chocolate Chunk**	1	220	10	5	100	30	<1	2
Cookie, Double Chocolate Chip**	1	210	10	6	170	30	1	2
Cookie, M & M®**	1	210	10	5	100	32	<1	2
Cookie, Oatmeal Raisin	1	200	8	4	170	30	1	3
Cookie, Peanut Butter**	1	220	12	5	190	26	1	4
Cookie, Sugar**	1	220	12	6	140	28	<1	2
Cookie, White Chip Macadamia Nut	1	220	11	5	160	29	<1	2
Pie, Apple	1 serv	250	10	2	290	37	1	0
Yogurt Parfait	1	160	2	1	75	30	2	6
DRESSINGS AND SPREADS								
Dressing, Italian, Fat Free	1	35	0	0	720	7	0	1
Dressing, Ranch	1	290	30	4.5	540	3	0	1
Mayonnaise	1 serv	110	12	2	80	0	0	0
Mayonnaise, Light	1 serv	50	5	1	100	<1	0	0
Mustard	2 tsp	5	0	0	115	<1	0	0
Olive Oil Blend	1 tsp	45	5	0	0	0	0	0

ITEM DESCRIPTION	Serving Size	Calories	Total Fat (g)	Saturated Fat (g)	Sodium (mg)	Carbohydrates (g)	Fiber (g)	Protein (g)
Ranch (on Sandwich)	1 serv	110	11	1.5	200	1	0	0
Red Wine Vinaigrette, Fat Free**	1 serv	30	0	0	340	6	0	0
Sauce, Chipotle Southwest	1 serv	100	10	1.5	220	1	0	0
Sauce, Honey Mustard, Fat Free	1 serv	30	0	0	120	7	0	0
Sauce, Sweet Onion, Fat Free	1 serv	40	0	0	85	9	0	0
Vinegar	1 tsp	0	0	0	0	0	0	0
PIZZA								
Cheese	1	680	22	9	1070	96	4	32
Cheese & Veggies	1	740	25	11	1270	100	5	36
Pepperoni	1	790	32	13	1350	96	4	38
Sausage	1	820	34	14	1420	97	4	39
SALADS								
Chicken Breast, Oven Roasted	1	130	2.5	0.5	270	9	4	19
Chicken Teriyaki, Sweet Onion	1	200	3	1	660	24	4	20
Chicken, Grilled w/ Baby Spinach	1	130	2.5	0.5	330	10	3	20
Ham, Black Forest	1	110	3	1	590	11	4	12
Roast Beef	1	140	3.5	1	450	10	4	18
Subway Club®	1	140	3.5	1	640	11	4	17
Turkey Breast	1	110	2	0.5	570	11	4	12
Turkey Breast & Ham	1	110	2.5	0.5	580	11	4	12
Veggie Delite®	1	50	1	0	65	9	4	3
SANDWICHES								
BLT	6 in	360	13	6	890	34	5	17
Cheesesteak, Big Philly	6 in	520	18	9	1370	52	6	39
Chicken, Barbecue	6 in	310	5	1.5	900	52	6	15
Chicken, Buffalo w/ Ranch Dressing	6 in	460	19	5	1390	47	5	27
Chicken & Bacon Ranch	6 in	570	28	10	1080	47	5	35
Chicken, Chipotle w/ Cheese	6 in	450	18	5	940	46	5	27
Chicken, Orchard	6 in	370	4	1.5	560	51	5	25
Chicken, Oven Roasted	6 in	330	7	1.5	790	45	3	22
Chicken Pizziola w/ Cheese	6 in	450	15	6	1250	50	6	31
Cold Cut Combo	6 in	410	16	6	1340	47	5	21
Flatbread, Chicken, Oven Roasted	1	330	7	1.5	790	45	3	22
Flatbread, Ham, Black Forest	1	300	7	1.5	980	44	3	17

ITEM DESCRIPTION	Serving Size	Calories	Total Fat (g)	Saturated Fat (g)	Sodium (mg)	Carbohydrates (g)	Fiber (g)	Protein (g)
Flatbread, Roast Beef	1	320	7	2	840	43	3	23
Flatbread, Subway Club®	1	320	7	2	1030	44	3	22
Flatbread, Sweet Onion Chicken Teriyaki	1	390	7	1.5	1050	57	3	25
Flatbread, Turkey Breast	1	290	6	1.5	950	44	3	17
Flatbread, Turkey Breast & Black Forest Ham	1	290	6	1.5	970	44	3	17
Flatbread, Veggie Delite®	1	240	4.5	1	450	42	3	8
Ham, Black Forest	kid	180	2.5	0.5	470	30	3	10
Ham, Black Forest	6 in	290	4.5	1	830	46	5	18
Italian B.M.T.®	6 in	450	20	8	1500	47	5	22
Meatball Marinara	6 in	580	23	9	1420	69	9	24
Pastrami, Big w/ Cheese	6 in	580	28	9	1700	49	5	31
Rib Patty, Barbecue	6 in	430	18	6	620	47	5	19
Roast Beef	6 in	320	5	1.5	700	45	5	24
Roast Beef	kid	200	3	1	410	30	4	14
Seafood Sensation® w/ Cheese	6 in	460	22	5	950	51	5	15
Spicy Italian	6 in	520	28	11	1720	46	5	22
Steak & Cheese	6 in	380	10	4.5	1060	48	5	26
Subway Club®	6 in	310	4.5	1.5	880	46	5	23
Subway Melt®	6 in	370	11	5	1210	47	5	23
Sweet Onion Chicken Teriyaki	6 in	380	4.5	1	900	59	5	26
Tuna	6 in	530	30	6	830	44	5	21
Turkey Bacon Avocado w/ Cheese	6 in	420	15	5	1200	49	7	24
Turkey Breast	6 in	280	3.5	1	810	46	5	18
Turkey Breast	kid	180	2	0.5	460	30	3	10
Turkey Breast & Black Forest Ham	6 in	280	4	1	820	46	5	18
Veggie Delite®	6 in	230	2.5	0.5	310	44	5	8
Veggie Delite®	kid	150	1.5	0	210	29	3	6
Veggie Patty	6 in	390	7	1	830	56	8	23
SIDES AND SNACKS								
Apple Slices	1 pkg	35	0	0	0	9	2	0
Chips, Baked Lay's®	1 pkg	130	2	0	200	23	2	2
Chips, Baked Lay's® Sour Cream & Onion	1 pkg	140	3.5	0.5	240	24	2	3

ITEM DESCRIPTION	Serving Size	Calories	Total Fat (g)	Saturated Fat (g)	Sodium (mg)	Carbohydrates (g)	Fiber (g)	Protein (g)
Chips, Doritos, Nacho	1 pkg	250	13	2.5	310	30	2	4
Chips, Lays® Classic	1 pkg	230	15	1.5	270	23	2	3
Chips, Sunchips Harvest Cheddar	1 pkg	210	9	1.5	240	29	3	4
Yogurt, Dannon Light & Fit®	1 pkg	80	0	0	80	16	0	5
SOUPS**								
Broccoli & Cheese	10 oz	180	11	5	990	16	4	5
Chicken & Dumpling	10 oz	170	5	2	810	23	2	8
Chicken & Dumpling w/ Rosemary	10 oz	90	1.5	0.5	810	14	1	6
Chicken & Rice w/ Pork, Spanish Style	10 oz	110	2.5	1	980	16	1	6
Chicken Corn Chowder, Chipotle	10 oz	140	3	1.5	900	22	2	6
Chicken Noodle, Roasted	10 oz	80	2	0.5	950	12	1	6
Chicken Tortilla	10 oz	110	1.5	0.5	440	11	3	6
Chicken w/ Wild Rice	10 oz	230	11	3.5	900	26	1	6
Chili Con Carne	10 oz	340	11	5	950	35	10	20
Clam Chowder, New England Style	10 oz	150	5	1	990	20	4	6
Cream of Potato w/ Bacon	10 oz	240	13	5	870	26	3	5
Minestrone	10 oz	90	1	0	910	17	3	4
Tomato Garden Vegetable w/ Rotini	10 oz	90	0.5	0	820	20	3	3
Tomato Orzo, Fire-Roasted	10 oz	130	1	0.5	410	24	2	6
Vegetable Beef	10 oz	100	2	0.5	960	17	3	5
TOPPINGS AND EXTRAS								
Avocado	1 serv	70	7	1	0	3	2	1
Bacon	2 pcs	45	3.5	1.5	190	0	0	3
Banana Peppers	3 pcs	0	0	0	20	0	0	0
Bread, 9-Grain Wheat	6 in	210	2	0.5	310	40	4	8
Bread, English Muffin	1	100	0.5	0	170	22	5	6
Bread, Hearty Italian	6 in	200	2.5	0.5	290	41	2	7
Bread, Honey Oat	6 in	260	3	0.5	330	48	5	9
Bread, Italian Herbs & Cheese	6 in	250	5	2.5	490	40	2	9
Bread, Italian White	6 in	200	2	0.5	290	38	1	7
Bread, Mini Italian	1	130	1.5	0.5	190	25	1	5
Bread, Mini Wheat	1	140	1.5	0	200	27	3	5
Bread, Monterey Cheddar	6 in	240	6	2.5	360	38	2	10
Bread, Parmesan Oregano	6 in	220	2.5	1	440	40	2	8

ITEM DESCRIPTION	Serving Size	Calories	Total Fat (g)	Saturated Fat (g)	Sodium (mg)	Carbohydrates (g)	Fiber (g)	Protein (g)
Bread, Roasted Garlic	6 in	230	2.5	0.5	1260	45	2	8
Cheese, American, Processed	1 serv	40	3.5	2	200	1	0	2
Cheese, Cheddar**	1 serv	60	5	3	100	0	0	4
Cheese, Monterey Cheddar, Shredded	1 serv	50	4.5	3	90	1	0	3
Cheese, Mozzarella, Shredded**	1 serv	40	2	1	100	0	0	2
Cheese, Pepperjack**	1 serv	50	4	2.5	140	0	0	3
Cheese, Provolone**	1 serv	50	4	2	125	0	0	4
Cheese, Swiss**	1 serv	50	4.5	2.5	30	0	0	4
Chicken Patty, Roasted	1 serv	90	2.5	0.5	330	4	0	15
Chicken Strips	1 serv	80	1.5	0.5	210	0	0	16
Cucumbers	3 pcs	<5	0	0	0	<1	0	0
Egg Patty**	1 serv	110	7	2	380	3	1	9
Egg White Patty	1	70	2	0	430	3	0	9
Flatbread	1	220	4.5	1	450	38	2	7
Green Peppers	3 pcs	0	0	0	0	0	0	0
Ham	1 serv	60	2	0.5	520	2	0	9
Jalapeño Peppers	3 pcs	<5	0	0	70	0	0	0
Lettuce	1 serv	<5	0	0	0	0	0	0
Meat, Cold Cut Combo	1 serv	140	11	3.5	830	2	0	10
Meat, Italian BMT®	1 serv	180	14	5	990	2	0	11
Meat, Subway Club®	1 serv	90	2.5	1	570	2	0	15
Meatballs	1 serv	310	17	6	570	25	4	17
Olives	3 pcs	<5	0	0	25	0	0	0
Onions	1 serv	<5	0	0	0	1	0	0
Pepperoni	3 pcs	80	7	2.5	400	1	0	4
Pickles	3 pcs	0	0	0	115	0	0	0
Roast Beef	1 serv	90	2.5	1	390	1	0	16
Sausage Patty, Breakfast**	1 serv	240	24	9	520	1	0	7
Seafood Sensation®**	1 serv	190	16	2.5	430	7	0	5
Steak, no Cheese	1 serv	110	2	1.5	550	1	0	16
Tomatoes	3 pcs	5	0	0	0	2	0	0
Tuna	1 serv	260	24	4	310	0	0	10
Turkey Breast	1 serv	50	1	0	500	2	0	9

ITEM DESCRIPTION	Serving Size	Calories	Total Fat (g)	Saturated Fat (g)	Sodium (mg)	Carbohydrates (g)	Fiber (g)	Protein (g)
Veggie Patty**	1 serv	160	5	0.5	520	12	3	15
Wrap**	1	310	8	2.5	610	51	1	8

A Registered Dietitian compiled this nutrition information from the following data: Nutrition analysis from Subway approved food manufacturers, an independent laboratory and the USDA National Nutrient Database for Standard Reference, Release #19. The nutrition information listed here is based on standard recipes and product formulations, however slight variations may occur due to the season of the year, use of an alternate supplier, region of the country, and/or small differences in product assembly.

** Regional and Limited Time Offer subs and menu items are only available in certain regions or at certain times of the year and ingredients and formulas may vary between restaurants. Nutritional information for these sandwiches is based on the most common formulas and ingredients.

1 The Exchange Lists are the basis of a meal planning system designed by a committee of the American Diabetes Association and the American Dietetic Association. While designed primarily for people with diabetes and others who must follow special diets, the Exchange Lists are based on principles of good nutrition that apply to everyone.

2 *** Values differ in California. See nutrition facts on milk container.

TACO BELL

BEVERAGES

ITEM DESCRIPTION	Serving Size	Calories	Total Fat (g)	Saturated Fat (g)	Sodium (mg)	Carbohydrates (g)	Fiber (g)	Protein (g)
Diet Pepsi**	16 oz	0	0	0	50	0	0	0
Dr Pepper**	16 oz	200	0	0	70	54	0	0
Fruit Punch, Tropicana**	16 oz	220	0	0	50	60	0	0
Frutista Freeze®, Mango Strawberry	1	250	0	0	10	62	0	0
Frutista Freeze®, Strawberry	1	230	0	0	55	57	0	0
Iced Tea, Lipton Raspberry**	16 oz	160	0	0	50	42	0	0
Limeade Sparkler, Cherry	16 oz	180	0	0	105	43	0	0
Limeade Sparkler, Classic	16 oz	150	0	0	80	39	0	0
Mountain Dew Baja Blast**	16 oz	220	0	0	60	58	0	0
Mountain Dew**	16 oz	220	0	0	70	58	0	0
Pepsi**	16 oz	200	0	0	40	56	0	0
Pink Lemonade, Tropicana**	16 oz	200	0	0	210	54	0	0
Root Beer, Mug**	16 oz	200	0	0	30	52	0	0
Sierra Mist**	16 oz	200	0	0	40	54	0	0

MAIN MENU

ITEM DESCRIPTION	Serving Size	Calories	Total Fat (g)	Saturated Fat (g)	Sodium (mg)	Carbohydrates (g)	Fiber (g)	Protein (g)
Burrito Supreme® w/ Beef	1	420	15	7	1140	53	9	17
Burrito Supreme® w/ Chicken	1	400	12	5	1060	51	7	21
Burrito Supreme® w/ Steak	1	390	13	5	1100	51	7	17
Burrito, 7-Layer	1	500	18	6	1090	69	12	17
Burrito, Bean	1	370	10	3.5	980	56	10	13
Burrito, Beefy 5-Layer	1	540	21	8	1320	68	9	19
Burrito, Cheesy Bean & Rice	1	480	21	5	1020	60	7	12
Burrito, Cheesy Potato	1	540	26	8	1430	59	7	19
Burrito, Chicken	1	430	18	5	870	48	3	18
Burrito, Chili Cheese	1	380	17	8	930	41	5	16

ITEM DESCRIPTION	Serving Size	Calories	Total Fat (g)	Saturated Fat (g)	Sodium (mg)	Carbohydrates (g)	Fiber (g)	Protein (g)
Burrito, Combo	1	460	18	7	1400	53	10	21
Burrito, Fresco Bean	1	350	8	2.5	990	57	11	12
Burrito, Fresco Chicken Burrito Supreme®	1	350	8	2.5	1060	50	7	18
Burrito, Fresco Steak Burrito Supreme®	1	340	8	2.5	1100	50	7	15
Burrito, Grilled Stuft Beef	1	700	30	10	1740	79	12	27
Burrito, Grilled Stuft Chicken	1	650	24	7	1580	76	9	34
Burrito, Grilled Stuft Steak	1	640	25	8	1670	76	9	28
Chalupa Baja, Beef	1	430	29	6	570	30	4	13
Chalupa Baja, Chicken	1	410	26	4	490	28	2	17
Chalupa Baja, Steak	1	400	26	4.5	530	28	2	13
Chalupa Nacho Cheese w/ Beef	1	390	24	4	540	31	3	12
Chalupa Nacho Cheese w/ Chicken	1	360	21	2.5	460	30	1	15
Chalupa Nacho Cheese w/ Steak	1	360	21	2.5	500	30	1	12
Chalupa Supreme w/ Beef	1	390	24	6	480	31	3	13
Chalupa Supreme w/ Chicken	1	370	21	4	410	29	2	17
Chalupa Supreme w/ Steak	1	360	21	4.5	450	29	2	14
Cheese Roll-Up	1	190	9	5	450	18	2	9
Cinnamon Twists	1 serv	170	7	0	200	26	1	1
Crunchwrap Supreme®	1	540	21	7	1150	71	7	16
Empanada, Caramel Apple	1	310	15	2.5	310	39	2	3
Enchirito® w/ Beef	1	360	17	8	1160	34	8	18
Enchirito® w/ Chicken	1	340	14	7	1080	32	6	22
Enchirito® w/ Steak	1	330	14	7	1120	32	6	19
Gordita Baja® w/ Beef	1	340	19	5	580	30	4	13
Gordita Baja® w/ Chicken	1	320	15	3.5	500	28	2	17
Gordita Baja® w/ Steak	1	310	16	3.5	540	28	2	13
Gordita Nacho Cheese w/ Beef	1	300	14	3.5	540	31	3	12
Gordita Nacho Cheese w/ Chicken	1	270	11	1.5	470	30	1	15
Gordita Nacho Cheese w/ Steak	1	260	11	2	510	30	1	12
Gordita Supreme® w/ Beef	1	300	14	5	490	31	3	13
Gordita Supreme® w/ Chicken	1	280	10	3.5	410	29	2	17
Gordita Supreme® w/ Steak	1	270	11	4	450	29	2	14
MexiMelt®	1	270	14	7	800	21	4	15

ITEM DESCRIPTION	Serving Size	Calories	Total Fat (g)	Saturated Fat (g)	Sodium (mg)	Carbohydrates (g)	Fiber (g)	Protein (g)
Nachos	1 serv	320	20	2	360	31	2	4
Nachos, Cheesy	1 serv	280	17	1.5	230	28	2	3
Nachos BellGrande®	1 serv	770	42	7	1050	79	14	19
Nachos Supreme	1 serv	440	24	5	680	42	8	12
Pizza, Mexican	1	540	30	8	910	47	8	20
Quesadilla w/ Chicken	1	530	28	12	1210	41	4	28
Quesadilla w/ Steak	1	520	28	12	1250	41	4	25
Quesadilla, Cheese	1	480	27	11	1000	40	4	19
Taco Salad, Chicken Ranch	1	910	55	10	1200	69	8	34
Taco Salad, Chipotle Steak	1	900	57	11	1480	69	8	27
Taco Salad, Express	1	580	28	10	1350	59	9	23
Taco Salad, Fiesta	1	770	42	10	1420	74	12	26
Taco Salad, Fiesta w/o Shell	1	460	24	8	1260	41	10	21
Taco Supreme®, Crunchy	1	200	12	5	350	15	3	9
Taco Supreme®, Double Decker®	1	350	15	6	710	40	8	14
Taco Supreme®, Soft Beef	1	230	11	5	560	22	3	11
Taco, Crispy Potato Soft	1	270	13	3	520	31	3	6
Taco, Crunchy	1	170	10	3.5	330	12	3	8
Taco, Double Decker®	1	320	13	4.5	690	37	8	13
Taco, Fresco Chicken Soft	1	150	3.5	1	480	18	2	12
Taco, Fresco Crunchy	1	150	7	2.5	350	13	3	7
Taco, Fresco Soft Beef	1	180	7	2.5	560	20	3	8
Taco, Fresco Soft Steak	1	150	4	1.5	520	19	2	9
Taco, Soft Beef	1	200	9	4	540	19	3	10
Taco, Soft Chicken	1	180	6	2.5	460	18	1	14
Taco, Soft Steak	1	250	14	4	550	19	2	11
Taquitos, Chicken	1 serv	320	11	4.5	770	37	3	18
Taquitos, Steak	1 serv	310	11	5	810	37	3	15
Tostada	1	250	10	3.5	550	30	9	10
Volcano Burrito	1	780	41	12	1660	80	9	24
Volcano Nachos	1 serv	980	60	9	1620	89	15	20
Volcano Taco	1	230	16	5	440	14	3	8
SIDES AND SNACKS								
Guacamole	1	35	3	0	85	2	1	0

ITEM DESCRIPTION	Serving Size	Calories	Total Fat (g)	Saturated Fat (g)	Sodium (mg)	Carbohydrates (g)	Fiber (g)	Protein (g)
Pintos 'n Cheese	1 serv	170	6	3	580	20	8	9
Potatoes, Cheesy Fiesta	1 serv	290	17	2.5	620	32	3	4
Rice, Mexican	1 serv	120	3.5	0	200	20	1	0
Salsa	1	5	0	0	80	1	0	0
Sour Cream, Reduced Fat	1	30	2	1	20	2	0	1

The Dietary Guidelines for Americans recommend limiting saturated fat to 20 grams and sodium to 2,300 milligrams for a typical adult eating 2,000 calories daily. Recommended limits may be higher or lower depending upon daily calorie consumption.

Product data is based on current U.S. formulations (based on zero grams trans fat canola frying oil) as of the date posted. Product formulations and nutritional values may differ for Taco Bell® Express and "multi-brand" (Kentucky Fried Chicken®/Taco Bell®, Taco Bell®/Pizza Hut®, and Taco Bell®/Long John Silver's®) menu items that may be based on a different type of oil, and for products outside the continental U.S. Although this data is based on standard portion guidelines, variation can be expected due to seasonal influences, minor differences in product assembly per restaurant, and other factors. Substitution of ingredients may alter nutritional values. Menu items and hours of availability may vary by location. Regional Menu items are available only at participating locations. Except for Taco Bell® Express, multi-brand menu items, limited time offerings, and test market menu items, single-brand menu products as of the date posted are included in this Nutrition Guide. For the most current U.S. nutritional information and for Taco Bell® Express, New York City and multi-brand menu items, see www.tacobell.com. If you have any questions about Taco Bell® and nutrition or are particularly sensitive to specific ingredients or foods, please contact us at 1-800-TACO BELL or visit our Web site at www.tacobell.com.

    * "Fresco Style" fat reduction varies per menu item and not all menu items will meet a 25% reduction in fat.

    ** Nutrition values for fountain beverages do not account for ice. Depending on the sodium content of the water where the beverage is dispensed, the actual sodium content may be higher or lower than the listed values.

    † ¼ lb. claim for Beef Combo, Beef & Potato and Cheesy Bean & Rice Burritos is based on average weight. Individual product weights vary.

TIM HORTONS

BAKED ITEMS

Bagel, 12 Grain	1	330	9	1	580	52	6	10
Bagel, Blueberry	1	270	1	0	470	55	2	10
Bagel, Cheddar Cheese	1	220	2.5	1	410	41	2	9
Bagel, Cinnamon Raisin	1	270	1	0	350	55	3	10
Bagel, Everything	1	280	2	0	460	53	3	10
Bagel, Onion	1	260	1.5	0	460	53	3	9
Bagel, Plain	1	260	1.5	0	450	52	2	9
Bagel, Sesame Seed	1	270	2.5	0	430	53	3	9
Bagel, Wheat 'N Honey	1	300	3	0.4	600	60	4	10
Biscuit, Plain Tea	1	250	9	4	590	35	1	5
Biscuit, Raisin Tea	1	290	10	4	590	45	2	6
Cinnamon Roll w/ Frosting	1	470	25	12	380	59	2	4
Cinnamon Roll w/ Glaze	1	420	23	11	360	50	2	4
Cookie, Caramel Chocolate Pecan	1	230	11	5	290	32	1	3
Cookie, Chocolate Chunk	1	230	9	6	260	35	1	2
Cookie, Oatmeal Raisin Spice	1	220	8	5	200	35	1	3
Cookie, Peanut Butter	1	280	16	7	260	27	2	6
Cookie, Trail Mix w/ Fruit & Nuts	1	220	8	3	160	35	4	3
Cookie, Triple Chocolate	1	250	13	8	220	31	2	3

ITEM DESCRIPTION	Serving Size	Calories	Total Fat (g)	Saturated Fat (g)	Sodium (mg)	Carbohydrates (g)	Fiber (g)	Protein (g)
Cookie, White Chocolate Macadamia Nut	1	240	12	6	270	31	1	3
Croissant, Cheese	1	320	20	10	440	25	2	10
Croissant, Plain	1	270	14	6	370	31	2	6
Danish, Cherry Cheese	1	350	13	5	310	53	1	5
Danish, Chocolate	1	490	27	11	240	56	3	7
Danish, Maple Pecan	1	410	21	8	260	49	2	5
Donut, Blueberry	1	230	8	3.5	210	36	1	4
Donut, Boston Cream	1	250	9	4	260	37	1	4
Donut, Canadian Maple	1	260	9	4	260	41	1	4
Donut, Chocolate Dip	1	210	8	3.5	190	30	1	4
Donut, Chocolate Glazed	1	260	10	4.5	300	39	2	4
Donut, Honey Cruller	1	320	19	9	220	37	0	1
Donut, Honey Dip	1	210	8	3.5	190	33	1	4
Donut, Maple Dip	1	210	8	3.5	190	30	1	4
Donut, Old Fashion Glazed	1	320	19	9	230	35	1	3
Donut, Old Fashion Plain	1	260	19	9	230	20	1	3
Donut, Sour Cream Plain	1	270	17	8	230	27	1	3
Donut, Strawberry	1	230	8	3.5	220	36	1	4
Donut, Vanilla Cream	1	320	13	5	230	46	1	4
Donut, Walnut Crunch	1	360	23	10	320	35	1	4
Fritter, Apple	1	300	11	5	350	49	2	4
Fritter, Blueberry	1	330	10	4.5	340	55	2	6
Muffin, Apple Spice	1	390	15	2.5	520	57	2	5
Muffin, Blueberry	1	340	11	2	570	53	2	5
Muffin, Chocolate Chip	1	410	15	5	430	62	2	5
Muffin, Cranberry Blueberry Bran	1	340	12	2	460	54	5	5
Muffin, Double Berry, Low Fat	1	290	2.5	.5	500	59	2	4
Muffin, Fruit Explosion	1	360	11	2	580	56	2	5
Muffin, Raisin Bran	1	410	13	2.5	490	69	5	6
Muffin, Strawberry Sensation	1	360	11	2	560	58	2	5
Muffin, Triple Chocolate	1	450	16	6	430	67	2	5
Muffin, Whole Grain Blueberry	1	380	15	2.5	530	58	5	6
Muffin, Whole Grain Raspberry	1	400	16	4	490	60	4	6
Timbits®, Apple Fritter	1	50	1.5	1	55	9	0	1

ITEM DESCRIPTION	Serving Size	Calories	Total Fat (g)	Saturated Fat (g)	Sodium (mg)	Carbohydrates (g)	Fiber (g)	Protein (g)
Timbits®, Banana Cream	1	60	2	1	65	9	0	1
Timbits®, Blueberry	1	60	2	1	50	10	0	1
Timbits®, Chocolate Glazed	1	70	2.5	1	75	10	0	1
Timbits®, Honey Dip	1	60	2	1	50	9	0	1
Timbits®, Lemon	1	60	2	1	50	9	0	1
Timbits®, Old Fashion Plain	1	70	5	2.5	60	5	0	1
Timbits®, Sour Cream Glazed	1	90	4.5	2	65	12	0	1
Timbits®, Strawberry	1	60	2	1	55	10	0	1
BEVERAGES								
Café Mocha	10 oz	170	6	5	170	27	1	1
Coffee w/ Cream & Sugar	10 oz	75	3.5	2	15	9	0	1
Flavor Shot	1 serv	5	0	0	0	1	0	0
French Vanilla	10 oz	240	7	7	240	39	0	4
Hot Chocolate	10 oz	240	6	5	360	45	2	2
Iced Cappuccino	12 oz	310	16	10	40	40	0	3
Iced Cappuccino w/ Milk	12 oz	180	1.5	1	45	39	0	3
Iced Coffee w/ Cream & Sugar	16 oz	80	4	2	30	10	0	0
Smoothie, Mixed Berry, w/o Yogurt	1	160	0	0	35	40	0	0
Smoothie, Mixed Berry w/ Yogurt	1	210	1	.5	75	48	0	2
Smoothie, Strawberry Banana, w/o Yogurt	1	160	0	0	35	40	0	0
Smoothie, Strawberry Banana w/ Yogurt	1	210	1	.5	75	48	0	2
Tea w/ Milk and Sugar	10 oz	50	1	0	20	10	0	1
BREAKFAST ITEMS*								
Bagel BELT™	1	460	16	6	1020	59	3	21
Biscuit w/ Breakfast Sausage	1	420	27	14	580	32	1	11
Breakfast Wrap w/ Bacon	1	270	16	5	630	18	2	13
Breakfast Wrap w/ Egg & Cheese	1	220	12	3.5	550	17	2	10
Breakfast Wrap w/ Sausage	1	390	28	9	840	18	2	16
English Muffin w/ Bacon, Egg & Cheese	1	330	15	6	790	33	1	17
English Muffin w/ Egg & Cheese	1	280	11	5	710	32	1	14
English Muffin w/ Ham, Egg & Cheese	1	300	12	5	960	33	1	18
English Muffin w/ Sausage, Egg & Cheese	1	450	27	11	1000	33	1	19
Hashbrown	1	100	5	0.5	210	12	1	1
Oatmeal, Apple Cinnamon	1 serv	300	5	2	300	62	5	6

ITEM DESCRIPTION	Serving Size	Calories	Total Fat (g)	Saturated Fat (g)	Sodium (mg)	Carbohydrates (g)	Fiber (g)	Protein (g)
Oatmeal, Maple	1 serv	220	2.5	0.5	220	49	4	5
Oatmeal, Mixed Berry	1 serv	210	2.5	.5	220	44	5	6
Sandwich w/ Bacon, Egg, Cheese	1	440	25	14	860	35	2	17
Sandwich w/ Egg & Cheese	1	390	21	13	780	35	2	14
Sandwich w/ Sausage, Egg & Cheese	1	560	37	19	1070	36	2	20
DRESSINGS AND SPREADS								
Cream Cheese, Garden Vegetable	1 serv	120	11	7	230	3	0	2
Cream Cheese, Light Plain	1 serv	85	6	4	200	3	0	4
Cream Cheese, Plain	1 serv	130	12	7	180	2	0	2
Cream Cheese, Strawberry	1 serv	120	10	6	160	6	0	2
MAIN MENU								
Chili	1 serv	300	16	6	1210	18	5	21
Sandwich, BLT	1	420	18	5	830	47	3	17
Sandwich, Chicken Club, Toasted	1	390	7	2	1000	52	3	29
Sandwich, Chicken Salad	1	350	9	1	880	48	4	20
Sandwich, Egg Salad	1	360	13	3	760	45	3	16
Sandwich, Ham & Swiss	1	400	12	5	1310	48	3	24
Sandwich, Turkey Bacon Club	1	380	7	2	1340	55	3	20
Sandwich, Turkey Caesar	1	370	11	2	1320	48	3	18
Soup, Beef Barley w/ Portobello Mushroom	1	110	2	1	650	18	3	5
Soup, Chicken Noodle	1	110	2.5	1	650	19	1	4
Soup, Cream of Broccoli	1	160	9.5	4	710	15	1	6
Soup, Minestrone	1	130	1.5	0	660	25	2	3
Soup, Potato Bacon	1	230	13	6	770	23	1	6
Soup, Split Pea w/ Ham	1	160	2.5	.5	780	28	5	8
Soup, Turkey & Wild Rice	1	120	1.5	0	850	24	1	3
Soup, Vegetable	1	70	0	0	850	14	3	4
Wrap, BBQ Chicken	1	180	6	2	600	19	2	13
Wrap, Chicken Ranch	1	190	8	2.5	620	17	2	13
Yogurt, Creamy Vanilla	1	160	2.5	1.5	80	32	2	4
Yogurt, Strawberry	1	150	2.5	1.5	75	28	2	4

* All nutritional information is based on regular sized sandwiches and standard ingredient servings.
Timbits, Tim's Own, and Bagel BELT are all trademarks of The TDL Marks Corporation.

WENDY'S

ITEM DESCRIPTION	Serving Size	Calories	Total Fat (g)	Saturated Fat (g)	Sodium (mg)	Carbohydrates (g)	Fiber (g)	Protein (g)
BEVERAGES								
Coca-Cola®	sm	160	0	0	0+	44	0	0
Coffee	1	0	0	0	0	0	0	0
Coffee Creamer	1	20	2	1	10	0	0	0
Coke Zero™	sm	0	0	0	5+	0	0	0
Diet Coke®	sm	0	0	0	15+	0	0	0
Dr Pepper®	sm	160	0	0	40+	43	0	0
Fanta® Orange	sm	180	0	0	25+	49	0	0
Frosty™ Float, Vanilla w/ Coca-Cola	1	380	7	4.5	135	75	0	7
Frosty™ Parfait, Caramel Apple	1	400	9	5	180	71	1	8
Frosty™ Parfait, Oreo®	1	400	10	6	220	68	1	8
Frosty™ Shake, Caramel	sm	680	15	9	330	126	0	11
Frosty™ Shake, Chocolate	sm	610	14	9	260	109	2	12
Frosty™ Shake, Strawberry	sm	580	14	8	190	104	1	10
Frosty™ Shake, Vanilla Bean	sm	620	14	8	450	115	0	10
Frosty™ Shake, Wild Berry	sm	550	14	8	190	96	1	11
Frosty™, Vanilla	sm	260	7	4.5	125	43	0	7
Frosty™, Chocolate	sm	250	6	4	115	41	0	6
Hi-C®, Flashin' Fruit Punch	sm	170	0	0	15+	46	0	0
Juicy Juice®, Apple	1	90	0	0	5	22	0	0
Lemonade, Minute Maid® Light	sm	5	0	0	5+	1	0	0
Milk, Low Fat	1	100	2.5	1.5	125	12	0	8
Milk, Low Fat Chocolate	1	140	2.5	1.5	170	22	0	7
Pibb Xtra®	sm	160	0	0	25+	43	0	0
Root Beer, Barq's®	sm	180	0	0	40+	50	0	0
Sprite®	sm	160	0	0	35+	43	0	0
Sugar	1 pkg	15	0	0	0	3	0	0
Sweetener, Non-Nutritive	1	5	0	0	0	1	0	0
Tea, Sweetened	1	100	0	0	10+	28	0	0
Tea, Unsweetened	1	0	0	0	10+	0	0	0
DRESSINGS AND SPREADS								
Dressing, Caesar Lemon Garlic	1 pkg	110	11	2	180	2	0	2

ITEM DESCRIPTION	Serving Size	Calories	Total Fat (g)	Saturated Fat (g)	Sodium (mg)	Carbohydrates (g)	Fiber (g)	Protein (g)
Dressing, Creamy Red Jalapeño	1 pkg	100	10	2	270	2	0	1
Dressing, French Fat Free**	1 pkg	40	0	0	95	9	0	0
Dressing, Italian Vinaigrette**	1 pkg	70	6	1	180	4	0	0
Dressing, Pomegranate Vinaigrette	1 pkg	60	3	0	160	8	0	0
Dressing, Ranch	1 pkg	100	10	1.5	150	2	0	1
Dressing, Ranch Avocado	1 pkg	100	10	2	210	2	0	1
Dressing, Ranch Light**	1 pkg	50	4.5	1	150	2	0	1
Dressing, Thousand Island**	1 pkg	160	15	2.5	290	5	0	0
Ketchup	1 pkg	10	0	0	95	2	0	0
Mayonnaise	1 serv	40	3.5	0.5	55	1	0	0
Mustard	1 serv	5	0	0	50	0	0	0
Sauce, Barbecue	1 pkg	45	0	0	120	11	0	0
Sauce, Honey Mustard	1 pkg	80	6	1	220	7	0	0
Sauce, Honey Mustard (on Sandwich)	1 serv	40	3.5	0	75	3	0	0
Sauce, Ranch (on Sandwich)	1 serv	40	4	0.5	55	1	0	0
Sauce, Ranch Heartland	1 pkg	120	12	1.5	240	3	0	0
Sauce, Sweet & Sour	1 pkg	50	0	0	120	12	0	0
KIDS MENU								
Cheeseburger	kid	260	11	5	570	26	1	14
Chicken Nuggets	4 pcs	180	12	2.5	340	10	0	9
Chicken Sandwich, Crispy	kid	330	13	3	700	36	2	15
Hamburger	kid	220	8	3	370	26	1	12
MAIN MENU								
Cheeseburger	jr	270	11	5	670	27	1	15
Cheeseburger Deluxe	jr	300	14	6	710	29	2	15
Cheeseburger, Double w/ Bacon	jr	440	25	11	820	26	1	26
Cheeseburger w/ Bacon	jr	350	19	8	750	26	1	18
Chicken Caesar Wrap, Crispy	1	430	25	7	950	35	2	17
Chicken Club, Asiago Ranch w/ Homestyle	1	660	33	9	1650	36	3	34
Chicken Club, Asiago Ranch w/ Spicy	1	670	34	10	1830	57	3	35
Chicken Club, Asiago Ranch w/ Ultimate Grill	1	540	24	8	1550	41	2	41
Chicken Fillet Sandwich, Homestyle	1	470	16	3	1190	55	3	26
Chicken Fillet Sandwich, Spicy	1	480	17	3.5	1370	56	3	26

ITEM DESCRIPTION	Serving Size	Calories	Total Fat (g)	Saturated Fat (g)	Sodium (mg)	Carbohydrates (g)	Fiber (g)	Protein (g)
Chicken Go Wrap, Grilled	1	260	10	3.5	730	25	1	19
Chicken Go Wrap, Homestyle	1	320	16	4.5	770	30	1	15
Chicken Go Wrap, Spicy	1	330	16	4.5	860	31	1	16
Chicken Grill Sandwich, Ultimate	1	360	7	1.5	1110	42	2	33
Chicken Nuggets	5 pcs	220	14	3	460	13	0	10
Chicken Sandwich, Crispy	1	350	16	3.5	730	38	2	15
Chili	sm	210	6	2.5	880	21	6	17
Chili	lg	310	9	3.5	1330	31	10	26
French Fries***	med	420	21	4	460	55	6	5
Hamburger	jr	230	8	3	470	26	1	12
Hamburger, Baconator®	1	620	35	15	1370	41	1	35
Hamburger, Baconator® Double	1	930	58	25	1840	41	1	59
Hamburger, Bacon Deluxe	1	640	36	15	1520	43	2	35
Hamburger, Bacon Deluxe Double	1	850	51	22	1690	43	2	54
Hamburger, Double w/ Everything & Cheese	1	770	43	19	1430	43	2	50
Hamburger, Double Stack™	1	360	18	8	740	27	1	23
Hamburger, Single w/ Everything & Cheese	1	550	28	12	1270	43	2	30
Hamburger, Triple w/ Everything & Cheese	1	1030	62	28	1800	44	2	71
Potato, Baked	1	270	0	0	25	61	7	7
Potato, Baked w/ Sour Cream & Chives	1	320	3.5	2	50	63	7	8
Salad	side	25	0	0	30	5	2	1
Salad, Baja	1	550	33	14	1650	34	12	32
Salad, Baja	half	280	17	7	840	18	6	16
Salad, BLT Cobb	1	450	25	11	1610	9	3	46
Salad, BLT Cobb	half	230	13	6	810	5	1	23
Salad, Caesar	side	60	3.5	2	115	5	2	4
Salad, Chicken Apple Pecan	1	340	11	7	1150	28	5	35
Salad, Chicken Apple Pecan	half	170	6	3.5	580	15	3	18
Salad, Chicken Caesar, Spicy	1	460	25	12	1410	27	6	33
Salad, Chicken Caesar, Spicy	half	240	13	6	710	15	4	17
TOPPINGS AND EXTRAS**								
Apple Slices	1 serv	40	0	0	0	9	2	0

ITEM DESCRIPTION	Serving Size	Calories	Total Fat (g)	Saturated Fat (g)	Sodium (mg)	Carbohydrates (g)	Fiber (g)	Protein (g)
Bacon, Applewood Smoked	1 pc	30	2.5	1	100	0	0	2
Bun, Premium	1	190	2	0	360	36	1	6
Bun, Sandwich	1	120	1	0	240	24	1	4
Buttery Best Spread	1 serv	50	5	1	95	0	0	0
Cheese, American	1	40	3.5	2	200	0	0	2
Cheese, Asiago	1	50	4	2.5	100	1	0	3
Cheese, Shredded Cheddar	1 serv	70	6	3.5	110	1	0	4
Chicken Fillet, Homestyle	1	240	11	2	770	13	1	16
Chicken Fillet, Spicy	1	250	11	2.5	950	17	1	19
Chicken Grill Fillet	1	120	1.5	0	670	1	0	26
Chicken Patty, Crispy	1	200	12	2.5	460	13	1	11
Croutons	1 serv	80	3	0	220	12	0	2
Hamburger Patty****	1/4 lb	220	15	7	170	0	0	19
Hamburger Patty, Jr.	1	90	7	3	70	0	0	8
Ketchup	1 pkg	10	0	0	95	3	0	0
Lettuce Leaf	1	0	0	0	0	0	0	0
Onion	2 pcs	0	0	0	0	0	0	0
Pecans, Roasted	1 serv	110	9	1	60	5	1	1
Pickles, Dill	4 pcs	0	0	0	150	0	0	0
Saltine Crackers	1 serv	25	0.5	0	80	5	0	1
Seasoning, Hot Chili	1 serv	5	0	0	270	1	0	0
Tomato	1 slice	5	0	0	0	1	0	0
Tortilla	1	130	3.5	1	280	21	0	3
Tortilla Strips, Seasoned	1 serv	80	4.5	1.5	105	11	1	1

* Toppings and Salad Dressings listed separately. ** Not available in all locations. ***Recommended portion sizes. French fries are individually portioned at every restaurant. Variations will exist from restaurant to restaurant.

To determine approximate nutritional information for a Kids' Meal size soft drink, multiply by 0.6; Value soft drink, multiply by 0.8; Medium soft drink, multiply by 1.5; Large soft drink, multiply by 2.0. To determine approximate nutritional information for a Jr. Frosty, multiply the small by 0.5; for a Medium Frosty, multiply the small by 1.3; for a Large Frosty, multiply the small by 1.7.
+ The sodium value will vary based on the level of sodium in your city's water supply.

**** Approximate weight before cooking.

** Note: For your custom sandwich order, add or subtract the nutritional value of any of the toppings to the totals above.

WHITE CASTLE

BEVERAGES

ITEM DESCRIPTION	Serving Size	Calories	Total Fat (g)	Saturated Fat (g)	Sodium (mg)	Carbohydrates (g)	Fiber (g)	Protein (g)
Apple Juice, Minute Maid***	1	100	0	0	15	23	0	0
Big Red***	sm (21 oz)	220	0	0	5	53	0	0
Cherry Coca-Cola***	sm (21 oz)	220	0	0	10	60	0	0
Coca-Cola Classic***	sm (21 oz)	210	0	0	15	57	0	0
Coffee	med (16 oz)	5	0	0	10	0	0	1
Coffee, Decaffeinated	med (16 oz)	0	0	0	10	0	0	0
Coke Zero***	sm (21 oz)	0	0	0	60	0	0	0
Crave Cooler Coke***	sm (21 oz)	110	0	0	10	29	0	0
Crave Cooler Fanta Wild Cherry***	sm (21 oz)	110	0	0	10	29	0	0
Cream Soda, Barq's Red***	sm (21 oz)	240	0	0	40	66	0	0
Diet Coke***	sm (21 oz)	0	0	0	20	0	0	0
Diet Coke, Caffeine Free***	sm (21 oz)	0	0	0	20	0	0	0
Fanta Grape Soda***	sm (21 oz)	260	0	0	65	70	0	0
Fanta Orange Soda***	sm (21 oz)	240	0	0	75	74	0	0
Fanta Strawberry Soda***	sm (21 oz)	260	0	0	65	70	0	0
Half & Half	1 serv	15	1.5	0	15	0	0	0
Hi-C, Flashing Fruit Punch***	sm (21 oz)	220	0	0	20	60	0	0
Hi-C, Orange Lavaburst***	sm (21 oz)	240	0	0	0	64	0	0
Hi-C, Poppin' Pink Lemonade Pink***	sm (21 oz)	200	0	0	85	51	0	0
Hot Chocolate	med (16 oz)	240	6	1.5	300	41	2	2
Iced Tea, Gold Peak Black Sweetened	sm (21 oz)	160	0	0	20	45	0	0
Iced Tea, Gold Peak Black Unsweetened	sm (21 oz)	0	0	0	15	0	0	0
Iced Tea, Gold Peak Southern Style	sm (21 oz)	210	0	0	15	57	0	0
Iced Tea, Gold Peak White Citrus	sm (21 oz)	180	0	0	15	47	0	0
Iced Tea, Sweetened	sm (21 oz)	80	0	0	10	20	0	0
Iced Tea, Unsweetened	sm (21 oz)	5	0	0	10	1	0	0
Lemonade, Raspberry Minute Maid***	sm (21 oz)	230	0	0	5	64	0	0

ITEM DESCRIPTION	Serving Size	Calories	Total Fat (g)	Saturated Fat (g)	Sodium (mg)	Carbohydrates (g)	Fiber (g)	Protein (g)
Orange Juice NTC, Minute Maid***	1	140	0	0	0	33	0	2
Orange Juice, Vita Fresh	1	140	0.5	0	15	34	1	2
Pibb Xtra***	sm (21 oz)	210	0	0	60	55	0	0
Powerade, Mountain Blast***	sm (21 oz)	140	0	0	115	36	0	0
Root Beer, Barq's***	sm (21 oz)	240	0	0	50	64	0	0
Sprite***	sm (21 oz)	210	0	0	45	55	0	0
Tea, Hot	med (16 oz)	0	0	0	0	0	0	0
Tea, Hot, Orange Pekoe	med (16 oz)	5	0	0	0	0	0	0
Vault***	sm (21 oz)	230	0	0	20	60	0	0
BREAKFAST ITEMS								
Bacon & Cheese Sandwich	1	150	9	3.5	460	12	1	7
Bacon & Egg Sandwich	1	200	11	3.5	400	12	1	12
Bacon Sandwich	1	130	6	2	330	12	1	5
Bacon, Egg & Cheese Sandwich	1	190	11	4	430	13	1	12
Bologna & Cheese Sandwich	1	240	15	6	760	14	1	10
Bologna & Egg Sandwich	1	290	18	6	690	14	1	15
Bologna, Egg & Cheese Sandwich	1	310	20	7	830	15	1	16
Cinnamon Roll (Awrey)	1	420	20	8	460	56	2	6
Danish, Apple (Awrey)	1	450	24	6	390	52	1	6
Danish, Apple (Haas)	1	470	22	10	520	62	1	6
Danish, Cheese (Awrey)	1	450	24	6	390	52	1	6
Danish, Cheese (Haas)	1	490	25	11	550	62	1	6
Danish, Cinnamon (Haas)	1	490	25	6	380	60	2	6
Danish, Strawberry (Awrey)	1	480	21	8	400	67	2	6
Donut, Plain Old Fashioned (Haas)	1	385	21	9	403	51	2	5
Donuts, Chocolate Frosted (Haas)	2 pcs	460	24	12	760	120	4	12
Donuts, French Twist (Haas)	2 pcs	460	24	10	580	58	2	6
Egg & Cheese Sandwich	1	160	8	3	330	13	1	10
Egg Sandwich	1	140	6	2	190	12	1	9
French Toast Sticks	1 serv	460	31	4.5	410	39	2	5
Hamburger w/ Egg	1	200	11	4	210	12	1	13
Hamburger w/ Egg & Cheese	1	230	14	6	350	13	1	14
Hash Rounds	med	600	46	6	760	42	4	4
Huevos Rancheros w/ Bacon Slider	1	190	11	4.5	500	14	1	12

ITEM DESCRIPTION	Serving Size	Calories	Total Fat (g)	Saturated Fat (g)	Sodium (mg)	Carbohydrates (g)	Fiber (g)	Protein (g)
Huevos Rancheros w/ Sausage Slider	1	310	23	9	710	14	1	15
Sausage & Cheese Sandwich	1	250	17	7	570	13	1	9
Sausage & Egg Sandwich	1	290	20	7	500	13	1	14
Sausage Sandwich	1	220	15	6	430	12	1	8
Sausage, Egg & Cheese Sandwich	1	320	22	9	640	13	1	15
DESSERTS								
Cookie, Chocolate Chunk	1	170	8	4	130	23	1	2
Cookie, Oatmeal Raisin	1	160	6	2.5	115	23	1	2
Cookie, White Chocolate Macadamia	1	180	9	4	125	22	1	2
DRESSINGS AND SPREADS								
Butter	1 pkg	30	3.5	2.5	30	0	0	0
Cream Cheese	1 pkg	100	10	6	110	0	0	2
Dressing, Ranch	1 pkg	150	17	2.5	210	1	0	0
Jam, Strawberry	1 pkg	40	0	0	0	10	0	0
Jelly, Grape	1 pkg	35	0	0	0	9	0	0
Ketchup	1 pkg	10	0	0	100	2	0	0
Lemon Juice	1 pkg	5	0	0	0	1	0	0
Mayonnaise	1 pkg	60	7	1	55	0	0	0
Mustard	1 serv	0	0	0	85	0	0	0
Mustard-Horseradish	1 pkg	5	0	0	65	0	0	0
Sauce, A1 Thick & Hearty	1 serv	20	0	0	230	5	0	0
Sauce, Barbecue	1 pkg	35	.5	0	390	8	0	0
Sauce, Cinnamon	1 pkg	110	4	.5	85	20	0	0
Sauce, Garlic Mushroom	1 serv	10	.5	0	125	1	0	0
Sauce, Hamburger	1 serv	0	0	0	75	0	0	0
Sauce, Honey Mustard, Fat Free	1 pkg	50	0	0	120	13	0	0
Sauce, Hot	1 pkg	5	0	0	170	1	1	0
Sauce, Marinara	1 pkg	15	0	0	260	4	0	0
Sauce, Nacho Cheese	1 serv	50	4	1	400	3	0	0
Sauce, Seafood	1 pkg	30	0	0	340	7	0	0
Sauce, Spicy Hamburger	1 serv	0	0	0	45	1	0	0
Sauce, Tartar	1 pkg	90	8	1	220	4	0	0
Sauce, White Castle Zesty Zing	1 pkg	120	11	1.5	190	4	0	0
Syrup, Maple	1 pkg	120	0	0	25	31	0	0

ITEM DESCRIPTION	Serving Size	Calories	Total Fat (g)	Saturated Fat (g)	Sodium (mg)	Carbohydrates (g)	Fiber (g)	Protein (g)
MAIN MENU								
Cheeseburger	1	170	9	4	550	15	1	8
Cheeseburger w/ Bacon	1	190	11	5	550	13	1	9
Cheeseburger, Bacon Jalapeño	1	190	12	5	560	14	1	9
Cheeseburger, Jalapeño	1	160	9	4	460	14	1	8
Chicken Breast Slider	1	360	26	3.5	510	20	1	11
Chicken Breast Slider w/ Cheese	1	390	28	5	650	20	1	13
Chicken Ring Slider	1	350	28	4.5	320	16	1	8
Chicken Ring Slider w/ Cheese	1	380	30	6	460	16	1	10
Chicken Supreme Slider	1	420	31	6	750	20	1	14
Double Cheeseburger	1	300	17	8	940	20	1	15
Double Cheeseburger, Bacon	1	350	22	10	1050	21	1	18
Double Cheeseburger, Jalapeño	1	280	17	8	860	21	1	15
Double Fish w/ Cheese	1	610	48	9	700	25	23	19
Double Fish, no Cheese	1	550	43	6	420	24	23	17
Double Original Slider®	1	240	12	5	660	21	1	12
Fish Slider	1	310	22	3	270	18	12	9
Fish Slider w/ Cheese	1	340	24	4.5	410	18	12	11
Original Slider®	1	140	6	2.5	360	13	1	7
Pulled Pork Barbecue Slider	1	170	4.5	1	460	25	1	9
Surf & Turf w/ Cheese	1	540	38	11	990	27	13	22
Surf & Turf, no Cheese	1	480	33	8	720	26	13	19
Traditional Bun w/ Cheese	1	90	3	1.5	260	12	1	4
SIDES AND SNACKS								
Apple Sauce	1 pkg	100	0	0	10	24	2	0
Chicken Rings	6 pcs	530	47	10	610	12	0	18
Chicken Rings	20 pcs	1760	158	27	2020	41	2	58
Chicken Rings, Buffalo	6 pcs	540	48	8	870	14	1	18
Chicken Rings, Buffalo	20 pcs	1790	158	27	2940	47	2	59
Chicken Rings, Ranch	6 pcs	540	48	8	820	14	1	18
Chicken Rings, Ranch	20 pcs	1790	159	28	2760	46	2	60
Clam Strips	med	210	17	2	620	5	0	8
Fish Nibblers	med	320	16	2.5	700	28	1	16
French Fries	med	370	25	4	50	33	3	3

ITEM DESCRIPTION	Serving Size	Calories	Total Fat (g)	Saturated Fat (g)	Sodium (mg)	Carbohydrates (g)	Fiber (g)	Protein (g)
Mozzarella Cheese Sticks	3 pcs	440	33	8	850	22	1	12
Mozzarella Cheese Sticks	5 pcs	740	55	14	1420	36	2	21
Onion Chips	med	670	50	8	970	46	8	5
Onion Rings	med	340	22	4	310	33	3	2
Onion Rings, Homestyle	med	480	33	4.5	580	40	2	6
Sweet Potato Fries	med	480	30	3	380	47	6	4
TOPPINGS AND EXTRAS								
Bacon	1 pc	30	3	1	105	0	0	2
Bologna	1	150	12	4	500	2	0	6
Bun, Traditional	1	70	1	0	120	12	1	2
Cheese, American	1 pc	30	2	2	140	0	0	2
Cheese, Jalapeño	1 pc	20	3	2	140	1	0	1
Egg	1	70	5	1.5	70	0	0	6
Hamburger Meat	1	70	6	2.5	15	0	0	4
Hashbrown	1	310	28	5	250	14	3	1
Sausage	1	150	14	5	310	0	0	5
Toast, Wheat	1	130	2	0.5	260	24	2	6
Toast, White	1	130	2	0.5	250	25	1	4

* Sodium values may vary depending on restaurant preparation and on the water used for beverages.
  ** Sandwich weight based on the weight before cooking.
  *** Nutrition based on 1/3 cup of ice for beverages.
  Nutrition Information on all Coca-Cola products provided by the Coca-Cola Company. FDA Rounding Rules used.

NOTES